The Memory of Health

My Journey to Mindful Living & Conscious Consumerism

Edie Summers

Media High ™

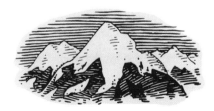

This book is a meditation and conversation on well-being.

*It is surprising how contented one can be with nothing definite – only a sense of existence. My breath is sweet to me. Oh how I laugh when I think of my vague indefinite riches...If the day and the night are such that you greet them with **joy**, and life emits a fragrance like flowers, and sweet-scented herbs –is more elastic, starry, and immortal – that is your success. ~Thoreau*

dedicated to my Pop who fought to live,
and worked on his own book
until the day he passed

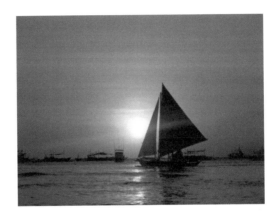

*"For years I never knew whether the twilight was the ending of the day
or the beginning of the night.
And then suddenly one day I understood that this did not matter at all.
For time is but a circle and there can be no beginning and no ending.
And this is how I came to know that birth and death are one.
And it is neither the coming nor going that is of consequence.
What is of consequence is the beauty that one gathers
in this interlude called life."*

~W.O. Abbott

Dear Friend,

If you have faced illness, then you are, in my eyes, a hero or heroine. There is little more daunting than the horizon of suffering. The odds are likely that you are reading this book because you have some type of health or other type of challenge, or you know someone else who is seeking answers.

You may be searching for a glimmer of hope that this current storyline will end. I wish I could tell you that you will find everything you are looking for in these pages. It's entirely possible that you will. It's also possible that your journey may continue beyond what you read here.

In any case, I can offer you this wish to carry with you along your path:

Whatever else happens, keep reaching for your goal of feeling better.

Whatever challenge you may be facing, it can feel like a lonely road, and we often have to wander off the path to find what it is we truly seek.

This is both a terrifying and ultimately liberating experience ...

While it can be daunting to face a challenge – health or beyond - it is also an opportunity to wake up to the bright light of awareness ...

Know there is support, even in the most unlikely of places, and know that you are not alone. Use any judgment to build a shield around you as you head toward the light. Whatever you do, don't give up. You are closer than you believe. And as you believe, so shall you set yourself free.

Wishing you much light and love...
This is your time. Step into the Flow...

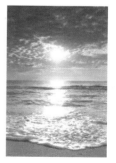

Be well,

Edie Summers

Table of Contents

Gratitude

To my beloved, cherished parents: Pop, you are my hero. Mom, you are my inspiration. Thank you, Mom, for all of your support. You have always loved and supported me unconditionally. I'm forever grateful and love you dearly. Thanks for the calls and for never giving up on me. To my dad who passed away August 31, 2008, thank you for believing in my gifts. I love you now and always.

Thanks to my dear friend Rhonda for the idea to write this book and for your faithful friendship and strength of heart. Your courage and devotion never fail to inspire and lift me up. Thank you for your love and support even when times were the toughest for you.

To Randa, my true friend, I thank you for your never-ending support and ideas. Thankfully you were in Portland to see me through the toughest times and to endure late night phone emergencies. Thank you for your wonderful cooking, for bringing me soup, and for all of your endless insight/intuition: physically, emotionally, and spiritually. You are the definition of true beauty. Love to your family as well.

Thank you to my sister, Sarah, for believing me when I told you I was sick, and for all the telephone talks, bringing sunshine to my life.

Thank you to my wise, high-spirited sister, Kate, for defending me when I was down and for believing in my worth by showing me yours.

Thanks to my brother, Billy, and my sister, Mary, for paving the way and for being so endlessly strong, brave, funny, and far cooler than us.

To my cousin, Janie, who passed away in 2015: I miss our four-hour lunches. Strength and beauty come in many forms. The amazing spirit and bright light of Kevin, lives on, too: "All my relations…"

To my cousins: Joe, Lisa, John, Margaret, Marcia … so happy we're family. Thanks for your love, light, humor, and for making me feel at home, literally. I am so blessed to know my extended family.

Thank you, Cousin Ann, for letting me stay with you while I received medical treatment in California. Margaret, thanks so much for your gracious hospitality and for reminding me about the comfort of family.

Love to my family & yoga tribe: old, new, extended, furry…family is home

To my nephews Connor, Gavin, Jacob, Zachary, and Trajan: we finally have more boys than girls! Love to Ken & Andy for the talks!

Thanks to my cousin John for building me that amazing, healing deck and for all the great conversations. You helped me so much.

Thanks to Joan P. for seeing my gift as a writer. Your whole family is like a second family. Love to Carol and your beautiful poetry.

To all the people who attended my wedding way back when, thanks for creating a magical day and evening that carried my soul for years to come through a long, dark night…

Thanks to the special family of Tobi, Pyper, Fred, and Doris for sharing all of your stories, inspiration, ideas, and your friendship. Thanks to Fred and Doris for taking me out to eat when I was sick and for offering me such great advice. Love to Justin, Mahala, Juniper, Elizabeth, and the rest of your amazing family, here and in heaven.

Thanks to Aimee for always showing me compassion and love. Your exquisite spirit helps me heal and gives me eternal hope.

Thanks to Karen K. for being the definition of positive energy. You are such an inspiration. Love to Bob, Jeff, Christine and the kids.

Love and thank you to Katherine, Lloyd, Ben, and Steven T. for being there, for asking questions, and for listening to the answers.

Stephen, thank you for your amazing, magical music that heals and inspires my soul. I still remember when Roni and I met you at the U. of U. You were then and are now a RockStar.

Thanks to Oren for the serenades. Thanks to Sonaljit for your sublime, inspiring music. There are no words … that's why it's music.

Thanks to Teri and Stephanie for your caring friendship. The zoo was magical, naked mole rat, baby birds, and all.

Thanks to Janice for inspiring me and reminding me of the bigger, metaphysical picture. And thanks to sweet Trajan for reminding me of the innocence and wonder inside myself. I had a blast. Super Dog and Superflex have defeated Rock Brain, I'm sure of it. But Harry Potter scares the hell out of me …

Thanks to Jakie for being adorable, and to all the amazing Utah people.

Aloha to Josh for reminding me to look people in the eye and for staying true to yourself. *Love to M. for the hug and loving me as I am …*

Thanks to Kathy for your big, brave, beautiful heart, and for creating true community, hope, and healing. *Thanks to Judith for believing in me.*

Love to Eve, Meg, Saif, Natalie, Ronnie, Barrie, Sayan, Manoj, Susan, Lilly, Roohi, Elahe, my ASU cohort, and *new/old friends* on and offline.

Thanks to Grant and the Harris's for holidays spent on the coast, etc.

Roni and Leena, thanks for seeing the light in me. I see it in you too. *Love to Porsche for your radiant energy, fierce love, and beautiful artistic soul...*

To Sandy in Salem, thank you for being a bright light at a dark time.

To Christy, my long lost Utah friend, your kind words healed my heart.

To the wonderful colleagues I have met along the way: Tas, Matt, Carol F., Susan B., Kerri, Linda, Debra, Danielle L. Porsche, Angela, Braxton, Tiffany, Diana, Martin, radiant Mariko, Adam, Julie, Jasmine, Edward, Dr. Tran, Elisa, Amy, Erin, Dianne B. J., Diane, Susan, PoP.

Love to Kristen P., Kristen H. and my New Frontiers, Wild Oats tribe. Much gratitude to my Smashon family and *The Art of Living Foundation.*

To Mel, Katie, Sonia, Danielle and those who suffer: I believe (in) you.

Thank you to all of the amazing, empowered, tireless advocates I have met in the Social Justice world: Choya, Amanda, Megan, Natalie...I am in awe of your tireless efforts to educate, eradicate, and empower.

Thanks to these medical professionals who helped me along the way:

To Ebu at Berman Skin Institute who treated me expertly, regarded me like an equal, gave me the benefit of the doubt as a patient, and encouraged me to write this book. Thanks for sharing the story of your mother's illness and for giving me faith in the medical community.

To Dr. Daniel Newman M.D., N.D., M.S.OM., for solving one of the greatest mysteries of my illness after 15 years in the dark.

To the emergency team at Alta View Hospital in Salt Lake City, Utah. Everyone took great care of me and I knew I was in expert hands the entire time. Thanks for calming me down on the ride there.

To the Center for Environmental Medicine team for uncovering part of the riddle. Thanks to Steve for lending an ear and reminding me about miracles.

To Gonzo at Groundspring for reassuring me I was not at the mercy of my illness and for all the amazing acupuncture. Thanks to Elisa and the rest of the Groundspring staff for being so friendly. It goes a long way when you're not feeling well.

To Dr. Carrie Jones N.D. for truly listening to me, and for going the extra mile.

To Deborah at the Hand Institute for teaching me to go with the flow above all else.

To Dr. Christian Vallejos for investing time and energy to talk to me in detail about my health.

To Carol, Joey, Cari, Rae, and everyone in the M.E./M.S./CFS communities and beyond: we will never give up.

Thank you to all my friends and family who have assisted me in any way you could. I know now that love comes in many forms. I am blessed by all of it.

Thanks to Deepak Chopra, Martha Beck, Barbara Brennan, Wayne Dyer, Oriah Mountain Dreamer, Louise Hay, Carolyn Myss, Marianne Williamson, Tony Robbins, Danielle Lin, Alberto Villodo, Marilyn Tam, and Oprah Winfrey among other luminaries for lighting the way.

For Greg, who always wanted to be a writer ...
To Eric for being so brave and for sharing your tremendous story ...
To those who came before me and before all of us: I honor you.

Thank you to the angels who sang to me at night by my bed in the darkest hours. Love to my sweet angels in heaven...

To all of the writers, authors, scholars, philosophers, wellness professionals, activists, and publishers who allowed me to print your brilliant words and wisdom, I graciously thank you...

To all those who believed in me, believed me, supported me, comforted me, defended me, tried to help me, inquired about me, or took care of me when I was sick:

~ Thank you. I love you all ~

Introduction

There are *eight major topics* in this book that may be of importance:

1. Childhood Stress and Chronic Illness

2. White Matter, Microglia, & Chronic Inflammation

3. Dysregulation of the HPA Axis

4. Microbes, DNA, and Your Health

5. PNI & Feedback Loops of Energy

6. Neuroplasticity, Epigenetics, & Resilience

7. Dynamic Balance: Rest, Eustress, & Well-Being

8. Becoming a Conscious Consumer

To you, dear reader, who have picked up this book and are looking for answers, but may be too tired to know where to read or look first, I'm going to give you a brief overview. Here is a highlight of some of the most relevant topics, as well as what has contributed to my positive recovery along the way.

Diet/Supplements ~ see Chapters Three and Four. This is some of what healed my body: deep nutrition and a more diverse microbiome, live, organic and unprocessed foods, and avoiding chronic stressors (irritating stimuli to my body). Supplements helped me greatly as well.

These also helped: low refined sugar, low stimulants, yoga, changing my relationship to stress, time, mindfulness, and sunshine: "Vitamin D regulates about 1,000 different types of genes in the body, [and] about 5 percent of the entire human genome" (Rutberg, 2015). I have a new normal, and I always refining and practicing my well-being, but I considered myself healed. Staying well is a conscious practice.

Memory is truly about being mindful of your life: see Chapter Three.

Becoming a Conscious Consumer ~ In the process of seeking answers to my health challenges, I became a conscious consumer.*
*See "Highlights" at end of book for information on how you can become a conscious consumer.

Yoga ~ It has helped restore my vagal tone, which is what heals and mediates your parasympathetic nervous system. This cultivates *The Relaxation Response* (Benson, 1975) where healing occurs. Most people who are exhausted are in a chronic state of fight or flight. Also, figure out what your stressors are, and reduce, remove, or reinterpret them.

Yoga also encourages *brain plasticity*, I believe. Brain/neuroplasticity is turning out to be a huge component of healing in general, for many conditions. Stress can affect your brain, but you can literally create neural pathways that make you stronger. This is a huge breakthrough in understanding in the realms of healing, well-being, and medicine.

Personal Connections ~ Love, family, friends, community – stay connected any way you can. Nurture the threads of connection in your life. Have faith that you are interconnected with all living beings.

Energy Connections ~ Your body works on exquisite feedback loops of energy. Your job is to bring awareness to this system. This is one way to cultivate well-being. Reinterpreting stressors are key too.

Body Systems Connections ~ The field of psychoneuroimmunology (PNI) shows us that the psyche, brain, immune system and possibly more systems are connected. What we do and think affects our whole body, and reverberates throughout our entire being, like touching a web. Everything in our bodies and the universe is interconnected.

Stress Connections ~ Research has proven that early exposure to stress or trauma can affect the stress response in vulnerable individuals. It also points to CFS as possibly being an auto-immune condition, or an activated immune system, as well as being influenced by genetic polymorphisms (see Chapter Three for in-text citations).

Microbe Connections ~In addition, the role microbes play in our health and even the onset or remission of chronic illness may be a major factor. Microbes are even part of our DNA. Also, the majority of our immune system is in our gut, and science has renamed the immune system the *microbial interaction system*.*

* We are exploring the microbiome for causes of SEID, etc. Please see "Highlights" for a discussion.

Brain Connections ~ A Stanford research team recently published data indicating bilateral white matter atrophy was present in CFS study patients (Zeineh et al., 2015). Also of potential major relevance is research by neurologists David Pleasure and Charles DeCarli regarding white matter inflammation. White matter is what "enables your brain to function" (UC Davis, 2014). When white matter in the brain is inflamed, it can lead to a host of other issues in the rest of the body, due to the blood-brain barrier becoming compromised.

According to Pleasure, "The blood-brain barrier becomes partially ineffective, and peripheral immune cells and antibodies can enter the central nervous system" (UC Davis, 2014). **This may lead to chronic activation of the brain's immune system and neuroinflammatory disorders.** Scientists have discovered lymphatic vessels in the brain, meaning part of your immune system is literally in your brain (Wernick, 2015). According to Jonathan Kipnis, lead author of the original research (published in *Nature*): "In neuro-inflammatory disorders, the communication between your brain and immune system is mediated by these blood vessels" (Flatow, 2015).

Primary Focus ~ Here is what has worked for me:* I fortify my body with real and deep nutrition, and use a small amount of stimulation when needed (acai, superfoods, Korean Ginseng, etc.) I reconditioned my nervous system by finding a dynamic balance between downtime and positive eustress (and learning how to interpret stress differently), thus raising my vitality over time.

What I found works for me is to *work within my energy envelope*, cultivating calm energy. It's about applying the opposite energy to what happened and **finding that sweet spot between rest, eustress, and raising your vitality.**

If it was severe stress of some kind that threw you off balance, apply the opposite energy of calm, balanced, restorative energy. Consider removing irritants (which are stressors), raise your nutrient levels, and learn to reinterpret stressors and opportunities to grow. Remove what you are sensitive to, amplify what fortifies you, and *find a place of dynamic balance.*

Consider placing your *primary focus* on *raising your vitality and relaxing deeply into the present moment.* When you put your energy into raising your chi levels - your level of natural vitality - through diet, mindset, restorative exercise, faith, connection, and community - you may naturally raise your energy levels.

Although it can useful at times to know the origins of our illness, we can't always know. What we can do, however, is focus on **feeling as good as we can in the present moment.** This action is always available to us.

*This is not a simplistic solution to a potentially complex condition. Please read the book for context.

The Relaxation Response ~ A huge factor in healing is cultivating what is known as The Relaxation Response. This response was discovered and researched by Herbert Benson in 1975.

The Relaxation Response is the opposite of the stress response. It activates the parasympathetic nervous system, and releases hormones and neurotransmitters such as oxytocin, endorphins, and dopamine that enable our bodies to heal. The Relaxation Response brings back our appetite so we can digest and absorb our food, and gives us the opportunity to harness our bodies' natural healing powers.

By simply by engaging in slow, rhythmic breathing, relaxing thoughts, relaxing movement, music that relaxes you, or anything else that helps you relax and engage in a slow, steady rhythm, you may literally harness your ability to heal. We can slow down and relax our way back into vibrant well-being and the *flow of life*. I believe this is how the placebo effect also really works. See Chapter Four for more details.

A definition of suffering is *resisting what is*. When we resist being tired, guess what persists? Instead of resisting low energy, I encourage you to put your energy into what raises your vibration, your natural vitality, and *live dynamically between rest and growth. These are not simplistic solutions to potentially complex conditions. I encourage you to read the whole book for context on these hard-won insights. And, ultimately your path and journey are your own.*

I encourage you to not focus too much on what caused your condition. Instead focus on creating awareness of the delicate but powerful feedback signals and loops of energy in your body that communicate with you, and *seek dynamic, blissful balance in both your mind, body, and life.*

When we bring awareness to the feedback loop systems in our body, we close the gap between symptoms and well-being. This is always at our fingertips, through the power of awareness and mindfulness.

Resilience is allowing challenges in our lives to be a *source of growth, and healing, instead of what depletes us*. Stress is inevitable. Living at our growth and healing edge is a choice. This is how I reached positive recovery. We can:
progress instead of stress…

I wish you the best on your healing journey…

Wishing you love, light, and healing… be well …

Some Things to Ponder...

The sun is on your side,
the moon is on your side,
your body is on your side...

Mindfulness closes the gap
between symptoms and well-being
and increases neuroplasticity.

What would your day be like
if driven by positive emotions and awareness
instead of by (unconscious) anxiety?

Who would you be
if you were all
and only love?

Preface

Journal Entry/1994 - The Terrifying Healing

I come from a dark forest, a deep, dark fairytale. I don't know where the path is that leads me out of the forest. I am in the maze: the terrifying and exhilarating landscape of healing. I only hope I emerge on the other side a happy, healthy heroine.

I ask myself this question often: Where is this place I come from and journey to? Sometimes it seems I am forever going in circles. Maybe this is what I'm meant to do: travel, spiral in or outwards depending on what's required of me: the journey with no real destination, but one that finds hope, gains ground, and finds some peace and healing along the way.

I heal because I have to. It is my solitary responsibility to bring myself to the world as whole and as full of courage as possible. There is a quote by Gaston Bacheland that says "What is the source of our first suffering? It lies in the fact that we hesitated to speak. It was born in the moment when we accumulated silent things within us." (as cited in Metzger, 2009).

Let me tell you about my silence. It is difficult, because what is silent in me is what defines me. The deep spaces I side-step around, don't tell anyone about ... these silent spaces haunt me. Yet in these spaces I have found my voice. It tells me to get off the main road, follow those blue highways, and see where they wish to lead me...

*I was reading about archetypes and I read something about the wounded healer that resonates with me. Deena Metzger says the **wound is one means by which we reach compassion**. I can see that, how illness is really such fertile ground for spiritual growth.*

Illness is a fire that has burned away my identity. In the aftermath, I have begun to write and find my true voice. I write to heal myself, to experience my inexorable pain perhaps through the eyes of the heroine who walks the unknown path toward the dawn...

Metzger says stories heal us because we become whole through them, "[and that] all suffering is bearable if it is seen as part of a story." So here is where I am, suffering in such a way that only makes me wish to grow stronger. Suffering no longer in silence, but in story

Chapter One - My Story

In My Shoes

Illness is a fire that burned away my identity.

"Considering how common illness is, how tremendous the spiritual change it brings, how astonishing, when the lights of health go down, the undiscovered countries that are then disclosed ... it is strange indeed that illness has not taken its place with love and battle ... among the prime themes of literature ... [it] does its best to maintain that its concern is with the mind; that the body is a sheet of plain glass through which the soul looks straight and clear."~Virginia Woolf

Story

Finally, so many of my untold stories have found a home in this book that I write. I could not tell some of my stories to anyone. Either I was too afraid, or I didn't have anyone to tell them to. So I am telling them here instead.

What are you afraid to tell about yourself?

Maybe you, like me, can whisper them here to a captive audience, the pages of this book, and they will bear witness to what you could not bear to say on your own.

Tell your story. Release your soul...

My story. At first, this was the easiest part of the book to write. Now, in the final stages, I cringe at the idea of it being shared.

What is worse than shame, pain, judgment, or blame? Being stuck in a story that is no longer yours or one that no longer serves you.

So I release my story to you, to the wind, to the waters, to god. It is what it is. For whatever reason, whatever it is, this is what transpired.

But before I tell you mine, what is *story* anyway?

We love stories because we love the process, the journey itself. We want to know how it starts and how it ends, and what was overcome in between.

We are the heroes and heroines of our own lives, whether or not we can see it.

Sometimes the stories we tell ourselves and others are different than the stories our bodies tell. But your body never lies, cannot lie to you, nor can you lie to your body. Every story you tell others or yourself about who you are shows up verbatim in your body.

Your body's story is the one you should listen to, especially if you are on a healing path. The path of healing leads you to your authentic self. It is a true gift and a direct path.

What does it mean to tell your story? Why do some people say to embody your story, and others say to leave it behind? What is the truth?

First of all, it's what is your truth. What works for you? This is the truth if there ever was one. If nothing else, I hope you take this away from this book:

What *works* for you? What truths lie in your heart that you find the courage to express and embody without an ounce of fear?

Here is my truth…

I believe it is helpful, if not essential, to embody your story at some point in time, to acknowledge it, to feel it … but then, ultimately, to let it go, let it fall away down the river, float downstream and join your perfectly alchemized, serendipitous past.

What lies ahead?

The radiant, magical presence where "story" is a beautiful, blank page filled in by the joys and sorrows of the day, and then washed away by the medicine of the night.

What we inhabit - like our bodies - deep down we know and can feel. What we release, releases us, and allows us to be truly free.

What can you know and then release? Your habits, your fears, your body, your life, your love, your wishes, your *story*…

Letter to My Body

Dear Body,

I feel you. I know your secret pain and loss.

I feel your suffering...

I know you feel weak and sick and exhausted ...

I feel you trying to talk to me. I feel the breaking of your (our) heart...

I feel the density of emotions that linger in your cells and muscles.

But what you may not know about is the inexhaustible light that burns inside of you. It is not tied to food, or sleep, or hurt, or people...

*It is pure, unwavering **light**...*

I want you to know that there is a place where there is no pain or fatigue.

I want you to know I care about you, love you, and that you are already whole.

In the year 2006, I wrote a book of poetry. It was about my experience both with getting sick and the loss of love. It was about redemption of spirit, too.

What matters is not what happened to you. What matters is what comes out of it ... how you come out of it ... eventually, ultimately, inevitably ... at some point in the storyline ... near, far ... whether here in your lifetime, or somewhere in the trail of stars in the eternal heavens above ...

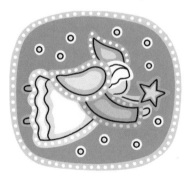

The story of my illness is just that: a story just like any other. No better, no worse. It's not mine, nor yours, to be judged. It's an experience of time that traveled with me for a while, like water that travels down a rock or river ...

13

The pain of my body is not a clear sheet of glass. It is a stained glass window. When you're sick, your body feels like shattered glass, like shards of glass have broken into jagged pieces that may inadvertently pierce you and slice your soul open.

Illness shatters your sense of self. You begin to feel like a ghost traveler on the planet. You begin to feel like you are disappearing, one splintered hour or day at a time. You feel yourself falling through the cracks in the floor in your room and house. You sense the smell of sickness on everything, like a stain that won't lift. You feel the black mark on your body and soul.

I became the ghost of a former self I couldn't even remember. I became The Lady of Shalott, floating on the river, searching for love or herself before she finally drowned. With the mark of abuse, trauma, and an illness I couldn't shake, I became lost in deep sorrow itself. I became my illness. This was the identity I could identify.

I could not shake the words, and feelings, and experience of sexual abuse and domestic violence that haunted my head, heart, and body. I felt tortured by harsh words and brutal actions that were 1000 years old. I tried to set myself free. But, my heart, head, and body felt like prisoners to other people's careless words and actions.

And then, it slowly occurred to me that these people were long gone, and weren't thinking about me at all. I was only perpetuating the pain.

And this continuation of pain became unacceptable to me.

It's not to say that CFS or chronic illness isn't real. It is. But, the story I live in is up to me.

What do I wish my story to be?

I'm not the Lady of Shalott. I'm not someone who is sick. I *am* a modern-day heroine. I'm sensitive, kind, wise, whole, aware, and awake to the possibilities of my life.

I'm pure white light and I'm good enough just as I am right now, right here, in this clear moment of being

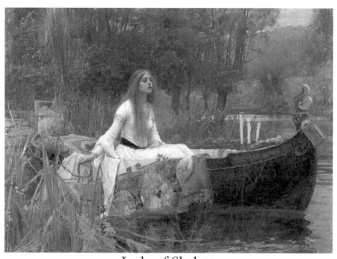

Lady of Shalott

I've peered into your fiction world
a thousand times. It becomes, on occasion,
demystified when I try,
not too hard, to catch your gaze.
That Look -- of somewhat searching,
yet somehow knowing, already,
why you're sitting there

   Among the shadow-green of leaves both conceal
and, sometimes, when you least expect, reveal the ripe, unattached
      lily-pads that just float there
         in your private pond.

I've seen this, on occasion, when I'm only
half-looking at your curious stare, avoiding
what could be mistaken for eye contact.
And, I must admit, I too, felt at times
as though I belonged there -- alongside you
in your wooden boat, before my courage, too,
was sunk, in unclear, jaded water.

      I've had a sense of timing.

From Frozen Light: A Collection of Poems
by Edie Summers

What does it mean to be *sick*? Is it about losing your spiritual power? What about your personal power? What does it mean to be well anyway?

Journal Entry/June 2006

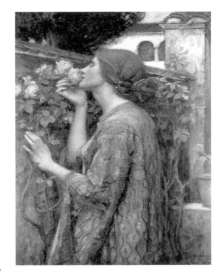

I'm sick. And although saying that may define me for now, it is not ultimately who I am. But for what has seemed an eternity now, I have been existing just outside of the living. I have been sick and exhausted for the last 5 years, and tired and/or exhausted on and off for the last 20 years. I've had good years and bad years. There have been times when I was so sick I thought I'd lost my health forever and my will to live.

I have not known until very recently what it was that made me so sick to begin with. To make matters worse, I've had to turn down many wonderful job offers, endured countless criticism and judgment from others, and even lost my marriage due, in part, to my chronic condition. It's been a difficult journey to say the least.

But I am optimistic beyond measure that I can regain my health fully and completely. I believe beyond a shadow of a doubt that all of this pain happened to me for a reason and telling my story is a part of me getting healthy again. I want to not only help myself, but to help others heal as well.

One thing I know for sure is this: what happened to me is real, and is a result of living in this modern, and in many ways, toxic world. But I am not a victim of my circumstances. And, ultimately, the way out of this vicious cycle of sickness is up to me.

I am my own cure.

My incredibly strong will, spirit, and desire to be live and be happy is what is pulling me slowly, but surely, out of this devastating web of illness. I am not a doctor. What I am is a beautiful, talented person whose life has been deeply and painfully altered and affected by circumstances initially beyond my control.

I don't know what the future holds, but I do know for sure that I have never wanted to be alive or live more. I am sick of being sick.

We all want to tell our story. We need to tell it, to set our lives free from the past. But the truth is, most of us are too afraid to take the risk. Fear of incrimination from others is overwhelming, defining, and deflating. But who are we if we don't tell our stories?

Living authentically means being brave. There is no other way. But it is liberating as well. It is when we are truly ourselves that our life begins. No matter what your life circumstances, your life is interesting, and matters to someone, somewhere.

Telling your story is part of getting well. The path of healing and health leads you to yourself. Telling your story is healing. Releasing it sets you free. Make of this what you will. Here is my story.

Health Journal

6/6/08

My nervous system feels shot today. Worries me a little…
I have a cold too. Sleep felt really good. I need more. My thumb still hurts. It hurts to write on this page.
Tired but hopeful … Writing feels good.

6/7/08

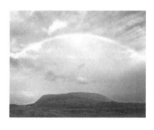

Woke up very tired…
Decided to go out anyway, and felt better toward end of day.
Had sugar though. Feeling a bit hopeless.
Trying to stay positive - xo

6/9/08

Have stomach flu today. No appetite (again).
Maybe this is why I can't seem to climb out of this hole.
Not sure about going to Utah, although I really want to go.

6/19/08

Utah was amazing. It broke my spell. I felt myself heal there. Something kicked in: the sun, exercise, my friend's wedding … all three?
Had a great time at Ruth's Diner too…
I feel different. Much, much better… I feel invincible. Almost like myself again

6/20/08

Sick today…Too much sugar … I will be well again soon, I know.
I'm craving nothing or super healthy foods only. Life still feels good.
I have been writing too. I feel on track and positive…xo

6/22/08

Feel lonely today. As I often feel. Almost unbearable, but holding my own…
Feel almost good. Trying to write…
Had an amazing dream about sharing a house with my two friends…
Very powerful…Wishing myself health and happiness…xo

11/10/2008

I don't know how to make my body work…

Looking back on it, I was drowning in my own fear. I had no anchor for joy and no rudder for how to cope with stress in a positive way.

The First Time

Morning. Light. Hopeful. I check in with my body. Maybe today is the day I will feel good again and get my life back. Rivers of pain run down my back and my legs. My body feels heavy like thick snow in the dead of winter.

Morning. Light streams through the curtains. How did I wake up drowning in quicksand? I am so tired I can barely force my lungs to breathe. How will I make it through the day, let alone the morning? God or someone help me. And so the day begins…

A Fateful Turn

It was March at Snowbird, spring, but an overcast day, and the slopes were icy. I was there with my family for our annual timeshare ski vacation. I was young, nervous, i.e. jacked up on coffee, and ready to ski with my dad.*

I was using either my mom's boots or skis for some reason, and not mine. In either case, I neglected to check the bindings. My family warned me to check them, but I felt invincible and young. Nothing would happen, I was more or less sure of it. I brushed it off. Let's go.

My dad and I hit the slopes, headed for one of his favorite runs: Regulator Johnson. It was a grey and cloudy day and I was skiing in my typical fashion: somewhat paying attention, somewhat checked out. We had just started, and I was still warming up.

*I realize now I am an HSP, and that was probably why I was overstimulated by caffeine. See pg. 204.

As I started to turn, my ski caught on the edge of the icy snow and did not turn with me. Worst of all, the bindings did not release. I felt my knee twist and break as I fell. Do I remember the pain? Not sure. But I remember the break and the subsequent fall. Did I wish I had listened to my family or my intuition that was sputtering along at the time? You bet.

Do I regret what happened as a result? For years, I would say "absolutely." One careless decision, and one fateful turn impacted the next 20 plus years of my life. Do I regret that day? No, because it led me to become who I am…

Fighting for My Health

I've had to fight for my health for about half of my life. Illness has been like walking through a maze blindfolded. Occasionally the blindfold would come off and I could see where I should go next, but then it was put back on again, or I put it back on … How do you walk through a maze blindfolded? *You trust your gut.*

The first time I experienced extreme, on-going fatigue I was 22. Up until that point I never had any major health issues and had a lot of energy. However, I can remember even from a young age being "bothered" by certain chemical smells and not feeling right. When my family fumigated our house for ants, I felt pretty sick. The first time I smelled formaldehyde on a frog in junior high, I almost passed out.

I did have some chronic stomach aches when I was young which I now realize was probably a combination of general anxiety (I was very shy), and too much sugar in my diet. But I was a happy go lucky girl until puberty hit. Then I started having trouble with depression. I now realize my depression was due to my body's inability to process estrogen and general poor nutrition. You can read more on these subjects in Chapters Three and Four.

But in general, I was blissfully in great health, active with dance classes, horseback riding, skiing, running, gymnastics, hiking, and going to the gym. I started working when I was 10 or so, delivering newspapers on foot before school started.

In high school I was in a very time consuming and demanding dance company and worked after school every day as well. I got great grades, went for jogs, and took walks late at night with my sister.

In my early 20's I was active in dance both in school as a dance major, and outside of school with various student dance projects. Sometimes I rehearsed for up to six hours a day, five days a week. I also worked as a busser, housekeeper, and hostess while going to college full time. I had a 3.7 G.P.A. in my major. I wasn't necessarily a *Type A* personality, but I was a passionate person in general. I juggled it all and didn't bat an eyelash. In short I had energy to burn.

When I was 22 I had my ski accident. I tore my ACL and severely damaged a number of ligaments in my right knee. I underwent arthroscopic surgery and spent the next few weeks souped up on the painkillers Codeine and Demerol. Since I had been told to wait three weeks before starting rehab, there was extensive scar tissue in my knee, and I could not bend it. It was straight as a stick, frozen like cement, and incredibly painful.

I was told to take six ibuprofen tablets a day in order to reduce the swelling in my leg. My therapists told me this was the only way to get the inflammation down and recover at least partial movement in my knee. They did not ask me if I was taking any other medications or inform me about the possible risks or side effects of taking NSAIDS (ibuprofen, etc.), in combination with anything else.

I was in physical therapy for eight months. Some of it was successful, some of it not. They used ultrasound on my knee every day which was helpful. I did all of the exercises and gained some ground.

At the eighth month mark, and still taking six ibuprofen tablets daily, I was able to bend my knee to 90 degrees. My therapists determined that the six ibuprofen tablets were not enough and switched me to a prescription drug: Naprosyn (now available over the counter as Aleve.)

A few weeks into taking Naprosyn I fell into a deep depression, and didn't get out of bed for a week. This was the first time in my life I had experienced such depression. It was foreign to me and it scared me to death. I had extremely dark thoughts.

Only once did I go to school, at night, to pick up some homework. Otherwise, I was literally lying in bed in the dark. It felt like I was falling continuously down a dark, black hole.

My knee remained "frozen" at 90 degrees. In fact, I think I lost some flexibility. The scar tissue wouldn't budge. They told me this was probably as far as I was going to get. I was devastated. I was a dance major at the university and had been dancing since I was five. I was informed I'd probably never dance again.

There was a retired policeman in therapy with me. He had been in therapy for nine years after crushing his knee in a high speed car chase on the job. He was still trying to get his knee to 90 degrees like mine so he could ride his motorcycle again. I looked at him and wondered if this was my fate too.

In addition, ever since surgery, I'd been extremely tired, and slept for 10-12 hours every day. Even with that much sleep, I felt tired often, and didn't feel right, like I used to before the surgery. I just assumed I was still healing from surgery and the trauma of it all. Regardless of the reason, I didn't feel like myself and I was even more exhausted than before. Nor did I look like myself. I was 20 pounds overweight and my skin was yellow.

After the week in bed, I took myself off of Naprosyn and made an appointment with a naturopathic doctor. I'd read about this type of doctor, and I was desperate. Something had to work. This couldn't be my fate, I decided. This was my first step into the world of alternative medicine, and it changed my life forever.

A New World

Walking into the naturopath's office was like walking into a foreign country, but it was also like a breath of fresh air. It even smelled different, due to the herbs and vitamins. I felt a sense of hope.

I was nervous after my last experiences with the medical community. Although overall my physical therapists were great and I'm grateful for the help they gave me, I felt slightly abused by the system. I can see now this is a victim mentality. However, I did have the impression that their way was the only way.

The doctor who had performed my knee surgery was skilled and capable, but there was coldness to his demeanor and his treatment of me. These feelings lingered in me, although I was very young at the time and wasn't really able to articulate them until years later.

The naturopath talked to me for an hour and a half. He quizzed me on my symptoms and health history. He reassured me that we would indeed be able to work through the remaining scar tissue, no problem.

He explained how the herbs and supplements he recommended would help reduce and eliminate the rest of my scar tissue. He shook his head when I mentioned how much ibuprofen I had been taking and said it was probably making the inflammation worse. He gave me a bottle of arnica gel that he had prepared himself to rub directly on my knee daily. He told me to take Devil's Claw (an herb) and papain (an enzyme) between meals to reduce scar tissue and swelling in my knee.

At a nearby health food store I bought Devil's Claw and papaya enzyme. Being in the health food store was another relatively foreign experience to me. In fact, it may have been one of my first few times in a health food store. I felt at home. The staff was helpful, and I found what I needed.

I began to use the naturopath's recommendations and noted significant results in about a week. I was able to work through the rest of my scar tissue pretty quickly and the therapists and I were surprised and happy.

Besides building up muscle again, that was the end of my knee chapter. I thought it was just a bump in the road. But my fatigue and poor health continued. I was 20 pounds overweight, breaking out for the first time in my life, tired, had lost half my hair, and felt *off*. I was confused by the way my body was behaving, but tried not to think about it and hoped for the best. I was 23.

In terms of my body, not much changed in the next few years. I was able to dance again, thank god, but all the other problems remained. I continued to shop at the health food store and did my best to eat well. But I was still sleeping 10-12 hours a night. If I got less, I didn't feel well. I noticed every time I drank coffee, I felt horrible. I could tell something was different in my body but I had no clue what it was.

I fell into some strange patterns. I was having trouble sleeping, so I would end up falling asleep very late at night or early in the morning. I discovered the popular overnight host, Art Bell, on the radio and learned all about alien sightings.

I got the only job I could get while still in school - delivering Chinese food - and the hours were from 4-11 pm every day. This only made my sleep habits worse. I would get home from work around midnight and often was not be able to fall asleep until four in the morning.

During this time, a disturbing incident happened during final exams. Before my ski accident I had started to drink coffee around the age of 19 or 20 like most college students. Sometimes I would feel a little shaky after an iced coffee or two but I didn't think much of it. So, although I had noticed a change in my tolerance for coffee after my accident, when things were super busy I still turned to caffeine. During final exams at the university I pulled an all-nighter finishing up a few papers. I drank coffee and had a few No Doz. The next day, I had a dance final as well. I finished my coffee and had one more No Doz. A few hours later, during my dance final, I began to feel funny. I felt dizzy. I drove home and the feelings continued to worsen.

My heart began racing so I lay on the floor because I could not move. It was a very strange feeling not being able to move and to have my heart racing a hundred miles an hour. I started getting scared and I was home alone. I got to the phone and called poison control. I asked if it was possible to overdose on No Doz. They said it absolutely was and I should go to the emergency room immediately. With no one home to drive me, and with my heart racing, I somehow made it there.

The emergency room doctor examined me and said it was too late to pump my stomach. They made me drink a quart or more of charcoal. It tasted awful. Later the doctor came back and told me that I had almost gone into cardiac arrest. He asked if I had done this on purpose. In other words, he thought I had been trying to kill myself. I told him no, that I had final exams, nothing more. He didn't seem to believe me, and kept pressing me to confess. I think now the reason he wouldn't let up is because I had come very close to accidentally killing myself. The charcoal passed through my system six hours later and I was in agonizing pain the rest of the afternoon and evening.

There are a few things relevant from this part of my story.

As it would turn out, I could not properly methylate the NSAIDs and caffeine I had been ingesting for eight months or more. I discuss this in great detail in Chapter Three. In addition, my liver and nervous system had been affected greatly by the stress and drugs of the surgery and rehab. Something in me had shifted and not in the best way.

Another relevant part of the No Doz story is that if it is possible to overdose from something as innocuous as No Doz, which only contains caffeine as an active ingredient as far as I know, then it is no wonder people are accidentally overdosing and/or experiencing significant damage from drugs, both prescription and non-prescription. Also, it has been shown that in the last few years people are 50% more likely to overdose from prescription drug use than from street drugs.

The human body is extremely intelligent and adaptable, but we still have to work within its natural framework. Go outside of this framework and consumer beware.

A drug is a drug is a drug.

Also, this experience was a foreshadowing and warning of the fact that I may have developed a sensitized nervous system early on. For further exploration of this topic, please see in Chapter Three the section on *Early Stress and Chronic Illness*.

But at the time, I simply resolved not to take caffeine again in any form. It took me about a month to break my addiction. I was extra tired and lethargic at first. I also felt my body *relax* and I slept much deeper.

By cutting out caffeine, I felt my fatigue levels improve as well. However, even though my fatigue levels were somewhat better, I noticed I had a new *sensitivity* not only to caffeine, but to perfumes, chemical smells, carpeting, etc. I became aware of scents I had never noticed before. I had to avoid some people's houses because the chemical smell from furniture and carpeting were too strong for me and the smells made me not feel well. I was also still breaking out badly, and sleeping more than normal.

I honestly didn't think much about any of these symptoms except for the excessive sleep. I was young - these were the years from ages 23-25 - and busy. I just hoped somehow I would feel completely like myself again.

At the age of 25, I was hired by New Frontiers, a small, independent, chain health food store in Salt Lake City, Utah. My job was to be a consultant, working in the supplement aisle for $4.25/hour. This may sound like slave wages, but this is where I wanted to be, and it had been difficult to get my foot in the door. I wished to learn more about this world. My intuition told me to pursue this job and this was the beginning of my first career. It was also where my true healing and a whole new life began.

My first six months on the job were a huge learning curve, as I lived and breathed the world of supplements and herbs. There was melatonin, just out on the market, St. Johns Wort in standardized form was just getting big buzz … there were literally hundreds of supplements and theories to memorize and learn how they assisted the body in healing and maintaining health.

I helped answer customer questions and was in charge of ordering several different lines. We had many trainings on vitamins, herbs, amino acids, essential fatty acids, superfoods, and natural HABA care (health and beauty aids) as well. I began to implement what I was learning into my health routine and started to notice changes right away.

Some of the changes I made included eating more organic foods, and foods made without synthetic/and or harmful ingredients such as hydrogenated fats, pesticides and herbicides, artificial flavors or preservatives like MSG, etc.

I also started taking superfoods - particularly Hawaiian spirulina - and added essential fatty acids to my diet, like flax oil and evening primrose oil. Slowly but surely, I started to notice a change in my energy levels, my vitality, and my body overall. I was still sleeping a lot, but my health was better. I also noticed that I was having reactions to chocolate, so I cut it out as well.

Over the next year or so, I cut out sugar, dairy, and wheat, and alcohol. I was never really able to tolerate alcohol, but now it really affected me adversely. I stopped eating meat for the most part as well, although not entirely. This was more for ethical reasons though. But, in general, my body was still extra sensitive, so anytime I noticed even a slight reaction to something I ingested, I cut it out. My vitality continued to increase.

However, I couldn't seem to make any significant improvements in my sleep patterns. Those patterns were inconsistent, and I would crash on the weekends after a long week at the store. We were on our feet for at least eight hours at a time. I was still falling asleep pretty late and waking up around noon. I had trouble sleeping as well. I used melatonin to knock myself out, although I felt funny the next day.

Something else I should mention that was going on was that at the age of 25 I was in my first relationship. Unfortunately, it was not a very good one. He was an alcoholic, pot smoker, and manic depressive.

He ended up verbally abusing me. A few months into our relationship he started yelling and calling me names. I knew some of his outbursts were tied to when he was sober, in withdrawal. But it seemed that some were just random.

On top of it, he snored. I had to wear earplugs. It is no wonder my sleep problems continued. I will address the connection between relationships/negative energy and health later in this book. Suffice it to say, the professional part of my life was wonderful, but my personal life was a mess.

One day I locked myself in the bathroom while he was yelling at me. He threatened to hurt me physically when I came out. I left him shortly after this since I had finally realized what was truly happening. But there was trauma there to be sure.

Trauma and negative energy are in no small way connected to poor health as I would discover down the road. This time around, I was able to shake it off or so it seemed. I chalked it up to lack of experience and bad luck and resolved never to be involved with an alcoholic again. End of story, or so I thought.

Starting around the age of 27, I was feeling and looking the best I ever had in my life. Although my sleep and fatigue issues still existed, they were somehow more manageable, although I still felt very tired often. But, when I wasn't super tired, I felt really good, consistently. I knew this had a lot to do with my diet and lifestyle.

I continued to work at New Frontiers, remaining in that position for about three years, and continued to learn more and more about alternative health, applying what I learned to myself. I felt better and better. I lived and breathed the alternative health lifestyle and it worked well for me.

As I mentioned, part of my job at New Frontiers was to place product orders for our department. One of the companies I ordered from was Gaia Herbs, based in North Carolina. I had the privilege of flying to Brevard, N.C. to attend a weekend-long training. I learned so much about the powerful nature of herbs and their medicinal and practical uses. We were fed amazing organic meals, I took walks in the mountains, and attended seminars on all aspects of the healing power of herbs. Later, I visited Gaia's $3 million dollar eco-friendly facility.

This was 1997. During this period of time when I felt the best I ever had before I was injured –from the ages of 25-32 - I consumed almost no stimulants of any kind, particularly coffee and chocolate. I felt my fatigue was linked to stimulants and sugar, so I was very strict about avoiding them. Yes, the link was there, but what I didn't know at the time, was that I had to support my body with deep nutrition as well.

Although I still struggled with fatigue, I did the best I could. But I did have to cut back on my work hours.

I also had one other problem at work: I was constantly catching something due to all the sick people walking in through our doors seeking help. I got sick in ways I had never been sick before, like a really bad case of bronchitis. I had never had bronchitis in my life. It was such a bad case I literally couldn't breathe sometimes due to congestion. It was horrible. Around the end of my third year there I started to get frustrated - and worried - that I was always getting sick. I decided it was time for a change.

Around this time, New Frontiers was bought by Wild Oats. My boss asked if I was interested in management. I knew I did not have the energy for it, even though it interested me. So, I left the health food store. I had some money saved up and I planned to travel for a bit and get my bearings.

A few months later, my old boss from what was now Wild Oats let me know there was a broker in town looking for someone to work with her natural foods brokerage. My boss told me she had thought of me and wondered if I would be interested. Of course I was and I was soon hired to work for Bolder Brokers out of Colorado.

My new job was the start of an exciting, amazing time. I was an independent broker representing over 14 lines and servicing around 50 independent and chain health food stores and integrative pharmacies in Utah. I felt blessed and lucky to have the challenge of a job that continued to teach me so much about alternative health and allowed me the flexibility to work more or less as my body allowed.

During this time I did work for Wild Oats again as a health consultant, filling in for people when they were sick or out of town, but I did not have the same exposure to sick customers like I did before. I had the best of both worlds.

As a broker, I had deep exposure to developments in alternative health through cutting-edge trade shows, company trainings, and one-on-one trainings. I learned so much during this period and my vitality continued to improve. However, some days I was beyond exhausted since I used no stimulants of any kind if I slept poorly - which was still often. Nevertheless, I was thrilled to soak up what I considered invaluable knowledge.

The companies I had the privilege of working for were: BHI, Herb Pharm, Nutribiotic, Weleeda, Ginco, Nutrex, Nature's Secret, Renew Life, Greens Plus…I worked for the *best of the best*.

I visited Herb Pharm's organic herb farm in Williams OR at the beginning of my new job. We had wonderful herb walks there, amazing organic meals served with fresh herbs and edible flowers, and I slept in a tent in one of their fields at nights. I was in heaven.

Little did I know that the very companies I was working for and learning so much about their products, would be the very supplements and healing modalities that would help me recover further down the line when I got sick the second time around.

I invested four years with Bolder Brokers and moon-lighting as a part-time consultant for Wild Oats. As a broker, I also gave many lectures at health food stores on how I had recovered my health, and I did trainings, as well, for the employees of the health food stores and the pharmacists of the integrative pharmacies.

Some of the companies I brokered for offered me corporate positions along the way. Unfortunately, even though I wanted to accept the opportunities, I felt compelled to turn them down. I did not feel I had the stamina to work full time in a corporate environment. But I was happy working for Bolder Brokers and grateful for all the exposure and training I received.

Plus I had one more part-time job I loved. I was a professional dancer. I had been with International Dance Theater since the age of 23. Between all three of my part time jobs, I had just enough energy to get by. I could not imagine doing more, even though I wanted to.

The nagging issue of fatigue was the only thing I did not have any answers for. It had occurred to me over the years after learning so much about the body, that maybe I had a bad reaction to the anesthesia from my surgery. I had read in numerous different sources that anesthesia can stay in the body for up to 10 years. What I realize now is that my fatigue may have stemmed from the **stress** of surgery, anesthesia, and painkiller use itself.

So I did a few liver cleanses, hoping they would clear up my fatigue. I tried taking ginseng from one of my lines (Ginco), which was supposed to help with fatigue. I tried both Siberian and American.

I tried NADH which was popular, along with other supplements meant to help energy levels. I had some success, but not a lot. The only supplement that consistently helped was organic spirulina from Hawaii. This product was from one of the companies I represented - Nutrex. I took it religiously, a tablespoon or more 6-7 times a week.

I began working with a different naturopathic doctor. He noted my low progesterone levels and put me on bio-identical progesterone. It helped significantly with any PMS I had, but did not touch my fatigue or sleeping problems much. So I used valerian and Calms Forte at night but often had to sleep in until late morning to get any sleep at all. No matter when I went to bed, I often couldn't fall asleep until three or four. I used to think it was because I was a night owl, but I knew my sleep patterns were more than just being naturally awake at night.

By the time I was 31, I had pretty much resigned myself to being tired on and off for the rest of my life. I had become very good at coping with fatigue much like it was chronic pain or something similar. I found ways through superfoods, supplements, exercise and just eating super, super well - or not eating much at all during day time hours - to deal with most of it.

The rest of it was sheer will. I was extremely disciplined. I had a stellar diet, or so I thought. In any case, I felt mostly great and was at the top of my game. Life was good. I felt happy and hopeful.

The Second Time

Right before I turned 32, I returned from Peru where I had been studying shamanism. Settling back into Utah, I attended a spiritual retreat called *The Awakening* at Solitude Ski Resort at the nudging of my friend Robert. It was a retreat that used modern shamanic techniques

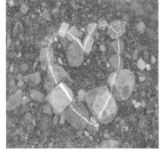

to help release the past and step onto a path of self-actualization.

In addition to eating well, I was into learning about alternative thought and its relationship to healing. I had participated in a soul retrieval workshop with Alberto Villodo before I went to Peru, and I felt that *The Awakening* was a continuation of this journey. It was at *The Awakening* that I met my future husband. We both had gone to the workshop to work on "intimacy," we later told each other. It seemed like destiny that we should meet.

We fell in love quickly and were married even quicker. Things were intense and romantic between us in the beginning. It was a huge change for me as I had been single for six years before we met.

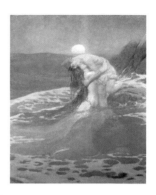

As I mentioned, the last and only other significant relationship I had been in was terrible and I had resolved never to be with someone again unless they were amazing, and most certainly not an alcoholic.

My future husband smoked cigarettes and drank beer, but for some reason I did not see these as red flags. He said he had attended AA for six months before we met and had struggled with drinking before but not anymore.

I choose to believe him and fell so in love that I forgot about anything other than I wanted to be with him. I gave notice to all three of my wonderful part time jobs, and we moved to Portland, Oregon to start our new life.

Love Poem

Evergreens at night in the fields.
In the evenings the fireflies glow and gather in the meadow grass.
Let it be by this light that we seek one another
while the earth turns silently on its steady course.
At dawn the silver is replaced with soft gold.
Sun and moon alchemize the day and we swoon --
Touching you is placing my hand on warm, moonlit sand

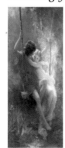

and sinking, falling into something quite possibly incalculable,
and most certainly irretrievable…
Still I follow you down paths I was not meant to take,
from which I feel no need to return…
until you are gone, and I have forgotten from where I came.
But the ache remembers, and rises to wake me every morning.
And I think to myself sometimes that illusion is good enough
to get me by, endure the nights, relish in what lives at odd hours.
The summer's calm that reels me in, leaves me breathless,
so in love, and hardly waiting for the placated day.

From Frozen Light: A Collection of Poems by Edie Summers

When we first lived in Portland, things were okay. We had some amazing times together, but in many ways, I was a very young 32, and this was also only my second relationship. My husband continued to drink beer and chain smoke and I began to have trouble with it, subconsciously.

As much as I didn't want to be reminded of my first troubling relationship, I was. On some level I knew he was checking out when he used substances.

For my part, I had relaxed my strict eating habits mostly because I felt so good and so in love. I felt super healthy, and I assumed that something had shifted in my health. I just wanted to be normal, do normal things, and have a normal life like everyone else. I felt that fate was on my side, finally in terms of health and love.

But I was experiencing some anxiety that I could not put my finger on, that only increased with time, and became very deep-rooted as our marriage progressed.

I began to be somewhat casual about my diet. Basically this means I was eating chocolate (mostly sugar-free) occasionally on days when I felt super tired. This initially helped with the fatigue that I had been struggling with so painfully for the last seven to ten years.

I felt invincible for some reason, because I was so healthy otherwise. I didn't seem to have the same reaction to chocolate that I did years before. Plus, I had read that chocolate did not contain caffeine, but rather a cousin to it: theobromine. I knew I had trouble with caffeine, period.

But I thought maybe theobromine was okay. I thought that for sure something had shifted in me again, although I didn't know what exactly. Beyond that, I still ate super well, including organics, and no preservatives, etc.

I was eating some meat at this time as well. My husband was a great cook, and he made many wonderful meals including some meat-based dishes. I felt strong and healthy overall. However our marriage was not very stable, even early on, despite supposed profound love.

Secret Beach

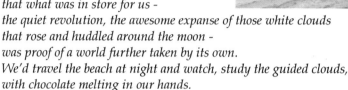

On some days it came down to this,
what to make of the spinning world.
The way it continued to travel
in a near perfect ellipse -
The drugstores we'd frequent
at nights in search of chocolate,
were tempered by an inkling,
that what was in store for us -
the quiet revolution, the awesome expanse of those white clouds
that rose and huddled around the moon -
was proof of a world further taken by its own.
We'd travel the beach at night and watch, study the guided clouds,
with chocolate melting in our hands.

Some days we got up early, when joy was still a figure of light.
When you said you loved me, we created the morning in rapture
even as the sun disappeared into the sky.
There was a call forth to commitment, what was still clear in us:
the eyes of infants and the arc of the whale,
the cadence of laughter, a beach linked with shells.
Some days we got up early because the tides beckoned us to come,
and the numinous clouds parted ways.

When is what was secret no longer so?
When winter came and froze the fruit on the trees,
and the sand was icy and sharp beneath our feet?
When winter came what was holy parted ways,
and all concept of faith was like an ethereal dream.
When what was secret was no longer so, when dreams die, in afterglow,
like seafoam that is washed upon the shore,
I called your name, and sent it out with the breaking waves.
If love dies, where does it go?

Come sleep on the beach with me tonight under the milkyway's infinite light.
Where the pull of my heart is stronger than the moon's:
I remember you, I recollect you...
Remind me of stories we once did believe,
of light from dead stars and the songs they still sing,
to recover what one would hope are not abandoned epiphanies.

From Frozen Light: A Collection of Poems
by Edie Summers

From the very beginning of my marriage, I still had major sleep problems and a growing, nagging feeling of resentment over the fact that my husband spent so much time smoking cigarettes and drinking beer. However, I knew he adored me – we adored each other – and he was very good to me at first.

But I could not help how I felt, subconsciously. I resented his constant drinking and smoking. I was passive-aggressive with him, due to my previous experiences with a chronic drinker/smoker/verbally abusive man from my first relationship.

There was some fighting and tension even from the beginning with us although we both hoped for the best. I even yelled at him during our first fights – which I am not proud of – a retaliation/reflex from being yelled at for a year and half by my manic-depressive ex-boyfriend.

It was all I knew to do when things heated up between me and a romantic partner. I seriously regret this behavior and I stopped most of it once I realized what I was doing. But there was some damage done between us, which would catch up with us further down the line a hundredfold over.

My husband loved me so much in the beginning of our marriage, and cared so deeply for the fact that I could not sleep well, that he did his best to figure out how to help me. His sister had trouble sleeping as well, and we took her advice on sleep aids. I began to take Benadryl at night, and occasionally took Xanax if my anxiety was particularly bad. Later down the road I tried Ambien as well.

I was also on the mini-pill for the first time in my life. I had told my husband that I was pretty sure I had some sort of liver thing going on because I had tried the pill before and did not react well to it. There was also the issue of anesthesia that I was pretty sure, at the time at least, that had maybe affected the health of my liver.

But my body seemed to tolerate everything pretty well, and I still felt and looked healthy. Moreover, I was sleeping better than I had since before I was 22 which was a godsend. I was hopeful for the future and felt like maybe all areas of my life were finally coming together.

And for a brief, blissful period of time they did.

I got hired part-time at a call center and was quickly promoted to supervisor. I also worked occasionally at my husband's office as a corporate secretary. A dance company hired me and we rehearsed tirelessly for eight months before our show opened.

My husband was in a rock band and spent long hours there as well. He was a gifted singer who was recruited by the opera at age 16.

And even though I had explained to my husband that I had never been able to tolerate working full time due to chronic fatigue, he asked if I could work full time to support us so he could focus on his music. I should have realized then that he lacked understanding of what was my current reality.

It hurt me very much when I got sick the second time around and he did not support me through it. The fighting between us was increasing although we had some great times too.

Unfortunately, early on in the marriage, there were some control issues that quickly manifested themselves as physical violence. It started out on our honeymoon, a red flag to be sure.

My husband had a difficult childhood in some respects. His father, unfortunately, was emotionally, verbally, and physically violent with him from the age of 14 until he left home at 17. He started drinking at age 14, to compensate, I'm sure … although I know now that having suffered abuse is not an excuse for hurting someone else.

Violence is a choice someone makes, plain and simple.

Unfortunately, I had one more abuse history in my past as well. At the age of 5, I was physically and sexually assaulted by a group of kids. I don't remember the details very well, but it is a big part of why I remained a virgin until the age of 25, and my first relationship was abusive as well.

Suffice it to say we were both primed to be sensitive to abuse of any kind; we were both the recipients of abuse, as well as instigators.

Noticing Signs of Abuse

I had several bruises that were pretty obvious during rehearsals with the dance company I joined in Portland. I know other dancers saw them. They did ask me if I was okay. I wish they had been more persistent, and I wish I had said I wasn't okay. They made a general comment that someone in the group had body odor. It was me, from a congested liver and stress, I believe. My sister had visited Portland in the beginning of my marriage and witnessed the bruise around my eye from the first time my husband hurt me. I told her I ran into a wall.

When I was younger, I had somehow hit my head on my own while working, and gave myself a black eye. My boss at work spoke up and asked me if there was anything wrong.

If you notice someone is not doing well, take a risk, speak up and be persistent.

You could literally save a life.

On our honeymoon, my husband got drunk the first night we were there. I was sick due to being worn down from an amazing yet exhausting wedding weekend and an extremely long plane flight from the states to Portugal. He left me in the hotel room and went out to party with a stranger.

A few days later, he became severely intoxicated again, and, during an argument about him drinking on our honeymoon, he aggressively pinned me down on the bed. It was the first time he was physically violent with me. It scared me so much, and he was so drunk, that I had to get another hotel room to sleep in that night.

Nothing of an abusive or violent nature happened again for quite a while. However, when it did occur again, and each time it did, the ante was upped. It went from pinning/wrestling me down, to strangling me, to knocking me out of bed, to much worse.

As a new wife, I assumed his abusiveness was a learned behavior since that was how he claimed to have been treated by his father. I'm not making excuses for him, just explaining how I believed the behavior originated.

As the violence grew worse and more frequent, my anxiety increased and my sleep problems re-surfaced. In addition, I was experiencing nights where I was awake all night due to fighting, violence, and/or extreme stress.

I relied more and more on sleep aids. I went from one Benadryl a night to two. The Xanax and Ambien bothered me from the very beginning, so I had stopped taking them. But the doctor we were both seeing at the time recommended Elavil for me. It was a mild anti-depressant that supposedly made you drowsy. She said it was very easy on the liver, which was my concern.

 I had gone off the mini-pill over worries about my liver as well. I just didn't feel right on the mini-pill, Xanax, and Ambien. Actually, I had felt very groggy when I first started taking Benadryl. But I ignored the feeling and it soon went away. Plus it worked so well for sleeping that I willed it to work and it did.

I started taking one Elavil nightly. It worked like a charm. Over time, as the fighting and violence escalated I took more and more of it. I started out around 15 mg, and was up to maybe 100 mg or more a night by the end of my marriage.

I felt like I was caught in a viscous cycle that kept getting worse and worse until the bottom, suddenly, fell out beneath my feet.

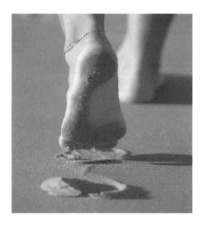

Holding Sand

It's bittersweet this meeting of minds
this coercion of bodies.
Eyes so double-edged; blunt or ready for battle,
but there is a sweetness that circles, that emanates
it circles the air slowly... looking for a place to land.
If only what is lost can be found.
Let the rooms become familiar again
so they radiate a certain something
like a surreptitious moment or touch
a blinking eye or two.

Washed up and spit upon the shore
we are stranded on this beach,
full of future glass.
Like a wounded panther
that cannot defend her cubs,
we are waiting, merely waiting
for the wounds to find their scars.
Time passes. We find ourselves well-traveled,
yet further along a dangerous highway,
anticipating a time of repose, as in a safe sleep.
A place where shields are burned,
when the flames stop licking...
What a head game with which to tempt ourselves,
this fawning over safety and the need for revelation.

My love, you are so precious
but something is faltering.
It is almost irretrievable, this image of twin stars
crystal, silver shards, splintering...
A rainbow, translucent and pure, but the distance has no earthly access.

But I am hanging onto something:
a string, a web, some light.
Holding onto your grace because I know it's there,
circular, inevitable, radiant...
Like the connection that we have,
I just can't find the switch.

From Frozen Light: A Collection of Poems
by Edie Summers

I mention the violence in my marriage because it is significant, and one of the reasons I got sick the second time around. I do not wish to persecute my ex-husband. However, there are many things he did that one could view as unforgivable toward the end of my marriage. I felt angry and betrayed for many years afterwards and had trouble forgiving him.

But, in the end, forgiveness is key to health. And trauma of any kind, as well as negative energy, is extremely destructive to health.

So I mention these incidents because they are relevant. I have fought long and hard to get well this last time around and I've had to recalibrate and release my negative feelings toward many people, not just my ex-husband. But the last two years of my marriage were an especially difficult time in my life.

Toward the end of 2004, my husband and I took a trip to the Oregon Coast. It was peaceful trip. The only catch was that my husband had been having snoring issues for a while, primarily when he drank too much, which made it even more difficult for me to sleep.

Sometimes at home when he had been drinking heavily, I would ask him to wear Breathe Right nasal strips. If those didn't work I would have to ask him to sleep on the couch.

This, of course, did not help things in terms of intimacy between us, but there wasn't much of a choice sometimes. At the coast, we stayed overnight and I ended up having to sleep on the floor with earplugs due to his snoring. Even then, it was too loud in the room in general, and I was not able to sleep. I was up all night – again.

The next morning, as we drove back, we enjoyed the beautiful scenery and I got a hot chocolate. I was tired but happy. It was the last time we were truly in love that I remember. I was able to sleep that night when we got home.

But when I awakened the next morning, I was exhausted and sick. I felt the same way the next day, and the next, and the next. Before I knew it, a month and a half had gone by. There had been a dramatic change in my body. I knew something was again wrong.

I felt so tired every day and it seemed like I had a mild case of the "flu." I would somehow make it through work and then come home and crawl into bed. I had zero energy.

I consulted with a few acupuncturists and a naturopath. They weren't able to tell me anything I didn't already know. I was too tired to pursue any more practitioners for a while. I was lucky to make it to work. As the months progressed, my husband became increasingly frustrated and even criticized me for being lazy and always watching TV when I was home. I told him I didn't feel well, but it didn't seem to faze him. He had never responded well to me being sick. When he was sick or under the weather he expected me -- and I went out of my way -- to take care of him, but it was rarely reciprocated.

I have never understood why, since he claimed to have loved me so much at one point. I wonder to this day if it was due to alcoholism in some way, or narcissism.

In any case, I believe my health condition was the final tipping point. He lost all sympathy for me. He became cold and callous for the most part from this point on in our marriage. Additionally, our fighting became worse and more violent.

In March of 2005 at Snowbird Utah, my family met for our annual reunion. His father had planned on being there too for some reason. My husband was extremely nervous. He became intoxicated the night before he was to see his father and was verbally abusive to me for a few hours in our hotel room. I finally got angry enough to verbally retaliate. He responded by punching my head and smacking my jaw with a force so hard it sent me flying onto the bed.

I lay there stunned, in pain, and in shock. He had physically assaulted me before this, but never like this. In the past he had knocked me out of bed several times, pulled my hair, roughed me up, slammed me against a wall, etc. to the point of pain and disbelief.

But this night the level of abuse was new. Afterwards, he told me I had to treat him better. I was so devastated I didn't know what to do. Here was someone who had claimed to love me more than life itself, who would never leave me, and who would love me forever.

All I could do at the time was cover the bruise with makeup. I was too traumatized to do or think anything else. The only person to comment was one of his sisters. She asked what happened to my chin. I lied about it. I found out later he had hit her in past years when he briefly lived with her. He had always told me that I was the only one he had ever hit, like I deserved it or something. I used to half believe him.

Not anymore.

We returned home and it was a dark time. I was beyond exhausted physically, emotionally, and spiritually. We continued to have bad fights, and the threat of physical violence was now part of the game.

He was drinking wine regularly, which is what he had drunk in Utah when he hit me, and I realized it was what he had consumed almost every time he was violent with me. However, sometimes he turned to hard liquor when at a club. I began to dread Fridays after work, when he would open a bottle of wine.

The days dragged by and many are a blur in some ways, as there was a lot of fear and fatigue involved for me.

I had learned to pack a small suitcase at the urging of my therapist and have it ready in case he started drinking. We had entered counseling together, in hopes of working on our marriage. But the therapist refused to treat him as long as he was under the influence.

I know I should have left immediately when the violence began and certainly when it escalated, but I think I may have been too sick to think clearly. A lot was happening all at once. And I was not perfect at all during this time. I was so hurt and so afraid and exhausted. I was verbally abusive with him at times as well as he was with me. So I felt partly responsible for the fights. He warned me that if I criticized him I would pay the price.

One of the worst evenings I remember ever was the night I tried to prevent him from going to a bar. We had had a fight after he got drunk on wine (the usual order of things). He said he was going to a bar to continue drinking. I knew he was taking his motorcycle and I was afraid for his life so I hid his keys.

He got raging angry. He towered over me with his fists and body (he was a large 5'10"; I am a petite 5'5") and screamed that he would do major physical harm to me if I did not give him his keys at once. I knew he was serious.

He returned in early morning and raped me. I had not been able to sleep all night I was so afraid for my life. After he was finished, I was up the rest of the night. It was truly a dark night of the soul.

The year 2005 was a blur of fear and fatigue. For some reason I held on probably with the hope that love was somehow alive. I know now I was the only one.

The next March, we went to Snowbird for the reunion. I had told no one about the previous year. I wasn't even thinking consciously about that previous year. I had just reached my limit.

The first day at Snowbird, he got drunk, during the day, on wine. At dinner, he drank even more wine flippantly in front of my family. I was disgusted and done. Back in our hotel room I told him he had to get into treatment. I told him it was the only way I would stay with him. He went out, angry, drank even more, and came home late at night. He attempted to force himself on me. I told him I wasn't feeling well and by some miracle he fell asleep.

In the morning, I told him again he had to go to rehab. He agreed that he needed help and would seek it. I was stunned. I did not know at the time that he was a compulsive liar on top of it all. He left the room. When he returned later that night, I sensed something was up.

We started to fight about drinking and rehab and I could feel the violence factor kicking in. He threatened me. I ran for the door and he blocked me from leaving. I tried again later but he grabbed me again.

As we sat on the bed, facing one another, he continued to sling insults. He verbally threatened me with violence and I knew I was in trouble if I didn't get out of there, and that this time would be different.

Worse.

In a moment of realization, I felt my soul rise up out of my body. It was then I was able to fall out of love enough to grasp the idea that my life was in serious danger. I needed to do whatever it took to protect myself.

I distracted him by asking him to look for my misplaced eyeglasses - luckily and thankfully - and I ran out of the room and down the hall, knocking on people's doors. Someone opened their door and I was safe for the time being.

All of this transpired around 2:00 in the morning, and I had no choice but to go to my parent's hotel room. I told them everything. We talked about it briefly, and then everyone went to bed. We would deal with it at first light.

But I was unable to sleep. I could not stop thinking about the surreal nature of my life. I felt like I was living a nightmare.

The next day, in a family meeting all of my family members confronted my husband. It was decided he would go home early from our trip with the understanding he would move out of our condo and get into rehab. He was polite to my family and acted remorseful. He said he would go to rehab because he could not imagine not being with me for the rest of our lives. He said this straight to my father ... and to me.

The day my husband left Snowbird was the day we separated. My marriage felt over. Despite all that had happened, I chose not to press charges for his abusive behavior, although I was counseled to do so many times.

When I flew back to Oregon a few days later, for some reason we had asked him to pick me up. He was over an hour late and acted rude and dismissive. We had little or no contact over the next months.

However, in late summer he came to our condo, and we spent the weekend together, thinking maybe we could fix things. I was saddened when he proceeded to drink. The next morning, while he was hung-over, he threatened me physically. The old patterns were still alive and well.

Soon it was September, 2006. Almost a year prior to that date, I had started having major fatigue problems. Again, he came over, so we could talk about it, and he threatened my physically again. In the middle of his tirade, he confessed he had never gone to rehab and that he had been seeing someone from work all summer. When we had spent that summer weekend together, I was under the impression we were trying to work things out. Now he was telling me he was no longer in love with me and that he had felt that way for about a year.

My father flew out practically overnight from Florida to Portland to literally protect me from unpredictable violence, and help me sort through divorce proceedings. Even with the calming presence of my father, my health deteriorated even more. There were lots of troubled and/or sleepless nights and severe, unrelenting stress.

This all sounds pretty dramatic. I'm a little embarrassed to write it. I have always considered myself a strong person. I have amazing friendships, and I'm easy going unless I experience injustice to someone else or myself. Perhaps that's why this was so hard to write.

I now know that there were red flags, if only I had been able to see them. In the beginning, when we were first getting to know each other at the spiritual retreat at Solitude, some of the people there were concerned that we were becoming a couple. He told me the reason they were trying to warn me was because they thought I was too stupid to know on my own that he wasn't good for me.

Hard to think it now, but I accepted what he said, and believed that's how they viewed me. I now know he fabricated those stories to keep me from talking to them. Manipulative, to be sure, and a portent of things to come.

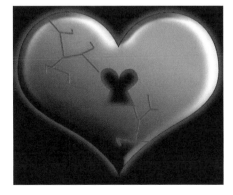

Pay attention to red flags, no matter how small they might seem. You can save yourself a lot of heartbreak, not to mention preserve your precious heart and health.

Writing this part of my story I realize how much it impacted my psyche and physical health. Yes, I'm strong, but I'm also sensitive. And my body, for better or worse, is sensitive, especially now.

Some people are born with strong constitutions. I consider them lucky because the modern world demands a lot of the body. In my case, I am sensitive all the way around, I suppose. My body seemed strong before my surgery, but my constitution has been different ever since.

Some practitioners call my type of person: the "clinical ecology patient." Founded by Theron Randolph, MD, the clinical ecology movement is controversial. Its primary theory is that a number of physical and psychological illnesses may be based on exposure to chemicals in the environment and possibly in foods. Please see Chapter Four for further discussion.

Despite my sensitivities, my spirit is strong, which is why I fought back when my husband became violent. Neither of us wanted to get hurt, of that I'm sure. But, in the end, I was fighting a losing battle with someone who had no business being in a marriage.

From my point of view, I never should have been fighting anyone or anything at all, ever. Why? Because stress is one of the worst things for the body. Chronic stress is actually trauma for the body. It is one of the major silent killers, along with chronic inflammation.

Near the end of 2006, I was in a bad place, and in critically fragile shape. Little did I know, it was only the beginning of my health's major downward slide.

The bottom line was that I knew I had to focus on recovering my health.

I also had to let go of a toxic relationship.

But, why were my feet so deeply entrenched in what felt like heavy, wet sand?

Crescent Moon

I had a dream about you again last night…
you came and put your hands on me.
And then you stood before me…
I knew you still loved me but you could not say it.

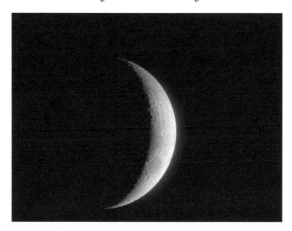

You stood there in silence, waiting for my consent…
until I told you to go away.
You said you could not be with me because you were not well…
you looked at me with unspoken longing
and then, with an empty stare, dismantled your gaze.
Here we yet reside where the river runs dark and deep,
where there is no sound or rippling of life to ascertain.
On the bank it is dry and hollow. The birds circle once and then fly
away…

Will I ever see you again? Maybe one day we will take that trip to Prague.
We would rent a house, play in the streets, kiss in the cafes,
make love after listening to Pucinni's encore and forget all the past
mistakes.
The crescent moon rises tonight. Its face is masked, it longs for the light,
the distant memory of the sun, dark star…remember when I was your
heart?
Come and paint the moon with me.
I am waiting for you here, before the strike of midnight.
Let's begin again before we go to the place where no green waters run.

From Frozen Light: A Collection of Poems by Edie Summers

Dark Angel

I find you in the graveyard,
dressed in black, with green wings.

What are you doing here?
Perhaps you wait for me
while my soul continues wandering.

You crouch behind the iron gate
and watch your silent dominion.
The cemetery otherworldly glows.

I wish you would speak,
for there's so much I would ask.

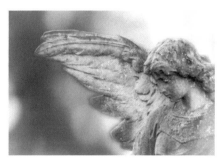

But the night is between us,
and my heart opaque.
And so I watch from a distance
and try to comprehend.
A world consumed by darkness,
and my soul that lies in wake.

From _Frozen Light A Collection of Poems_ by Edie Summers

Afterthought

Ancient ruin I am, my story yet untold…
Underneath my breath, I am holding it
ever so quietly so that you may not even notice
I'm only really half impressed,
a mere image or carbon copy,
an Aztec princess who may not have existed at all.
There's a rupture in the sky quietly susurrusing…
It's where the action is, the real unraveling.
The sun sinks then into such a lazy distance
that I can hardly trace its glow
or believe that it was really a sun at all.
And your kisses miss my mouth
by at least the distance of the nearest star.
In the evening there is a whispering…there are cracks in space…
I see the wind drive through them with the speed of shall we say sound.

From _Frozen Light: A Collection of Poems_ by Edie Summers

My father insisted I seek the help of a doctor again. I resisted as is my nature. I told him no one had ever figured out much of anything that was going on with me. But he persisted and I finally gave in.

We found an independent doctor who was also a naturopath, Dr. Daniel Newman, a student of Chinese Classical Medicine. Dr. Newman interviewed me for two hours. He listened intently and took notes on his computer the entire time. I never even filled out paperwork initially. I just talked, and he listened. I had never experienced such devotion, in terms of listening, from a health care practitioner, ever. Most of the doctors I had seen had me in and out of their offices in about 15 minutes except for the first naturopath I had seen when I was 23.

Dr. Newman asked all sorts of questions, starting with my history of health from the first time I started having health issues in my early 20's. He asked me about my diet, my lifestyle, my reactions to perfumes, chemical smells, everything.

After he was finished asking questions and listening to my answers, he looked up from his computer. "I think I know exactly what's going on with you," he said. My heart leaped in my chest. God, I hoped so. They sounded like miracle words to me. "I think you have a liver condition. We'll take a genetic liver test to be sure, but I think your liver may not be detoxing properly in *Phase II* ..." It all sounded like a foreign language to me, but I was very hopeful that we – I – was finally getting somewhere.

He also told me we would be checking for candida, and we would do an ASI test. This was an adrenal stress index test to see how my adrenals were functioning. He ordered a stool test to check for parasites, and lectured/asked me about my diet. He told me I had to start eating more meat and taking fish oil every day, along with high doses of Vitamin C (up to bowel tolerance.) He asked me to bring in my supplements when I returned for my follow-up visit to review my test results.

I left the office feeling hopeful, although I was unsure about the meat recommendation. (Please see the Box titled "Meet Your Meat.")

Meet Your Meat

My ex-husband and I had watched the PETA video "Meet Your Meat," which was horrifying. It showed the cruelty that factory farm animals endure. It was like viewing a holocaust. The video showed chickens and pigs being picked up by their feet and having their heads slammed into the ground, multiple chickens stuffed live into buckets, and downer cows (unable to walk) falling off slaughter-bound trucks, then left with to die in the road. I was profoundly affected by the video – I bawled when I saw it -- and had trouble with any kind of animal products afterwards for quite some time, especially meat.

After talking with Dr. Newman, my list of symptoms was significant and even strange. Besides chronic fatigue - CFS - which is what Dr. Newman diagnosed me as having, and therefore my insurance would not cover my visits, I had the following symptoms:

Constant runny nose,
Bloodshot eyes that continued to worsen
Nosebleeds
Mild headaches
Strong negative reactions to EMF's (electromagnetic fields)
Chemical smell sensitivity
Really bad body odor
And my teeth were turning black

Huh? You read that right, my teeth were black. Or at least there was a black filmy substance that kept re-appearing. It freaked me out - there are no other words. I later discovered the hair, mainly on top of my head, was growing in coarse, wiry, and black as well. And it itched. As time progressed, I began to lose my hair. It fell out in cycles, and it never really stopped for a few years. I used to have long, lustrous hair. Not anymore. Later when I visited yet another acupuncturist, he noticed my tongue was black as well. He was very concerned.

The black film on my teeth and black hair to this day is a mystery to everyone I have consulted. But it's entirely possible it was due to heavy metals my body could not get rid of. I found a little information on the web about cancer patients whose hair would grow back in the way I've described after chemotherapy and/or radiation treatments.

The possible connection between heavy metals and chronic fatigue will be further explored in detail in Chapter Three. All I know is that once my genetic test results came back, Dr. Newman confirmed that, indeed, several of my *Phase II* enzymes were contributing to inadequate detoxification, due to what is known as *genetic polymorphisms*.

In addition, the test gave me a list of chemicals to avoid. They are chemicals my liver cannot process – or process very well – again due to *genetic polymorphisms*. Number one on the list is Elavil. Naprosyn and caffeine are on the list as well. Go figure.

I stopped taking Elavil and Benadryl immediately. I did not want to mess around with my liver anymore and I was shocked that my worst fears in some ways were being confirmed. But at least I had some answers finally.

For reference, there are two phases in liver detoxification. My genetic liver test, performed by Genova Diagnostics Laboratory, revealed the following:

In *Phase I,* I have a polymorphism detected in one enzyme. Sadly for me the decrease in this enzyme's ability to do its job means that toxins that pass through *Phase I* can actually become more toxic than in their original form.

These toxic intermediates are then accumulated in the body and passed on to *Phase II.* The toxins this particular enzyme breaks down include: PAHS, which are basically exhaust fumes, charbroiled meats, etc. It also breaks down estrogen, nitrosamines, nicotine, coumarin, prilosec, sulfonureas, anticonvulsants like Valium, fifty percent of prescription drugs including tricyclics (like Elavil), MAOIs, SSRIs, opiates, beta-blockers, and most steroid hormones. No wonder I didn't tolerate synthetic drugs!

As luck would have it, my *Phase II* detoxification is much worse than my *Phase I* detoxification function. I have three enzymes where both of my chromosomes carry genetic variations, and one gene that has nil to poor functioning, according to my test. *The latter one, with nil to poor function, is one of three genes that make glutathione.*

Glutathione is a powerful liver detoxifier and antioxidant, (please see Chapter Three.) Basically, the very enzymes and glutathione that I am short on *act to break down* many water-soluble environmental toxins, including certain solvents, herbicides, fungicides, lipid peroxides, and heavy metals like mercury, cadmium, and lead.

One of the enzymes I am low on is responsible for interrupting the effects of the neurotransmitters dopamine, epinephrine, and norepinephrine. Thus I may be left potentially at risk for depression, anxiety, and, ironically, alcoholism.

And here's a really relevant fact: the *lack of glutathione can contribute to fatigue syndromes* and to oxidative stress, and various cancers as well.

Eat Your Greens
What is one of the best ways to detox your liver, especially if you don't detox properly, which actually is true for a significant portion of the population? Eat your leafy greens. There are a whole lot of reasons to eat your greens, including better digestion, but enabling your liver to detox more efficiently is a major bonus. Find a way to eat your greens consistently. Please see Chapter Three for a detailed discussion.
Your body and liver will thank you!

The genetic liver test I took produced results that were supposedly 99.7% accurate. However, the test is not approved by the US Food and Drug Administration, and Dr. Newman told me that very few doctors order it. In my opinion, genetic tests are a resource we should utilize, always keeping in mind that these genetic tests *indicate genetic predispositions, not guaranteed outcomes.* For me, I have no intention of letting my genetic pre-dispositions rule my life any more than they already have.

My candida test came out highly positive, meaning I had candidiasis – an overgrowth of yeast – throughout my body. Some doctors dismiss this condition, but candida overgrowth can be very serious if it is systemic. It may even be a major contributing factor to CFS. It can even lead to death in elderly patients. Dr. Newman advised me that candida feed on sugar, so I cut out sugar immediately. Our plan was to starve the candida.

I was not able to complete a few of the other tests due to extreme reactions to the chemicals used in some of them. My reaction to chemical smells was horrible at that time. Even small exposure to perfumes or detergents made me feel awful and could affect me for days. It sounds extreme, but I even had to stop reading any magazines, which contained perfume scratch ads. Most perfumes today contain 500-600 substances, including formaldehyde, petroleum products, etc. For a short, informative post titled *What's in My Perfume?* click on this Jurgita link: http://www.jurgita.com/articles-id111.html

Dr. Newman sent me home with a kit to test my adrenals. I was disappointed in myself when I could not tolerate the wax on the film paper I was supposed to hold in my mouth four times a day for 10 minutes to extract saliva for the test. I had to wait to take this adrenal test until much later, down the road. Note: while testing one's adrenals can be useful, it is the whole HPA axis that is involved. See Chapter Three for a detailed discussion of hypocortisolism, etc.

At any rate, my main concern at the time was the health of my liver. Dr. Newman told me to take as much milk thistle as I could stand. I was to drink it in tea, eat it, and take it as a supplement.

The problem was, my liver was in such poor shape that taking even a small amount of milk thistle sent my body into a tailspin. Milk thistle is a potent liver detoxifier and regenerative (although, I believe it works best in combo with other herbs). I had taken it before in my late 20's and had never noticed any side effects from it. Not so this time.

My body was so weak that I was in no condition to be detoxing. First, I had to build myself up. I had started divorce proceedings, sold the condo we had both lived in, and moved into a new place. So there was a lot of external stress going on in addition to my own internal stressors.

In fact, my life had been hectic for years. I had moved five times in five years, got married, left my old jobs, started new jobs, moved to a new state, had a rocky marriage, got sick and started the process of divorce. It was a lot to sort out. The stress factor in my life was a10 out of 10 and had been so for a long time.

After I moved into my new condo, my father took me to the coast to celebrate my 36th birthday that November. I think we both assumed this would be the end of this chapter in my life and that things would get better. My divorce did not finalize until February of the following year. But it did feel like it was, hopefully, a new chapter for me.

It was also a new chapter for my dad. That previous summer of 2006, he had been diagnosed with *stage three esophageal cancer*. We didn't know it then, but his destiny was to fight his disease for two years and then pass away in Florida. What I did know was that when he said good-by to me that November, I felt more or less alone in Portland with little or no support at first, dealing with chronic illness and unable to work.

I started to settle into my new place and I assumed that things would change. They did, but for the worse.

I felt tired, even more than I had before. There were some days when I couldn't even get out of bed. My place smelled a little funny to me as well. When I had found the place, it had been late summer. So the windows were open when I was checking it out. I noticed it smelled the worst in my bedroom, which was small and didn't have a lot of air circulation. I looked over the papers again and I noticed it said my place had new carpeting and a new paint. Uh oh. I wondered how I had not noticed this before.

In addition, I had purchased a new custom-made chair for the living room. It was a chair and a half (I was hopeful for my personal life). After it was delivered, I could smell something funny coming from the chair's upholstery. My sense of smell had heightened lately. Plus it was now cold, so all the windows had to be shut to keep the heat in.

I felt out of sorts and exhausted most of every day. It seemed worse than before. I wasn't sure if it was depression or what. I just felt bad.

My world was drowning in fog. And every time I tried to take milk thistle I felt awful. I was so tired I couldn't even finish unpacking the boxes from the move. One time my friend came over to water my plants while I was out of town and she was shocked at the state of my condo. It was in complete disarray. I had been too tired to even load the last batch of dishes from the sink into the dishwasher before I left.

At the end of December 2006, I traveled to Florida to be with my family. I felt immediately better when I got there and took long walks on the beach.

But a strange thing happened. My brother's girlfriend used sunscreen with an intense, chemical scent. I was even in the other room when she was using it, and the scent was so strong, that I was immediately affected negatively. I started feeling panicky and dizzy, and did not feel well at all. It was bizarre but real. I had a reaction to a chemical perfume from another room. Actually, I thought she was wearing perfume since I react the most intensely to those ingredients. Unfortunately, I had to ask her not to use that sunscreen for the rest of the trip. It was embarrassing, but I had no choice. Any kind of chemical odors were absolutely intolerable.

Overall, in Florida, I felt better and had more energy. When I returned to Oregon, I thought for sure I would get better. Instead, I soon started to feel overly tired again, and lost any energy and feeling of well-being I had gained from the trip.

I quickly descended into physical hell.

There is no denying that much of what happened to me was physical. I know that without a doubt. But a pattern I also noticed was that anytime in the next four years that I was essentially alone, my health slid, even during periods when I was on the mend. I absolutely believe that human connection - genuine connection - is essential to health.

In wellness coaching there is a quote that says *connection is the currency of wellness, (John Travis)*. No matter how much of my unrelenting fatigue and illness was due to exposure to drugs and stress, an equal amount was due to loneliness and the breach of trust and faith when my marriage ended.

The contracts I had with people – especially the marriage vows I had made with my husband – were broken. My friendships were tested and so was my relationship with my family.

When I was at my sickest, I was alone.

It is no wonder it took me so long to climb out of the hole. If you are currently alone and sick reading this, I urge you to seek and make real connections. It is the quickest way to get well and stay well.

I understand that the last thing you may want to do is reach out when you are down and out, sick, depressed, or all of the above. You may have to force yourself to reach out. If that's the case, do it. Force yourself to reach out and connect with others.

Any shame or any other feelings you may have are not as important as having real, genuine tethers in your life. When we are around or in close proximity to others, including familial and social connections as well as romantic bonds, helpful chemicals such as dopamine and oxytocin are released. These are powerful immunomodulators and help to enhance our immune system. Find a way to get and stay close to others to save your health and life.

When I got back from Florida, I fell off a cliff. Unfortunately, my liver had not healed/detoxed enough. In addition, the new chair I had bought was still in my condo.

When I walked in, I was immediately overpowered by a chemical odor. I now understand that it was the off-gassing from the chair's fire retardant. I started to feel sick and tired almost immediately. I made a mental note that I had to get rid of the chair a.s.a.p.

Of course, very quickly my sense of smell adapted to the chemical smell, and I convinced myself that I would be okay. A number of days later - I lost sense of time - my body crashed. I felt so awful I literally could not get out bed. I started to feel extremely funny in my body, including my head.

The neurotoxins created from the fire retardant (fire retardants are more toxic than ever now), were affecting my brain as well as my body. I knew I was in serious trouble. I literally felt myself fall into serious illness. It was one of the worst feelings in the world.

I felt so debilitated that I started having suicidal thoughts. I tried telling people, but I did not get the reaction I hoped for, which was *help*.

I asked several people to help me remove the chair. The chair weighed probably close to 300 pounds. I even called my ex-husband out of desperation. He told me to fuck off, he was watching a football game.

I was so sick I was in bed most of the time. I could barely function. I did not know what to do as I could not think straight. I called the suicide hotline. They told me to call my friends or family. I tried my ex-husband again as I knew my body was in serious danger and getting sicker. He called me a fucking bitch.

I could tell even in my haze that he was drunk. I called several other friends and no one picked up. Finally I was able to reach my friend in Utah. I felt so sick I was panicked. She talked me through it and brainstormed with me. Later that night my friend in Portland returned my call. It was hell day for me, the day I felt my body descend into true sickness. It was one of the worst days of my life.

I bought a ton of plants like ferns and spider plants that I had read could absorb toxic fumes. They helped a little, but not much. It occurred to me finally after some research on the net, to order an air filter.

My friend in Portland had told me that she and her husband used them in their home. I read online how they were used in offices to pull VOC's out of the air in airtight office buildings. I found the website AllerAir through a search on *multiple chemical sensitivity* (MCS.) AllerAir was founded after a close relative of the president of the company was diagnosed with MCS. Sam Teitelbaum researched and found technology developed by NASA using carbon filters that were very effective in true air purification, not just pulling dust out of the air. AllerAir uses up to 40 different proprietary carbon blends and offers non-toxic material for the housing of the filters as well.

The AllerAir filters are designed for people who cannot tolerate any kind of off-gassing whatsoever. I was one of those people.

My tolerance at this point had gotten so low that I had to stay in a motel for almost a week until the air filter showed up. I could not handle being in my place for even a little bit any more. My body would not allow it.

Once the air filter arrived, I noticed a pretty significant change. I was able to at least function again. The air in my place smelled significantly lighter and cleaner. I ordered another air filter for my bedroom.

It occurred to me to call the place from where I had bought the chair. It had been a number of months but they were gracious. Even though it was a custom made order originally, they allowed me to exchange it for something else. It was the only help I could get in physically moving the chair out of my place.

The chair was gone, but I knew I was still reacting to the new carpeting and the new paint. My body was so worn down, I was reacting to any kind of synthetic scent, and there seemed to be a lot of them.

I had especially violent reactions to laundry detergents and perfumes. These types of scents seemed to be the biggest problem for me. Even something as innocuous as receiving mail that was scented could affect me negatively for days at a time.

For whatever reason, my body could not bounce back quickly from exposure to the scents. Some perfumes were worse than others. I figured out later that artificial scents made with synthetic estrogens were the worst offenders for me. This is because my liver enzymes - or lack thereof - could not properly break down synthetic estrogens.

Synthetic estrogens are some of the worst offenders in the chemical world, next to dioxins and then VOC's. VOC's are found in carpeting, paint, cosmetics, air fresheners, household cleaners, etc. They can cause fatigue, headaches, allergies, asthma, difficulties in concentration, etc. I will explain more about synthetic estrogens and synthetic chemicals in Chapter Two, coming up here.

While synthetic estrogens are a particular problem for me, I definitely noticed a pattern where I did not do well with most things synthetic. I remembered how I had trouble with perfumes and scents the first time I dealt with fatigue in my early 20's.

At any rate, I was feeling better since I wasn't exposed to quite so many fumes every day, but I was still exhausted and still felt sick. But at least the filters were working. I was grateful for that.

A month or two later my family got the news my dad was sick with Stage Three esophageal cancer. It was a devastating blow for all of us. I immediately got to work researching alternative treatments for his type of cancer. I also secretly wondered if all of the stress of my marriage falling apart, all of the lies my ex-husband told us, and the ongoing violence factor, had contributed to my dad getting sick. I knew it certainly had contributed greatly to my condition.

My mom later told me that my dad was far more greatly affected by the circumstances surrounding the end of my marriage than he had let on to me. I think I knew this already, but it was hard to hear. I felt responsible somehow for all that had transpired.

My ex-husband was not only violent, but had told all of us many lies, basically whatever he thought we wanted to hear. I will not go into all of the details, but his lying affected us greatly. We never knew where he was coming from or what he truly meant.

In addition, we endured extreme stress dealing with his alcoholism, violence, and untruthfulness, with my acute fatigue, and with the divorce, all of which affected the course of my life and my dad's life greatly. It was devastating and exhausting each and every day.

Beyond the stress of knowing my dad was sick and the fact that I was still unemployed, I was starting to feel at least somewhat better. Even though I was still very tired, I had just enough energy to test the waters with exercise.

I began taking a hip hop class since I was a former dancer and I knew it would lift my spirits. I could barely make it through class at first, but I felt my liver being cleansed even more (intense exercise is one of the best ways to clean the liver) and slowly but surely I felt myself start to recover.

I was still very tired, but I was eating well and the intense bi-weekly dance classes were helping with my chi, i.e. vitality.

As the summer of 2006 wore on, my father was in chemotherapy and radiation treatments. I still felt super tired but I was definitely stressing about money and work.

I also felt that something had not been addressed in terms of my health. Why was I still so tired? I was doing everything I was supposed to be doing to get well.

I saw Dr. Newman again, and he put me on Chinese Herbs. I have had some success with Chinese Herbs, but these were not working particularly well for me.

I looked around for another practitioner. I had done so much research on environmental illness lately, and I kept thinking that I needed to detox more due to all the synthetic chemicals I had been exposed to.

I was trying to figure out where my fatigue was coming from, where it originated. I learned later that fatigue is a sign of many illnesses; it is a general warning sign or symptom. At the time however, I was convinced it had one point of origin in me, one overriding health issue that was causing it (and, in my case, dysregulation of the HPA axis).

Many people deal with chronic fatigue: it may be up to 50 million people worldwide and growing. Chronic fatigue is, unfortunately, a bit of a Rubik's Cube. Why? Because the causes are varied and seemingly unrelated; it can be a symptom or warning sign for many different named illnesses; it feels different to each patient; and the ways to try and help oneself are so varied for each person. Each of the foregoing points shares the attribute of *multiplicity*. Chronic fatigue is like a complicated machine that no one understands.

The bottom line is, chronic fatigue is awful. It is difficult to think even how to describe it to someone who has not experienced it.

Chronic fatigue is feeling that you have no energy, absolutely zero energy - like you are at zero point energy - and even below that if it's possible. It feels like the main switch in your body that gives you energy has been turn off - or shorted out - and you can't turn it on.

At my worst times of fatigue, which are yet to be told in my story, I felt like I was being dragged through suffocating quicksand where I could not breathe because I did not have the energy to draw breath on my own. I was literally too tired to breathe. I have experienced some chronic pain as well, and I have heard that it is horrible to live with.

I once knew a young woman whose back was in constant pain after a car fell on her when she was a teen. I met her when she was in her late 20's and realized that she battled agonizing pain each day. No matter what she did, she faced on-going, excruciating pain, along with an addiction to painkillers that often left her incapacitated.

We met in group therapy. She hoped to deal with her pain on an emotional level at least. I am not comparing chronic pain and chronic fatigue except to note that both are seemingly unrelenting, and physically and emotionally agonizing, although in different ways.

Fatigue seems to manifest itself on many levels: physical, mental, emotional, spiritual, etc. In fact, I believe the issue of chronic fatigue on the deepest level is related to *fear, which activates the stress response.* It may also be related to power. There are also medical reasons for the multiple levels of fatigue and I will explore them in Chapter Three.

When we live in state of fear, our fight or flight system is activated, and this can drain us, especially if we stay in this state indefinitely. How does one become trapped in a state of fear? Trauma - early childhood and PTSD in particular - are two such ways. I examine both of these in Chapter Three. How does one move out of it a constant state of fear? Two ways are by cultivating the Relaxation Response and mindfulness … Please see Chapters Four and Five, respectively.

Many people who get sick easily also have boundary issues, meaning they easily let people with negative and/or toxic energy into their worlds, and thus into their energy fields. It's no surprise they then become ill. Again, this phenomenon may be related to trauma.

For better or worse, we are all like sponges. Our energy fields expand or contract depending on with whom or with what we interact.

By allowing people into your world who are energy demons or who have seriously unresolved issues such as substance abuse, or problems with anger and/or negativity, you are essentially playing Russian roulette with your health.

You are a sitting duck - unless you protect yourself.

The issue of power is one I will address throughout this book. It is a sublime, weighty, transcendental, esoteric, and extremely practical topic all rolled into one big word: *power*. Power, energy, empowerment …

Both *power and fear*, as they are related to chronic fatigue on the physical, mental, emotional, and spiritual levels, may be crucial to understand in order to truly heal and break free from the nightmare of chronic exhaustion.

Ideally, our bodies are so powerful - they have so much energy - they could light up the entire United States at night for a week if not more. On top of that, the quiet energy stored in our souls is so powerful that we know, on the deepest level of being, that *love* is the greatest power/energy in the known universe.

These are the levels of power I refer to when I mention the elusive, sought-after state of being called *empowerment* and *freedom from fear*.

Clearly at this point in my story, I was not there quite yet.

In late summer of 2006, I had an inkling that I was feeling somewhat better. I was eating well, sleeping well, and exercising. I felt my body begin to slightly recover. I still had bad days - most of them - but I could tell I was mending. In August, we had a three day heat wave where the temperatures were over 100 degrees. As I have described, I was living in my tiny second floor condo with no air conditioning.

Unfortunately during those particular three days, I was not feeling so well. I have had many days in the last 18 years where I felt like I had a slight, constant fever in the course of dealing with chronic fatigue. The feeling resembled a mild case of flu.

During the heat wave, I had those common *flu-like symptoms*, so I was in bed a lot. I tend to run cold and I used to do very well in the heat overall, so the extreme heat did not bother me too much.

On the second day, my head started to hurt. I went to see a movie and hang out in a cool theater until the heat abated. The third night, very late, when I was lying in bed, I felt something literally *pop* or break in my neck and travel down the left side of my leg.

I was immediately in pain from the left side of my neck to my leg, including an intense pain in my left buttock. My whole left side seized up as well. I could barely move that part of my body from my neck through my leg. My head was in a lot of pain on the left side as well where my initial headache had been.

For years, symptoms created by this injury would flare up mildly if I was exposed to chemicals, etc. For the longest time, I would get *head pain* and it even affected my motor control (my motor control can be affected if I am overstimulated in general).

Many people on my Facebook page - Chronic Fatigue Support – talk about how they have head pain or headaches. Some even have migraines, including some of my former wellness coaching clients.

As I mentioned, I used to love the heat, and I thrived in the summer months. I do pretty well now, quite a few years after my injury, but my tolerance is nonetheless diminished. Is my heat intolerance from a dysregulated nervous system (HPA axis) or is it something else?

People who have multiple sclerosis (MS) also have very low heat tolerance. It is lower than even mine. Nevertheless, could all of this evidence point to the fact that not only is CFS a condition of the central nervous system but also that it might be an *auto-immune condition* just like MS? Some people call it an energy disorder, but I think it's more realistic and accurate to call it a central nervous system disorder.

Cold and Hot
I know now the *cold feeling* is most likely related to sub-clinical hypothyroidism. It's also possible my internal regulating mechanism, the hypothalamus, which detects and measures body temperature, was dysregulated. For years, I've had trouble detecting my appetite, and I suspect this was the same mechanism in me that did not properly assess just how hot it really was, or rather how well my body was reacting to the intense heat. See Chapter Three for details. Of course, it's also related to self-esteem and how I valued myself at the time, since I did not leave my condo more quickly. See Chapter Five for details.

After my injury occurred that night, I was devastated and totally alarmed. In a panic, I called my only friend in town at the time. I had no idea what had happened, and I thought maybe I would have to go to the emergency room, one of my least favorite things to do. I explained to my friend about the sudden pain. I knew it sounded odd to say the least. We talked a bit until I determined that I did not need to go to the hospital.

But I still did not understand what the hell happened to me. Here was something else that seemed to be off the radar in terms of my health. The entire left side of my body was in extreme pain. I could barely move and walk, and then only with limitations. Instinctively, I knew it was tied to the previous day's headache. And the pain in my head was still excruciating. I was devastated.

In the morning, I noticed a number of large blue veins extending from my head down either side of my face. There were also new, blue veins spanning out from my bottom eyelids. Under my eyes were some burst capillaries. All of this shocked and worried me, to say nothing of the fact that I looked like a character out of a gothic movie or novel.

Something highly unusual had happened but I still did not know what to do to help myself. My mom recommended I see a specialist and request an MRI immediately.

The last thing I needed was this injury on top of not feeling great. I could no longer sleep on my side due to pressure in my head. The sensation felt like my head was *leaking* on either side and down the back. I also had intense pain on the upper left side where my headache had originally been. Much to my alarm, my head was swollen as well. I know this because the many of my sun hats I usually wore seemed way too small all of a sudden.

My situation quickly stabilized, but there was a dull pain remaining in my head and I was severely lacking in being able to walk normally without limitation in my left leg. To my amazement, I noticed a bulging on the left side of my inner thigh. I knew it was connected to the same vein - or the thing that had popped - in my neck. Ok, enough is enough. Time for action.

I realized I had to consult a neurologist but the problem was that it has been push/pull with me to see professionals ever since my experience with the knee surgeon. I associate traditional doctors with lack of compassion, and lack of listening skills, etc. I know this is not true across the board and I have had some positive experiences as well. The other hesitation I had is that it is frustrating to be told there is nothing wrong, even when there *clearly* is something wrong.

Finally, I made an appointment with a neurologist. My friend went with me since I dreaded trying to get myself across to doctors. Also, I could barely walk or open doors. The neurologist later told me that when he first met me he had been afraid I had multiple sclerosis. He scheduled an MRI. The results came back as normal.

The only abnormal result on the MRI report was that a gland on the left side of my neck was swollen and oversized about an inch. This is often the case in people with CFS. It may have indicated an overtaxed immune system, one that is always *on alert*, fending off pathogens, etc. My mom urged me to get a second opinion from another neurologist. I assured her I would.

For some reason, I did not feel a sense of urgency about it since my injury had stabilized, even though my head still ached. But I knew I had to make sure everything was okay. I think I also resisted because I did not want to receive any bad news. But knowing what I know now about head injuries I should have been in the second doctor's office the next day.

I'm thinking of Natasha Richardson, the actress, who hit her head while skiing. She was rescued and taken to the infirmary but she refused to stay there. She said she felt okay enough to walk back to her hotel. Unfortunately, she actually had sustained an epidural hematoma so that blood collected between her skull and her dura matter, or the covering that protects the brain. Ms. Richardson died a day or two after the accident.

I was lucky in the respect that although my head injury can still bother me today, apparently whatever happened, was not serious enough to impact my life like Ms. Richardson's.

Nevertheless, I was so frustrated to have to keep dealing with all of the horrific things that kept happening to my body. Certainly, I felt devastated by how the broken and enlarged veins in my head and on my face made me look.

I searched the web about blue veins on the face and found a doctor in California who specialized in getting rid of them through cool glide lasers. His establishment was the only place I found that promised they could erase of these unsightly large blue veins. So even though I was fighting exhaustion, I packed my car and drove to California, desperate for help with my veins.

I arrived at The Berman Skin Institute for my appointment with Ebu, an assistant to Dr. Berman. I told her what had happened to my head. She said she could get rid of the blue veins, but that I should see a neurologist because I kept complaining that my veins hurt. She said they should not hurt and that there must be something else going on.

She listened carefully to my story, even the part about my illness and on-going fatigue. She was professional, yet compassionate. She treated my blue veins and also did some laser work on spider veins on the rest of my body. The laser treatment for the rest of my body lasted for about an hour.

On the way home to Portland, I noticed my body had inflammation. It was making it challenging to drive, since I also had increased swelling in my head. I definitely knew that this was a new sensation: body-wide inflammation. I tried to brush it off and completed the trip home, although it was difficult as I had so much inflammation in my body, and I felt beyond exhausted.

When I was home again my inflammation went down, but I was feeling more tired than usual. I also noticed my blue veins had not been completely erased. So I called the Berman Skin Institute, and they told me I could come back for a free follow up visit which I eventually did. At the institute, Ebu gave me another hour long laser treatment, including the touch up on my face.

Afterwards, on my way to my cousin's where I was staying, I noticed an overall inflammation had returned to my body.

Suddenly, I felt awful and started having extreme reactions to perfume fragrances. But, where were those scents coming from? Were they on me? I figured out that in the waiting room of the medical office where I just had been, there were cosmetics and perfumes for sale, etc. Synthetic fragrances are so strong, and the fumes can linger for hours if not days in rooms, on bodies, etc.

I now know my HPA axis was overwhelmed again, and chronic stress was creating body-wide inflammation.

I drove to my cousin's with my windows rolled completely down because I noticed that my inflammation was better with the windows wide open (fresh air diluted the fumes from the synthetic scents). It seemed like I just couldn't win because with the windows down, I then had to deal with exhaust from all the vehicles caught in traffic.

My body could only tolerate the chemical scents so much if at all. My sense of smell was heightened and anything with a synthetic odor, smelled horrible to me and I felt my body react violently to it.

To top it off, I went over a large pot hole. The jolt to my body hurt my head all over again. I was just in constant, massive pain.

On the morning I set out for Portland, I had so much inflammation in my body felt like soft cement, like I could barely sit and was super inflexible. I was exhausted as well, like beyond exhausted. I knew something was horribly wrong with my body again. What the hell?

A couple of hours into the trip, the inflammation had risen to an even higher level in my body, so much so that I could barely sit in my seat. The inflammation was so bad that it was putting tremendous pressure on my injured head on top of everything else, making it nearly impossible to drive.

It is hard to describe what happened. You would have to experience it first hand to understand. My body literally felt like semi-soft cement. My body's reaction seemed unreal to me. I was in disbelief. I did not have the energy to drive very far. Around noon, the inflammation was so intense I had to get off the road. I pulled into a motel and got into bed. I was in absolute agony the rest of the day and night.

Nothing is perfect but the whole scene was becoming so much less than perfect, it was a nightmare. It didn't take long for me to also start reacting to the cleaning fluids they had used in the motel. Plus, I could barely watch television, because the radiation coming off of the TV was increasing my level and intensity of inflammation. It was a very long night.

The next morning, I knew I didn't have the energy to drive home. I was that tired. I called my cousin to see if I could return and stay with her a few more days. I was only about three hours from her place if I turned south, whereas Portland was at least 10-12 hours north.

My head was still hurting too and, again, my mom advised me to see a neurologist. But in order to see one, I had to have a referral. So instead, I went to the local hospital emergency room near my cousin's.

The smells of ammonia and other chemical smells in the hospital were overwhelming. I have never liked the smells of hospitals, but now it was almost unbearable. It made my inflammation even worse. I was definitely noticing a pattern that whenever I was around any synthetic scents or chemicals, my inflammation increased significantly.

The doctor on-call ordered a CAT scan. He said he did not see anything abnormal (of course.) I was so worried though, I made an appointment with a local neurologist as well, just to be safe. The neurologist told me I probably had a muscle pull. A muscle pull? That did not sound right to me. But with two doctors telling me I was fine, I tried to let my worries go, or at least put them on hold.

I stayed a few more days in California until I felt strong enough to drive to Portland. I couldn't understand. Why couldn't I have a procedure done like any other human being, drive home, and get on with my life? It seemed like everything happening in my life was just incredibly difficult and almost impossible to bear.

Upon arriving home, I was exhausted. I kept waiting for this new problem, inflammation, to go away. It did not. In addition, over the next six months, or even longer, my ability to move - both due to my injury and now this pernicious inflammation - was severely limited.

I gained 20 pounds and went from being underweight, due to an on-going lack of appetite, to overweight in a short period. This was not a good development. I know now how crucial movement is to getting and staying well. Movement *is* life force.

I read Lance Armstrong's book *It's Not About The Bike* and he said he knew he had to keep moving during his illness. Even when he was in bed in the hospital getting chemotherapy treatments, he would get up and walk or exercise as much as possible. He kept telling himself, *If I can move, I'm not sick.* How true.

These days, ever since I've been able to exercise again, I've noticed improvements in my overall health and energy levels. Yes, it is very much the case that some people's symptoms with chronic fatigue are made worse by exercise. That has certainly been true for me in terms of prolonged, intense exercise in the past. I had a few experiences where a long hike or intense exercise class could exhaust me for days. But, in general, I strongly believe that moderate exercise overall makes and keeps you well. The trick is to stay in the parasympathetic state – The Relaxation Response – and not in the sympathetic state (Fight or Flight or the stress response) while you are moving (see Chapter Four).

There is scientific basis for why movement helps us. Inside of every human cell are tiny bean-shaped systems called mitochondria. We all have mitochondria and we have the ability to produce more of them when we exercise. Mitochondria are energy powerhouses. **The more mitochondria we have, the more energy we have.**

Exercise also cleans out the lymphatic system, which is crucial for all of us, including those who do not process synthetic substances well. The lymphatic system cannot clean/detox itself. Foods and supplements like greens and organic lemons can help as well (and juicing citrus fruit helps my energy levels as well tremendously). Breathing is one of the best ways, and is a large part of what exercise is, involves the breath.

I believe this is one of the reasons yoga is so beneficial. Focused deep breathing is a large part of what makes us well. And, as they say, exercise is so good for you, it would be the *number one pill* prescribed by doctors – if indeed they could put it into a pill. Now that's a drug I'd be inclined to take, although there's nothing like the real thing.

When I was experiencing the massive level of inflammation in my body, not only could I not walk or move very much, but dance was pretty much ruled out as well. I tried a class, but the inflammation just aggravated my head injury, because the body is connected, and every move you make reverberates everywhere. Plus, my head had its own, localized inflammation around the injury.

When you're injured, your body freezes the part that's injured until it has healed.

We all know that the body tries to protect itself. But when you experience it firsthand, along with systemic inflammation, it is overwhelming. At least that's how it was for me. It was so frustrating after having been such an active person for so long. I was used to going and doing anything, even if I was tired. I almost always found a way to be active, exhaustion be damned.

But now I literally felt *trapped* in my body. It was the final straw for me. And thus I entered into the worst six months of my life…

My inflammation, called *cellular inflammation* or *chronic inflammation* by medical professionals, was so bad I was literally mostly bed-bound.

For at least six months, I more or less lay in bed, much of it in total darkness, with nothing but my thoughts about the excruciating state my body was in to keep me company.

I did watch TV or get online for maybe half an hour at a time a few times during the day. But for the most part, I could not tolerate lights, radiation from the TV, computers, the radio, etc.

My nervous system was completely shot. It was beyond shot. My body began behaving in ways that you normally couldn't imagine. I couldn't sit most of the time because the level of inflammation in my body was so bad. Again, imagine cement right before it dries. This used to be how my knee was after surgery. Now this was how my whole body was, and even worse.

It is very hard to describe what body-wide inflammation feels like. It's like I had *no flow* in my body. It was literally almost stiff.

Part of me knew it was because my nervous system was or felt completely out of whack. But I didn't understand too much about what was causing my body to behave that way. All I knew was that it was a very frightening place to be. I learned much more as time went on. What causes chronic inflammation, you might be wondering? *One factor may be chronic stress, which elevates insulin levels, and leads to a pro-inflammatory, even activated immune state* (see Chapter Three for details).

My immune and/or nervous system was activated to the point that when I did try to sit down, say at the computer, or worse, in the car, or God forbid, on an airplane, there was no guarantee I could sit at all. There were windows of time, usually in late morning, when my inflammation was at least somewhat better so I could actually sit comfortably. I now know that's because those hours are when cortisol levels are at their highest.* I finally figured out down the road that one of the reasons I was experiencing such massive, wide-spread inflammation was because my cortisol levels were extremely low.

When your body reaches the final stages of exhaustion, this is often what happens: at first cortisol levels usually rise when you are first experiencing exhaustion. But if the stressors in your life continue, eventually the bottom drops out beneath you, and your cortisol levels can plummet. This is called the exhaustion phase. Cortisol is one of the things that reduces and controls inflammation levels in the body.

The only way I could survive an airplane trip during this time and for the next six months as well, was to raise my cortisol levels or reduce my inflammation levels by taking ginkgo, certain types of homeopathy for inflammation, gota kola, or eating, ideally, sugar-free chocolate.

Otherwise, my inflammation would not have allowed me to sit for such a long period of time, or so I thought, at least. I endured one very long trip to Disney World in Florida. I was so sick, I don't know how I even made it there.

It was supposed to be a feel good trip. A lot of people who are sick go to Disney World, I noticed when I was there. There is definitely something magical in the air, and magic is certainly a part of healing. The daily parade they held really lifted my spirits and gave me hope for the future of my health and my life ...

*It can be useful to work with - and not against - your cortisol levels when consuming stimulants. Of course, your cortisol levels may be reversed, so listen to your body: http://u.pw/1MdJzZT

Some of the strange things that continued to happen to me included the following:

A raft of tiny spider veins were breaking. I could feel them burst due to the pressure of inflammation, as well as the condition of my adrenals and nervous system.

To this day I wonder about my head injury. Was it connected to the breakdown of my nervous system? Was my vagus nerve involved somehow? Hopefully someone will shed more light on this for me.

My toleration of TV waves, radio waves, or light waves, was super low. This was strange to experience. I believe most of it was due to my nervous system, which was shot. Perhaps it was also because my aura was weaker, and not strong and bright. Your aura is your electromagnetic shield, among other things. See Chapter Five more information on your energy body.

Another thing that occurred was I became acutely aware of the *inside* of my body. For instance, if I ingested a homeopathic dose of arnica I could feel it profoundly affect my head injury - I felt the arnica reducing the inflammation by working on the energetic and physical levels - in a positive way.

At the same instance, my body would have a violent reaction to the sugar pellet that carried the 200C arnica dose. I could feel on the energetic as well as physical levels, the healing mechanism of the homeopathy working on the energetic/vibrational level, as well as the detriment that even one sugar pellet had on my body. One promoted health in my body. The other promoted disease in my body.

My body had literally violent reactions to the sugar, and still does to this day. If you have seen a single, tiny homeopathy pellet, you know what I'm talking about. The amount of refined sugar in one pellet is not a lot, by any measure. But it was always plenty to upset my system.

I realized that despite the fact I was in physical hell, I was also getting an up close experience of the nature of healing and/or what creates disease, for me. I felt the processes unfolding in my body, depending on what I introduced to it.

This was a gift, I knew.

I also had a moment one day, when I felt so sick I felt like I was slowly dying, lying on my bed, unable to do anything. I felt a strong sense of intuition that what matters in this life is the connection we have with one another. Nothing else really matters.

Love and relationships are what you will think about and remember when it really counts. I felt this was a flash of insight I was receiving from, whatever you wish to call the Source. It was a profound moment. I will never forget it.

There are times in life when the mystical supercedes the practical. In times of joy, love, illness, or great turmoil…sometimes the veil is lifted, and we experience life from a different perspective. It was this time period when I began to hear angels singing. I often wondered, is it really angels singing? You might be wondering that as well. Was I imagining angels to make myself feel better? They were consistently there for so long, and the sound was so clear, that I doubt I made it up. I am not a religious person, but I am spiritual, and this was one of the most spiritual experiences I've ever had.

I had heard them before too when I was married and when I was younger as well. When I was sick in my marriage, I began to hear a very faint sound of angels singing - like a chorus of angels – often when I was lying down to go to sleep, or when I was waking up. It was a faint, distinct singing sound – an ethereal chorus - that I could distinguish. When I finally started to recover, the singing became softer again, and then finally disappeared altogether over time.

However, I've had several mystical experiences along the way: *turiya* - feeling like I was in the palm of God's hand – in the bathroom on airplanes, no less - *angels* whispering in my ear at two trying times in my life, my friend accidentally videotaping a ghost (discovered while he was putting in Sting's *Ghost in the Machine*, and, most importantly, profound, palpable, *divine love* (romantic, social, familial, animal, etc.) …

I don't know what the bigger picture is, but I remember much of what I have experienced, and I am grateful for all it.

Remember this always:

When you are sick, you definitely surrender to the mystery. It's far and away your best option for survival.

This was a hard time for me. I have a tendency to be a perfectionist, which is probably at least part of the reason I have struggled so much with my health. The intense inflammation lasted about two years, but I still struggle with it a bit. A year or so into it, I applied for a job, feeling pressure to work, even though I was still beyond exhausted.

I knew Whole Foods was opening a new store near me, and they were looking for buyers. I felt it would be irresponsible not try to get the job since it was in my field. So, regardless of my intuition, which told me I was in no condition to be working, let alone full time, I applied for the job and landed an interview. They hired me immediately. I was now a buyer in the supplements department. I went through an intense training for a month and half, and helped set up the store as well. I was excited to be doing what seemed familiar and natural.

Once the store opened, I worked full time until they let me go a few months later. I was floored. I had worked hard for them. It was a humiliating experience. I have never been "let go" before in my life. When I was an employee for New Frontiers and Wild Oats, I was a model employee.

Yes, there was a recession and my department was cutting back. And yes, I probably came across as strange in some capacity. But there was more to the story. I had a difficult boss who was a "partier" and who knows what else. He often showed up to work at noon with dark circles under his eyes. I have no idea how he got into the position he was in. He and I clashed, of course.

Why did I keep running into alcoholics and addicts? It was definitely a recurring theme in my life.

It reminds of my ex-husband, whom I loved dearly at one point, and, in the beginning, who loved and adored me, I think. When we loved each other, we burned brighter than the sun. When we didn't, it was the blackest hell on earth.

Dear Orion,

Like the flower bends with the rain, I fracture where you fall.

The moment you were born, my heart broke.
Like your mother or father, I loved you before you spoke.
I love you without limits,
and as far as starlight wishes to travel.
I love you like the snowflake loves to curve,
and the flower to unravel.

I am haunted by your eyes, haunted by the ghost of love.
I am troubled by the absence of the wings of the dove.
I look to the skies for some kind of solace,
but all I see is black, and all that is lawless.

If we meet again, I know it will be magic.
I will drop to my knees and forget all that was tragic.
But if we never do, I won't hold a grudge.

I'll wait for you in heaven, or wherever is eternal blue.

I know you have more traveling, and things left empty yet to fill.
If only we could do everything we need to do,
and not leave each other behind still.
I saw you when you were born, innocent and good.
And I know now that everything happens as it should.

Yet we never end up where we start,
and somewhere along the line, you broke my heart.
But I wish you safe travels as you continue on.
I wish you much love and light as you journey now into the dark.

love,

The Scorpio

From <u>Frozen Light: A Collection of Poems</u> by Edie Summers

Midnight Sun

Soulmates splitting everywhere like the atom

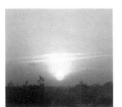

What do I do now since you were the one?
Sacred geometry, particles of light…
What did you see when you stared into the sun?
and turned your back on love…

Was it god or the golden ratio?
Perhaps it was your shadow you chased.

Darkness falls and I settle into incessant wait.
At night I pray that you'll be here when I awake.

I am waiting for your love
like an insomniac waits for the deep night to cease.
I am waiting for your reign of freedom to end its lease.

What endless beauty exists compels you to chase the flame…
If only you could see that love and freedom are the same.
I wonder when you've had enough of all you've known
And hear my voice again calling you home…

Because love, I swear, is calling my name.
And so I wait, a mermaid washed upon the shore.
What rapture I hold for you forevermore.

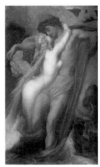

I'll wait for you forevermore…

I hear the angels, do you hear them too?
Perhaps they are too quiet for you.
They whisper where the static murmurs
And sing in praise the exalted views.

The waves crash in and devastate the shore
And wipe away the covenants we swore.
To keep forever nothing stays, remains the same
The coast is gone. It's been washed away.

But the whispers of divine energy call my name.
And the weight of the world breaks open my veins.
Darkness falls and spreads her wings…
The waves crash in and devastate the shore
And you can't see me anymore

From Frozen Light: A Collection of Poems by Edie Summers

Time moved on. More and more, my writing became part of my healing. I started outlining this book and brought my poetry together in my book _Frozen Light: A Collection of Poems_. I also created a wellness coaching website, www.Connektwell.com I studied and passed a wellness coaching certification course. I participated in many teleseminars and began to redefine who I was professionally.

Who you are _professionally, socially, romantically_, etc., all begin to lose focus during the challenge of illness. It can be so painful to lose all that used to define you. There were so many moments, days, months I went through where I had nothing but the constant reminder that I was sick.

For a long time, being sick **was** my identity.

Illness is a terrifying maze, and when you are in it, it feels as if there is no way out. Illness is a fire that burned away my identity and left a gaping black hole in my life and my heart.

Then again, from the ashes of nothing comes new life, and with new life there is endless possibility.

I finished my book of poetry in the fall. I was feeling somewhat better, but still had a long way to go so I decided to apply coaching techniques I had learned ... on myself.

I also revamped my diet, again. Eating well when you are sick is so important; I can't stress it enough. I went through many different versions of my diet from the time I first had trouble with my health in my early 20's to this last time when I got really sick. I watched cooking shows, like Rachel Ray. I learned the basics and taught myself to cook.

I read a ton of books on how to prepare food. Over time, I bought a Vitamix, a Cuisinart, a mini protein shake blender, and a spiralizer. I whipped up rice protein shakes with spirulina powder and berries. I created raw pasta with my spiralizer. I experimented with and continue to refine my diet to best suit my current wellness needs. See PortlandWellnessCoach.com for recipes and on-going support.

Improving my diet did improve my condition. But there was the nagging issue of fragrances. Whenever I left my place to go on a trip, I would feel better. Then as soon as I got home, my health would start to decline again.

There are a few possible reasons for this. My condo still had the paint and carpeting that had been bothering me all along. Yes, I got rid of the chair which had the fire retardant on it, and that was simply intolerable to my body. Yes, I had air filters, and a number of plants to help pull out the VOCS in the air. These all helped.

But every single time I would return after traveling I would walk into *smell*. It was hard to put my finger on exactly what the *smell* was that was bothering me, bothering my body. It often smelled like paint, or like some metallic something or other. But sometimes it was a combination of the two, or another odor. At any rate, my health would inevitably slide backward to at least some degree.

It also could have been due to the fact that I was so isolated where I was living. I had a cat at this point, and she provided me an enormous amount of love, comfort, and companionship. But beyond that, I had been living alone for quite a while.

I didn't have too much of a support system in Oregon either. I had a few friends, one of whom I saw sort of frequently. Beyond that, I didn't see anyone. I did not have a boyfriend either. I spent enormous amounts of time alone. In wellness coaching they say that "connection is the currency of wellness." I believe this 100%.

There is a saying that loneliness is poverty of self, and solitude is richness of self. I agree with this in many respects, and solitude has its purposes, but we are social creatures and we are meant to connect. There is no substitute for connection. I have spent long periods of my life either living alone or feeling alone. I have struggled with loneliness since I was a teenager.

I have isolated myself in the past due to trauma when interacting with other individuals. When you are alone, you think you cannot be hurt. Except that is not true. When we are alone, we can hurt ourselves sometimes, if we have been exposed to violence, trauma, etc.

My friends – the ones I had left – would tease me that I needed to get out more. Loneliness is no laughing matter, especially when it comes to the state of your health. Loneliness has been the greatest sadness and heaviness of my life, surpassing even trauma and chronic illness. It nearly broke me and my heart. *I urge you to connect.*

At times our own light goes out and is rekindled by a spark from another person. Each of us has cause to think with deep gratitude of those who have lighted the flame within us. ~ Albert Schweitzer

In January 2010, I enrolled in calculus. I needed it to finish my undergrad degree. Long story. I had attempted to take it before but was so exhausted I couldn't concentrate, and couldn't understand the professor to save my life. Then again it was calculus, and I am right-brained. I told myself I would take it as soon as I could.

I was hoping to go to grad school in the fall, so I knew it was now or never for calculus. Well, that calculus course took all of my energy and then some. I studied my ass off - up to 25 hours a week. I noticed early on that in order to even get my brain to work, I had to exercise, eat exquisitely well, and take certain neurotransmitters like L-Theanine.

I was extra, extra careful of my healthcare routine so I could have a shot at being able to concentrate enough to absorb the material and do the homework. I had not had math in more than 25 years - so this fact made it even tougher. Through very hard work, I passed the class.

Calculus taught me a number of things about what my body needed in order to function. *The brain controls the nervous system, for starters.* The more I took care of my brain, the better I felt and could concentrate on facts and figures. Calculus also taught me to stay in the moment, no matter what. More on what calculus taught me in Chapter Three.

Something else I noticed: I felt better. You could say this was a result of neuroplasticity. I explore the concept of neuroplasticity in Chapters Three, Four, and Five.

It could have been that I was using my brain a lot in calculus, and a result it influenced the health of my body. Brain health is crucial for all of us, and is perhaps very helpful, for CFS patients and beyond.

The Apple Falls Close to the Tree
Genetics, Environment, and the Human Will

Something has disturbed me and disturbs me to this day…
Most of the enzymes that have polymorphisms in me are carried
by both chromosomes, meaning both of my parents might have
some of the same health issues as I have.
Dr. Newman encouraged me to share my results with my parents
which I did.

In the summer of 2006, my father was diagnosed with
esophageal cancer. There are theories that this type of cancer is
at least in part caused by, or made worse by nitrates.

Of course the enzyme that breaks down nitrates was in my
Phase I polymorphism, and it did not indicate on my test whether
or not it involved both of my chromosomes.
However, it seems possible that my father had this issue as well.
He ate a lot of processed meat in his life.
And he had trouble with acid reflux. He took antacid pills for as
long as I can remember.

I also know for sure that my dad and one of my sisters suffered
from a great deal of generalized anxiety like me.

Genetics are powerful. But they're not everything.
Candace Pert, a neuroscientist who discovered the opiate
receptor, was once skeptical of the connection between
environmental toxins and cancer. Like many professionals from
different fields, and after years of research, she then came to
believe that environmental toxins are one of the primary causes
of cancer. *We're just as much at the mercy of the environment as we are at
the mercy of genetics.* But, even stronger, is the human will and our
powerful minds and spirits. This is the power of epigenetics.
See Chapters Three and Five.

As much as I wish I could have helped my father more, he lost
his battle with esophageal cancer on August 31, 2008. He fought
for over two years utilizing both modern methods like chemo
and radiation therapy, as well as alternative methods such as diet
and super food therapy, crystal healing, positive thinking, etc.
Perhaps this book will help some other people so they don't have
to suffer the way so many of us have.

In spring of 2011, I was no longer so tired and sick that I wanted to just die. There were many days, in fact, where I felt almost *normal*, more or less, whatever that means. That's not to say I didn't have to stay on top of it and that I didn't ever feel tired or sick sometimes.

Even with a stellar diet which excluded sugar, refined foods, and stimulants, I still had to stay on top of it all ... watching out for chemicals.

Take this example: One day, I decided to *experiment* and I bought an automatic toilet bowl cleaner, the kind you drop in the tank. Right away I knew I was in trouble. The chemical smell overwhelmed me. I started to get light-headed. I put a ton of plants in the bathroom. I couldn't even stand to be in the bathroom for more a few seconds. The next day I woke up feeling *sore*. My hair started falling out again.

Fast forward again to 2015 as I edit this book.

I moved to a new place four years ago, one that was a much healthier environment overall. Although it took my body about a year to stabilize after I moved out of my old condo, I noticed a pretty steady return to health in general, beyond my loneliness, which persisted.

I now work full time as a corporate wellness consultant and live in Silicon Valley. I am completing a Master's in Health Psychology. I also earned certification as yoga instructor.

How do I do all of this? Am I cured? Am I healed?

I live off of passion, motivation, and inspiration. This definitely helps me keep going. I also pay close attention to what I put in my body and the thoughts I think. I currently operate at about a 90-95% rate of feeling good.

Do I have bad days or hours? Sure. But I have an arsenal for combating fatigue on the physical level. In addition, I utilize powerful techniques to keep my fear and anxiety levels at bay through yoga, mindfulness, eating well, practicing deep self-care, etc. I explore all these techniques in Chapters Four and Five.

How do I know I was sick? Because over three-fourths of my hair fell out … because my eyes were bloodshot straight in a row for ten years … because I lost my appetite for years on end … because I kept getting sick every time I went to work or out in public … because I was persistently, devastatingly *exhausted* for five years in a row and on and off for 20 years …

The chronic fatigue alone is enough of a marker that something was off in my body. I do not understand how chronic, persistent *fatigue* could not be seen as a red flag and taken seriously.

If it happened to you, if your whole life were suddenly taken away, you would understand. If only you could *walk in my shoes* for even an hour.

I Am...

I am from Utah, which I never really appreciated until I grew up. It's a near perfect place, in my mind, at least …

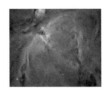 I am now a resident of Oregon. It's hauntingly beautiful and bittersweetly imperfect.

I am a writer, a dancer, introspective, and a middle child. I am not sure if any of these have to do with one another, but I can remember being all of them from pretty much the start of my story.

I am either trying to move away from my *story*, or sink deeper into it.

I am wondering what I AM means. I think it means *I am fully present. I am aware...*

I am wondering if this is how the universe started: with sheer awareness

I feel I am closest to or in this state of being when I stop trying, and just inhabit aliveness

I am a bit shy, but not nearly as shy as I used to be. These days, I am brave. I am too afraid not to be brave.

I am aware I am intellectualizing this poem, and that this is my defense.

I am aware that it is pure metaphor that allows us to dive deep into the heart of person or situation.

I am salt melted into snow ...

I am really an Aztec princess who may not have existed at all.

I am a high alpine meadow.

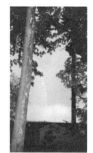 I am a glistening Northwest forest shrouded in fog heavy with water droplets - I am deep immersion in life.

I am a pod of dolphins feeding during a pink sunrise along the Florida coast at dawn.

I am white. I am Scottish, English, German, and maybe Basque or Jewish. I am sure I am more blended than I appear.

I am quite certain I have Latin blood somewhere, as I am moved by all things Latin and Native American….and ancient Celtic…and Indian…

I am moved easily...

I am secretly Black Raven with midnight hair that runs to the center of the earth, and whose courage is the wingspan of a thousand fields.

I am doing my best to enjoy life to the fullest, live in *flow*, and still fulfill my deepest dreams.

I am touching that point where life melts into a rapidly dissolving center with no ending or resolution ... and it is far more heartbreaking and incredibly blissful than I could have possibly imagined...

I am the soft heart of an artichoke

I am fast pure spirit. I am a rainbow with no (apparent) earthly access...

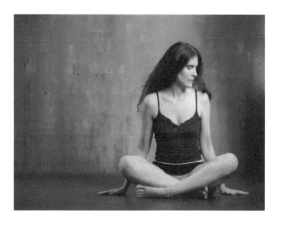

Chapter Two - Making the Connection
Body Burden

Disillusion is the last illusion. ~ *Wallace Stevens*

Calling 911 - Toxins in the Modern World

Why am I dedicating a whole chapter to environmental toxins and other toxic substances? Because they greatly affected the quality of my life and health.

As I have described in Chapter One, when I moved into my condo after my separation, I was exhausted. But after being in my condo for just a short period of time with its new paint, carpeting, and the new chair with the fire retardant, I became ill. I wasn't just super tired day after day: my body had descended into true illness.

Are all inventions of modern living bad for us? Of course not. *But we live in a complex world, and some of us are surviving better than others.* There are now close to 100,000 synthetic chemicals in our world, with only a fraction of them, about seven percent, having been fully tested.

Add to that the possibility that almost half of us may not detoxify properly. The more a person is genetically susceptible to poor detoxification, the more chance they have for developing health issues down the road, I believe.

For vulnerable populations, the inability to detoxify properly leads to a breakdown and state in the body called oxidative stress. This state is a breeding ground for chronic illness, a setup which may lead to chronic conditions such as Myalgic Encephalomyelitis (ME)/Chronic Fatigue Syndrome (CFS), auto-immune conditions, autism, asthma, diabetes, Parkinson's, liver conditions, Alzheimer's, cancer, kidney pain, etc. For more details and references on this topic, and the roles poor methylation and glutathione deficiency may play, please see Chapter Three.

The question remains: what does it take for us to make the emotional connection that the way we treat ourselves, each other, and the environment directly and undeniably affects the quality of our own lives and long-term health?

September 11, 2001 - When the World Changed Forever

September 11, 2001: That day changed the world in every imaginable way. It was a defining moment in history, of course. However, the aftermath carried with it a portent that perhaps didn't register with most of us. Not only did countless people suffer at the moment of the attacks, but the first responders and those who dealt with the aftermath paid an unseen price as well.

Thousands of firefighters, police, military members, civilian rescuers, emergency health personnel, construction personnel, and many more worked tireless 18 hour days for 10 months, seven days a week to clean up at Ground Zero. Many of these selfless folks are now plagued with respiratory illness, including a chronic, soot-laden hacking known as "World Trade Center Cough" or the WTC cough, according to The New England Journal of Medicine (Prezant, 2002).

The fine particles, called volatile organic compounds (VOCs) from the gases and vapor generated by the tower collapses included a toxic dust storm from burning asbestos and carpeting, as well as disintegrated office equipment. Such a compilation of dust may carry a reputation for causing multiple chronic health complications and even death.

Gases from this deadly soup were comprised of hundreds of different poisonous chemicals including dioxins, PCBs, asbestos, benzene, silica, polybrominated diphenyl ethers (PBDE), manganese, chromium, lead, mercury, nickel, oxides of nitrogen, and sulfur.

The unprecedented, massive, toxic exposures that led to the WTC cough also posed long term risks for people developing cancers (including throat and face), and multiple environmental illnesses. Additionally, they may face heart disease, respiratory disease, increased miscarriages, and neurological issues, to name some of the potential conditions which might be spawned by such toxic exposure.

Ultimately, in 2011, *The First Responders Bill* was signed into law. Most of the $4.2 billion allocated to the bill will provide medical coverage for the brave folks who gave aid to others during an overwhelming crisis. A smaller portion of the funds will be for compensation payments. So many years later, as some of the rescuers are *fighting for their own health and lives*, they are receiving aid and recognition on this level, finally, for what they have been through and continue to face.

If we choose to listen, this tragic event could serve as a wake-up call. Environmental toxicity has reached a new, extremely high level in our world, casting a deathly shadow over the general health of our bodies.

But there's more. September 11 is thought to have been instrumental in "widespread economic and social disruption" (Bruckner, 2010).

Yes, the vicious attacks on the World Trade Center affected many Americans physically. However, it affected most of us mentally and emotionally as well. I cannot begin to imagine what people went through who lost loved ones in that attack. September 11 was a collective mass trauma for the United States, and for many around the world as well. The effects of trauma can play a big role in the maintaining or losing of health.

> Research shows that just witnessing somebody else getting injured or killed can induce PTSD-like symptoms ... and that includes witnessing horrific scenes via television, says Dr. David Spiegel, a professor of psychiatry at California's Stanford University. (Mundell, 2006)

For me, witnessing 9/11 through TV broadcasts caused me feelings of deep grief, disbelief, and fear. It was a turning point in my ability to trust people in this world. Little did I know that September 11 would affect my life profoundly when coupled with personal tragedy. I had reached a breaking point regarding the way we treat each other as disposable, and as enemies.

It's not only how we treat one another, but how we treat our home on this planet. Again, what will it take for us to make the emotional connection that the way we treat ourselves, each other, and the environment also directly and undeniably affects the quality of our own lives and our long-term health?

We've made progress to be sure. But bias and stigma still exist when it comes to connecting the dots between *toxic, synthetic chemicals that have almost zero testing and regulation,* and the untold millions of people across the world whose health has been altered due to exposure to such chemicals. Those with chemical sensitivities continue to be subjected to ridicule or, even worse, ignored by health practitioners, insurance administrators, and even friends and family. An example of this type of dismissal is an attitude toward veterans who show symptoms of Gulf War Syndrome. A web article issued by the Associated Press was titled: *Study: Gulf War Syndrome Doesn't Exist.* This is the first line: "There is no such thing as Gulf War Syndrome" ("Study: Gulf War," 2006). Both Gulf War Syndrome and Chronic Fatigue Syndrome have been downplayed as not legitimate diseases, or *wastebasket diseases* as they are sometimes labeled. Yet there is abundant evidence to the contrary that these conditions are real. They both have symptoms that vary widely, but the symptoms are real.

As we gain knowledge, we change our minds about how to classify and treat disorders and disease. It wasn't long ago when doctors thought female patients with the disease we now call Multiple Sclerosis were experiencing female hysteria. Those patients were confined to mental institutions. Today we know the immune system attacks the central nervous system.

Body Burden
Connecting the Dots Leading to Chronic Illness

Body Burden is a term made popular by The Environmental Working Group in a report published by Houlihan, Wiles, Thayer and Gray (2003). The phrase could hold multiple meanings to be sure. But what does it mean to have a body that has been burdened by the assault of unchecked chemicals?

Body Burden means essentially that the tipping point has been reached in terms of the amount of synthetic chemicals and/or toxins the body can process. Beyond this point comes illness for many, including what is known as environmental illness. When one reaches a threshold of *bioaccumulation* of chemicals and toxins, then one has felt what it means to have a body burden. Believe me you know it when you feel it.

One of the first signs of chemical injury is fatigue, followed by adrenal stress, insomnia or waking up early, increased hunger, and weight gain. Other signs include headaches, sinus problems, flu-like symptoms, rashes, inability to concentrate, poor memory, depression, and anxiety.

Environmental toxins may be stored in your fat, lead to weight gain, cause inflammation, and even cause other serious, chronic symptoms. See Chapter Three on *Oxidative Stress* and check out this link: http://www.medscape.com/viewarticle/758210

In addition, weight gain happens due to unstable blood sugar levels caused by high or erratic cortisol levels. Your hair may fall out, as mine did. Fatigue, low energy, sleep disturbances, and sore muscles, are other potential symptoms of chemical injury. Consumer beware.

There are about 100,000 synthetic chemicals currently in use with about 1000 new chemicals introduced every year into our ecosystem. The European Union has registered 140,000 synthetic chemicals and counting (Lopate, 2009). Just one type of these synthetic chemicals - dioxins - belongs to a family of 222 related chemicals.

Agent Orange: An Early Wakeup Call

Agent Orange is a dioxin, and *dioxins are one of the deadliest classes of chemicals and poisons known to man.* There are three main types of dioxins, with some 419 different chemicals among the three types, each one with its own fingerprint. About 30 are considered extremely toxic.

We don't make dioxins intentionally. They are formed as by-products during any type of burning process under the right conditions. They also can be formed during the manufacturing of certain chlorinated chemicals. For example, a well-recognized dioxin is the discernible smell of *chlorine-bleached paper pulp.* Paper mills are infamous for polluting rivers, wells, etc. However, mills are converting their processes so they use less chlorine.

Once dioxins are produced, they become unstable environmental toxins in the form of air particles. We breathe those particles, inviting dioxins into our systems. Worse yet, the particles settle on the ground and in lakes and rivers where they are consumed by animals, fish, and other creatures. The particles are impregnated in the soil where we grow our crops. Thus, dioxins work their way up the food chain and are found in meat, fish, and dairy sources. We, in turn, consume those foods and the dioxins accumulate mainly in our fatty tissue, remaining in our bodies for seven to eleven years.

As mentioned, one member of the dioxin family was the primary contaminate in the wartime herbicide, Agent Orange. Just so we can identify this dioxin, it is known as 2,3,7,8 and it has the highest toxicity of all the dioxins and dioxin-like compounds. This specific 2,3,7,8 dioxin in Agent Orange is notoriously linked to several types of cancer and reproductive health problems.

Many veterans have been exposed to Agent Orange because it was the poisonous blend of herbicides used to remove foliage that hid the enemy. Millions of gallons were sprayed from trucks or by military personnel wearing backpack sprayers during Korean and Vietnam engagements. It has been used in other areas of the world, as well, for military purposes. Countless vets who served where Agent Orange was used, or near where it was used, have endured health problems and even chronic illness. Some veterans have developed cancers and some have genetically passed on the aftereffects of their exposure to their children. Some have suffered permanent damage to their lungs and nervous systems. Others have developed Type II diabetes.

Added to the existing list of twelve *presumed illnesses* already linked with Agent Orange are three additional diseases:

(1) Parkinson's, (2) hairy cell and other chronic B-cell leukemia, and (3) ischemic heart disease (VA, 2009)

Thankfully, additions like these make it easier for vets and their loved ones to have their claims taken seriously. To our shame, we've forced our Agent Orange veterans for years to battle the misperception that their chronic illnesses are not connected to Agent Orange exposure. But times are changing, finally. To file a claim, please see the *Resources* section near the end of this book.

In October, 2013, Congress acted to widen the definition of veterans who may be eligible for aid if their chronic diseases are linked to Agent Orange exposure. *The Blue Water Navy Vietnam Veterans Act of 2013,* was introduced by U.S. Congressman Christopher Gibson of New York ("The Blue Water," 2013).

This bill will *lift the burden from the individual veteran to prove direct exposure to toxic herbicides.* At the Veterans Administration (VA), it will also "reduce the backlog of claims for ... compensation from veterans who are suffering from diseases the U.S. government has linked to Agent Orange and other toxic herbicides" ("The Blue Water," 2013).

Regarding other theatres of war and other types of chronic illnesses, please note the VA *does* actually consider CFS, IBS, and Fibromyalgia (FM) as real conditions for veterans of Operations Desert Shield, Desert Storm, and Iraqi Freedom (Gulf War Veterans' Medically Unexplained Illnesses, n.d.).

The debate over the long-term impact of Agent Orange was one of our first serious wake-up calls to the dangers of synthetic chemicals on human health, yet for some reason we have been painfully slow to pay attention. In fact, we even went on to use *Triclosan,* a derivative of Agent Orange, on ourselves. Developed in the 1960s, by the 1970s Triclosan was used in doctors' scrub kits. By the 80s, we were using it as an antibacterial agent in toothpaste, hand soap, toys, clothing, furniture, body washes, etc. "Three-quarters of Americans are carrying traces of triclosan in their blood" (CDC, 2013). When are we going to wake up?

> Short-term exposure of humans to high levels of dioxins may result in skin lesions, such as chloracne and patchy darkening of the skin, and altered liver function. Long-term exposure is linked to impairment of the immune system, the developing nervous system, the endocrine system and reproductive functions. Chronic exposure of animals to dioxins has resulted in several types of cancer. *(WHO, 2014)*

Pleural mesothelioma is a malignant cancer which develops on the lining of the lungs called the pleura. It is the most common type of mesothelioma, accounting for 75% of all diagnosed cases and may be caused primarily by exposure to asbestos, a *naturally occurring*, toxic mineral. Yes, naturally occurring. *Dr. Brenda Buck*, professor of medical geology at University of Nevada Las Vegas, and geologist, Rodney Metcalf, were testing Boulder City soil near Las Vegas for arsenic when they found *actinolite*, a toxic mineral in the asbestos category. There it was in the dust, probably created millions of years ago in *plutons*, i.e., the roots of volcanoes. Boulder City is atop a pluton which explains the asbestos concentration. Read more: (Komak, 2013; "Naturally occurring asbestos," 2014).

But in our wisdom, we have manufactured products with asbestos in them. Remember when asbestos was commonly used in many industries in the 20th century, exposing laborers who worked in those companies, and exposing everyday consumers to lung disease? I recall asbestos being installed in attics and ceilings of homes.

U.S. naval veterans, especially those who served during peak asbestos years - 1940 to 1970 - account for many mesothelioma cases due to asbestos used in ships. In addition to enlisted and drafted personnel, anyone who worked on the vessels or in the shipyard was vulnerable to potential lung disease. http://www.mesotheliomanavy.org/out the vessels.

Seven Generations: Our Children

"Babies are born … with as many as 300 industrial chemicals in their bodies" (Environmental Working Group 2005).

Our children are our hearts and our biggest responsibilities. They also represent our most valuable resource on this earth. Yet who is the most vulnerable to our modern experiments with chemicals? Our children. In fact developing fetuses are the most sensitive of all.

Look around. Forty percent of children suffer from allergies (Wardrop, 2009) and childhood chronic illness is rising (Delaney & Smith, 2012). More kids than ever are diagnosed with asthma and bipolar disorder.

Also on the rise among children is Attention Deficit Hyperactivity Disorder (ADHD) which has been linked to pesticide exposure. And let's not forget autism. As you may know, due to wide-spread media controversy, autism has been questioned as linked to toxic vaccine preservatives (some say disproven, some say the debate is not over – either way, it's a hot-button issue). Autism may be connected to social and environmental conditions, as well. At any rate, it may be an epidemic, like childhood obesity, and we are still researching causes.

More kids are turning to prescription drugs now, the drug of choice of our modern era, and they may, in fact, be raiding your medicine cabinet. Prescription drugs are powerfully addictive. They are a gateway drug, and now the most common type of drug abused by the youngest members of our society.

Children are also exposed to convenient plastic products and consume foods every day which may be contaminated by three types of toxic chemicals. In a blog published July 2014 by the government of Westchester County, New York, every parent, and anyone expecting a baby, was warned to learn about the dangers of "everywhere chemicals" ("Bisphenol-A [BPA] & Phthalates," 2014).

Bisphenol A (BPA) is toxic, endocrine-disrupting, industrial chemical used to make unbreakable plastics such as those used in baby bottles and sippy cups. It is also found in the lining of canned foods. It has been linked to birth defects, infertility, cancer, diabetes, heart disease, and behavioral issues.

Phthalates are a class of chemicals used to soften and increase the flexibility of plastic and vinyl in hundreds of products such as rattles and teethers. However, they may interfere with reproductive development. Data is being gathered in on-going studies ...

Melamine is a chemical added during manufacture of infant plates, cups and other tableware, and was found in baby formula from China where six babies died in 2008 and thousands more became ill. If you have melamine ware in your home, never use it to heat food and avoid putting acidic food on it. Also, melamine has been turning up in pet food. According to writers on *Organicauthority.com*, high concentrations of melamine contamination can put people at risk for kidney stones, kidney failure and even death (Hudson, 2013).

Some natural food stores like Whole Foods are very strict about what they carry on their shelves in terms of food additives and chemicals. One of the many problems with these synthetic chemicals is that we store them in our fat which means they can linger in our bodies.

Environmental Illnesses/MCS

Please see MCS - Multiple Chemical Sensitivity in Chapter Three.

Fragrances and VOCs

Have you noticed how fragrances of perfumes and laundry detergents can make you dizzy? Hello, VOCs. Volatile organic compounds (VOCs) are gasses emitted from solids and liquids. An obvious one you would notice is fresh paint. Feel dizzy or like fainting? No wonder, because you are inhaling VOCs from the solvents in paint.

Do you know what you are putting on your skin and inhaling untold times per day? Coal, coal tars, and petrochemicals, for starters. These additives can lead to headaches, nerve damage, or even more. Sexy? Not so much. *Fragrances are hormone disruptors* which throw our body systems out of balance, leading to potential health problems. Our society favors commerce and innovation over *safety first*, it would seem.

Thankfully, there is a relatively new European agency, REACH, developed to register, evaluate, authorize, and restrict chemical substances that have received a free pass thus far. (Please see link in **Resources** at the end of the book.) In past years, DDT, lead, and cigarettes all were deemed as "safe." Yet today we know they are clearly not safe.

CVS Health Bans Tobacco Sales

As of February 2014, CVS Health (they changed their name) will no longer sell cigarettes even though they will lose $2 billion in sales annually from cutting tobacco sales. CVS is moving to become a health oriented chain.

Out of more than 100,000 chemicals on the market, about *60,000* of them or more have received a free pass thus far. The perfume industry is one of the worst offenders, and has almost no regulation.

All Is Not Lost

Thankfully *low VOC* and even *no VOC* paints like Aura are available.

Researchers have come up with a solution to the problem of plastic outgassing, or the toxic release of plastic chemicals into food and the environment. The new technology prevents chemical leeching from certain plastics by stopping polyvinyl chloride, a commonly used plastic chemical, from migrating to the surface of plastics and escaping.

Remember: houseplants can remove up to 90% of VOCs (*Claudio, 2011*). Some of the best plants include varieties of fern and *spider plants*. But there are many plants that do the trick if you look into it. Please see **Resources**, under *VOCs and Plants*, for tons of useful tips on VOCs, indoor air health and quality, and the best plants to use.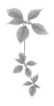

Cosmetics

Your skin absorbs so much more than you realize. What you put on your skin is just as important as what you put in your mouth. Do you know what you're consuming chemicals through your skin? What are you inhaling (hello hairspray)? Or swallowing? With lipstick alone, perhaps you've heard the disturbing news that the average woman consumes up to six pounds of lipstick in a lifetime.

The cosmetics industry is minimally regulated. Essentially only color additives and over the counter drugs (OTCs) are reviewed (*EWG, 2013*). This is why label reading is so important not only for cosmetics, but for food packaging. If you have sensitivities or allergies you have to be even more diligent.

The Environmental Working Group has an in-depth online resource – *Skin Deep* - for finding out about the safety of tens of thousands of cosmetics and personal care products. http://www.ewg.org/skindeep/

As I've mentioned, Whole Foods has strict rules about what products make it onto their shelves. They have identified more than 400 unacceptable ingredients including parabens, polypropylene and polyethylene glycols, sodium lauryl and laureth sulfates. For their premium body care line, Whole Foods examines the most recent research to determine if each ingredient in each product is truly safe, natural, effective, has zero to minimal environmental impact, and that there was no animal testing. The Whole Foods guide for suppliers is available in the **Resources** section, near the end of this book.

This is not a plug for Whole Foods. I used to work there, so I know about their high standards. They've done the research and the testing so that you don't have to, unless you wish to, of course. They take the word *natural* seriously and promise to only carry health and beauty aids (HABA) that are truly natural.

Since the term "natural" is not regulated – and marketers know everyone wants natural these days – well, you can see where all sorts of products, *natural or otherwise*, are turning up in many stores and on-line. "Natural" just like "green" can mean so many things. We have to ask the questions.

What do glycols, sodium lauryl sulfate, surfactants and chelators do to your skin and your body? Well, they can irritate your skin for one thing, like parabens. They can also impact the environment, as chelators can do. To find out more about skin care, visit **Resources** near the end of this book; then look for *Body Care, Cosmetics, Sunscreen* and also check out the FDA list of selected cosmetic ingredients.

We already mentioned anti-bacterial soap in the section on Agent Orange. You recall that the composition of such soaps include a derivative of Agent Orange. Triclosan (the derivative) is everywhere, including in toothpastes. I figured out it was in a toothpaste I received as a sample for gum health because the toothpaste smelled like soap. No wonder it fights gingivitis. It is derived from an herbicide.

Do you consume cosmetics? You bet you do, as this seminal study indicates: "Sixty-one percent* of tested lipstick brands contain residues of lead" ("Lead in lipstick," 2007). *Levels are higher now. See Resources

The most problematic of the sunscreen chemicals used in the U.S. is oxybenzone, found in nearly every chemical sunscreen (Calafat, Wong, Ye, Reidy, & Needham, 2008). EWG recommends that consumers avoid this chemical because it can penetrate the skin, cause allergic skin reactions and may disrupt hormones. (EWG, 2015)

One of my biggest reactions ever was to a chemical sunscreen I used at the height of my illness. Here's my account. Judge for yourself:

In My Shoes
Journal Entry

A day in the life…

So I was feeling pretty good and optimistic on Sunday. I had been having some trouble, but I was starting to feel a lot better in general. I definitely felt like getting some fresh air, sun, and most importantly, exercise. I knew it would help me keep the upswing going.

I had tried this particular sun block a few times, and had some trouble with it: the "fragrance" bothered me. I also seemed to get mild body odor the day after. But I was having so much trouble with sun sensitivity – it was the middle of summer – and I hadn't been able to find any other sun block that worked for me. I have fair skin to begin with and I've also experienced significant sun sensitivity for a few years due to illness and taking certain sleep aids (Benadryl and Elavil). So sun protection was an issue for me. But I really wanted to go outside, hike, and not worry about it. My soul needed it. So I put on the sunscreen and a sun protective hat, and did my best to forget about it.

I felt pretty awesome and relaxed for the first few hours. Even with SPF 30 on, the sun felt super intense – way more than normal – but I hardly thought about it. I was just so happy to be out among the living and hanging out in nature for the first time in a while. About 4-5 hours into the day, my facial skin started to itch. At first it was just annoying. Then it really bothered me. I also felt ever so slightly "off," but I brushed away the feeling, and ignored the sensation. I'd worn this sun block before I told myself, and I'd more or less survived it.

Looking back, I know I should've jumped in the river and washed the sun block off when it started to bother me as my intuition told me to do. It was my ego that wanted to plow on through. It's no wonder I got so sick to begin with. I may not be the classic Type A personality, but I do have a tendency to ignore suffering in myself. But when the body gets so sick, you're forced to do what it asks of you. I ignored the vague sensation that something was "off" since I felt okay in general and was having too much fun to think about anything happening chemical-reaction-wise. But by the end of the day I started to feel awful. My skin was screaming.

I remember looking in the mirror when I got home that night and barely recognizing myself. My face was pale and bloated. I could tell I wasn't doing well. I took off the sunscreen and hoped for the best. Maybe the feeling would just go away. I began to feel progressively worse. I slept for almost 12 hours and woke up feeling absolutely horrible. Despite having slept so long, I was super tired.

My body felt heavy, and I had body aches all over. This was my first experience with fibromyalgia symptoms. My lymph nodes were swollen, I felt like I had the flu, and I was mildly depressed on top of it all. In short, I felt beyond awful.

I was in hell all day. My mouth and face burned and stung. It was one of my worst reactions ever to chemicals. I couldn't believe it. I had been feeling so much better in general. I couldn't understand why my body was reacting so violently to something I'd only mildly reacted to before. It felt very overwhelming. I couldn't think straight, and even the simplest task seemed almost impossible to undertake. I could barely move, and I had zero energy. I was completely overwhelmed with fatigue and body aches all day, and so exhausted I had trouble finding enough energy to breathe. I felt like I had the weight of the world on me, literally.

There is a huge difference between sun block and sunscreen. Sun blocks primarily or exclusively use mineral like titanium or zinc oxide. Sunscreens use chemical agents as their sunscreen. But artificial fragrances can often be found in both, and many sun blocks these days also have some chemical sunscreens in them.

I have had the least problems with Oil of Olay's sensitive line in general and Nia-24. They seem to understand what "sensitive" skin really means. There are some pretty good sun blocks in the natural food stores too. I am also a huge fan of skin protective hats and clothing. Sunblock is important, but I use it mostly in sunny climates. Chemicals and I do not mix.

Mossville

Mossville sits adjacent to no less than 14 chemical plants that have been there since WWII. Many residents have been tested and their blood compositions show the same chemicals that are in the chemical plants such as vinyl chloride, benzene, and ethylene diochloride which are carcinogens affecting the liver and kidneys, and of course the nervous system. Mossville citizens now have numerous health conditions including cancer, Parkinson's, and heart disease.

> Thousands of pounds of carcinogens such as benzene and vinyl chloride are released from the facilities near Mossville each year, according to the EPA's Toxic Release Inventory. Vinyl chloride makers, refineries, a coal-fired energy plant, and chemical plants now operate in what was once rural country, rich in agriculture, fishing and hunting. (Gupta & Selig, 2010)

And who lives in Mossville? Mossville, Louisiana is a longstanding African-American community. Unfortunately many chemical plants are built in minority communities, leading to the new term of *environmental racism*.

In May, 2014 a coalition of three organizations, under the banner *Environmental Justice and Health Alliance for Chemical Policy Reform,* submitted an extensive report titled *Who's In Danger? Race, Poverty, and Chemical Disasters.* The list of authors, contributors, reviewers, and funding organizations for this comprehensive study is impressive. (Environmental Justice, 2014).

Perhaps the report just mentioned may become a catalyst for changes needed in the document called the *American Convention on Human Rights* (Organization of American States/Secretariat of Legal Affairs, 2012). This document was signed in 1969 at the Inter-American Specialized Conference on Human Rights held in San Jose, Costa Rica. However, in this document, there is no provision for the right to live in a healthy environment. Nothing in this document is equivalent to equal protection and the freedom from discrimination that is in our Declaration of Independence.

Mossville residents have joined together to lobby the Environmental Protection Agency (EPA) for stronger emissions rules for polyvinyl chloride plants. For some unspoken reason, those rules were set unusually low for the Mossville PVC producing plant.

Who knew that environmental oversight and racism might be linked? Then again, it doesn't surprise me. Just so you know, the EPA does not deal with individuals who get sick or need to relocate. We must look out for and stand up for ourselves and for our neighbors.

Gasland

There is on-going controversy regarding the subject of whether or not *fracking,* used to obtain natural gas, is environmentally safe. We need alternative sources of energy, that's for sure. But is fracking the answer? Here is information on the documentary films *Gasland and Gasland II.* Decide for yourself.

Josh Fox (2010) wrote and produced *Gasland*, a documentary about *80-300 chemicals* used in a process called hydraulic fracturing – or fracking – in order to obtain natural gas by drilling. For horizontal fracking, the number of chemicals used is even greater at *596*. The natural gas industry hasn't been required to disclose types of chemicals used to extract gas. In fact, many are proprietary chemicals. However, it *is* known that some of the chemicals include VOCs such as *benzene, toluene, xylene, methanol, ethylbenzene, glutaraldehyde, sulfuric acid and polynuclear aromatic hydrocarbons.* Kinda poetic, eh? It's estimated that up to 70% of the fracking fluid remains in the ground and is thought to be not biodegradable.

The Halliburton Loophole
In 1974, the *Safe Drinking Water Act* … was passed by Congress to ensure clean drinking water free from both natural and man-made contaminates. In 2005, the Bush/ Cheney Energy Bill exempted natural gas drilling from the Act. The Bill exempts companies from disclosing the chemicals used during hydraulic fracturing. Essentially, the provision took the EPA off the job. The Bill is now referred to as the Halliburton Loophole. (Gurule, 2013)

And there's another problem which has immediate consequences: Fracking is thought to contaminate surrounding water sources such as rivers and wells used for drinking water. Many residents who live in areas where fracking has taken place have contaminated wells. In some cases, the tainted water may be lit on fire as it flows from faucets.

> The average [natural gas] well is up to 8,000 feet deep. The depth of drinking water aquifers is about 1,000 feet. The problems typically stem from poor cement well casings that leak natural gas [and] fracking fluid into water wells. (Fox, 2013)

Gasland (Fox, 2010) received the special jury prize in the documentary category at the 2010 Sundance Film Festival. Josh Fox followed up with a second film on fracking issues, *Gasland Part II (*Fox, 2013*)*. I urge you to watch them, along with the film *Food, Inc.* (Kenner, 2008) to see where your food really comes from and how it is made.

Dioxins and Endometriosis

Endometriosis affects at least 6.3 million adolescent and adult females in the United States, according to the Endometriosis Association.

> It occurs when the tissue similar to the lining of the uterus is found elsewhere - usually in ovaries, fallopian tubes, abdominal lining, bowel, and bladder - which can cause chronic pelvic pain ... painful periods and bowel movements as well as difficulties with urination during periods, and pain during sex. (Chang, 2010)

It is often misdiagnosed, and can take some women years to finally get diagnosed correctly. Its origins are unknown. It may be genetic and it has been linked to *dioxin exposure*. Treatments include: laparoscopic surgery, pain medication, and hormone treatments.

Animals/Pets

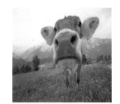

There is so much I could say about animals and our pets. I simply adore them. I think they are here to be our friends and not to serve our needs.

Much attention has been given to factory farming. There are so many issues at stake with factory farming, most of all for the animals themselves. Animals are fed hormones to make them produce milk faster, and to simply grow faster, so they can be *processed* more quickly (ugh.) These hormones end up in *your* body as well. Everyone has heard of rBGH at this point. It is simple: synthetic hormones are not good nor for you or the cows. Enough said.

As far as factory farming goes, the first video I ever saw on it involved watching what they referred to as a *downer cow* dumped off the truck, unable to walk on her own, and with the other cows on their way to the slaughterhouse stumbling over her.

A downer cow is too sick and/or weak to walk. This is no surprise if you take one second to look at the conditions most factory animals are raised in. I urge you to watch *Meet Your Meat* (Friedrich, 2002). This is the image that changed my mind and opened my heart to what *meat* really is, and the story about where it comes from.

Animals are not here for our uses. They have a life and a purpose that is all their own. *Nature knows and goes her own way. ~ Goethe*

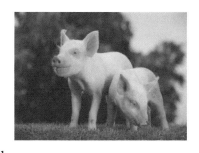

There is a massive disconnect with how we treat animals. It's the same disconnect that we have with how we treat ourselves and our own health.

Animals are works of art more wondrous than anything man is capable of creating. How can we be gentle in the way we handle our material possessions and careless with the precious life of an animal? Animals long to have faith and trust in us, and often do have faith and loyalty that far surpass anything in the human realm. ~ Dianne Hillier

Living creatures are interactive spiritual beings with whom we have a collaborative relationship. Our companion animals, creatures in the wild, and humans are all here to fulfill a sacred purpose. We're all part of the Divine and connected through time and space. I've always believed that animals have souls that are wiser and more authentic than us humans. They are teachers, guides, and healers with us. ~ Colette Baron-Reid, author of Messages from the Spirit

When animals express their feelings they pour out like water from a spout. Animals' emotions are raw, unfiltered, and uncontrolled. Their joy is the purest and most contagious of joys and their grief the deepest and most devastating. Their passions bring us to our knees in delight and sorrow.

~Marc Bekoff, The Emotional Lives of Animals: A Leading Scientist Explores Animal Joy, Sorrow, and Empathy - and Why They Matter

Pet Food Recall

Remember the pet food *recall* where wheat gluten was found to be tainted by the industrial chemical *melamine*? It caused kidney failure in many pets. Commercial animal food is made up, in part, of road kill. Many chronic conditions like arthritis can be traced to routinely feeding dogs and cats substandard commercial pet food.

What does it take for us to wake up to our beloved friends and companions' quality of life and well-being? I urge you to take a look at the pets and animals in your life and see them through new eyes.

Our bodies are ancient and should be fed as such. It is simple, really. Whole, real food, from unadulterated sources makes all the difference to your body in how it performs and how it heals.

Nevertheless, we realize that some of what is sold in supermarkets is far from real food. Most packaged food contains either corn or soy, both of which, in the United States, are predominantly *genetically modified organisms* (GMOs.) Are GMOs safe? There is a hot debate, currently. This is not to imply that only harmful things are synthetic/engineered. Far from it. Remember asbestos? Asbestos, we said, occurs naturally, yet poses significant threats to our well-being. And, some claim research shows that engineered food (GMOs) are safe and promote sustainable agriculture (Entine, 2013).

But safety is only one concern. We don't know the full impact on the microbiome or biodiversity, although research points toward impact on gut health (Meyers & Malterre, 2015). However, the fact remains that when it comes to assaults on our health, synthetic concoctions take the cake.

Speaking of cake, do you know that imitation vanilla is not vanilla at all? Quite the contrary. First of all, real vanilla comes from real vanilla beans which grow in pods on a type of orchid. Those beans contain a naturally occurring chemical called *vanillin* which gives the beans their flavor.

Since the worldwide demand for vanilla was so great, and the natural supply was so small, we developed imitation copies. There are two main sources of imitation vanilla: (1) lignin vanillin, a by-product of the paper industry that has been *chemically treated to mimic the taste of vanilla*, and (2) ethyl vanillin, which is a *coal tar derivative*. We are most likely today to find ethyl vanillin listed as an artificial flavoring on labels of foods like maple syrup and medicinal products. Yum.

Adding fuel to the fire are other artificial flavorings, artificial colorings, artificial sweeteners, preservatives, pesticide residues, sulfites, etc. Do you begin to see why much of our *food* isn't food at all? It's more like Franken Food as GMOs have been endearingly labeled.

Again, *Food Inc.* (Kenner, 2008) is a great film to watch to get educated about how the food supply is produced and the process it goes through to get to you. But this chapter is primarily about environmental toxins and your well-being. What do all of these modified or *artificial* ingredients do to your body, mind, and spirit?

Aspartame causes headaches, even migraines. *Corn syrup* (and no, it is not natural like ads on TV want you to believe) used to cause sores or irritation around my mouth every time I accidentally ate it.
Table sugar, which is highly refined, has the same density as heroin and is similarly addictive, (Garber & Lustig, 2011). Just like MSG, it can cause erratic behavior in some people.

Artificial ingredients and additives may potentially contribute to serious health issues which may include hormone disruption, cancer, and chronic conditions such as MS, CFS, Type II Diabetes, and heart disease (Lustig, Schmidt, & Brindis, 2012).

Food is supposed to be your medicine, not what you need medicine for after consuming it.

The Sugar Controversy

I highly recommend reading *The Sugar Controversy* (Vio & Uauy, 2007). It is one of several case studies presented in the book *Food Policy for Developing Countries: Case Studies:*

> Consumption of calories either as sugar or fat by sedentary populations promotes overconsumption of energy and thus may contribute to the "globesity" epidemic and associated chronic diseases. (Vio & Uauy, 2007)

Yes, evidence shows that sugar is one of several dietary factors contributing to obesity. Thus it may affect onset of some nutrition-related chronic diseases. It facilitates overconsumption of energy and may cause a hormonal/metabolic response (insulin/glucose) that may promote increased abdominal obesity, insulin resistance, altered plasma lipid levels, and hypertension (Poppitt et al., 2002). What may follow are diabetes, heart disease, and some forms of cancer (Schulze et al., 2004, updated as of 2010).

Chronic Disease and the Sugar Controversy

The *sugar controversy* has its roots in a 2002 conference held by the World Health Organization (WHO) and the Food and Agriculture Organization of the United Nations (FAO) on diet, nutrition, and physical activity for the prevention of *chronic disease*. The conference report focused on the dietary and physical activity determinants of major chronic diseases and helped establish the scientific basis for prevention of these conditions.
(WHO/FAO, 2003)

> As part of the response to the global epidemics of diabetes and obesity *(diabesity)* - major threats to the lives and well-being of all populations – the report TRS 916 recommended limiting the mean intake of added sugars to 10% or less of total energy supply.
> (Nishida, Uauy, Kumanyika, & Shetty, 2004)

> Sugar producers and sugar-exporting countries raised concerns about the consequences of this recommendation for future markets. They challenged it on strength of evidence, scientific merit, and assumptions made; it became the focus of debate between the nutrition community, the sugar industry, and agricultural policy experts. Their positions contrasted health gains with the economic implications of limiting sugar consumption. (Vio & Uauy, 2007)

GMOs
Gene Revolution/Genetic Splicing

GMO stands for *genetically modified organism*. The subject of GMOs is an enormous topic that is highly controversial. It can fill a book on its own. I urge you to learn more, beyond what you will read in these pages, including following legislation like the DARK Act. *Food, Inc.* (Kenner, 2008) may be a great place to start as well.

GMOs are living organisms, first and foremost. This is an important fact to grasp. These organisms have DNA, just like we do, and *their DNA has been altered* by the insertion or deletion of certain genes into the crops. The purpose of alteration is to improve pesticide or disease resistance, or to enhance flavor. Thus, the alteration process is actually *genetic modification*. Now you can see why they are called *GMOs*.

According to the World Health Organization, "Genetically modified foods are derived from organisms whose genetic material (DNA) has been modified in a way that does not occur naturally, e.g. through the introduction of a gene from a different organism" (WHO, 2015).

The general idea behind GMOs is to make it easier to grow a crop, or to enhance certain characteristics of a crop. For example, the *FlavrSavr tomato* was genetically engineered to cause ripe fruit to remain firm longer. Demand for the FlavrSavr tomato was high, but the product was never profitable.

Another example of gene manipulation is ***putting a flounder gene into a tomato cell*** so that the tomato will better survive the cold.

Organisms and micro-organisms that have been modified by means of genetic engineering include plants, fish, insects, mammals, yeast, viruses, and bacteria. Are you worried yet?

GMOs are in most foods sold in most supermarkets. In fact you have to watch it if you *don't* want them. They are everywhere, in everything. The reason? *Corn and soy.* It is very hard to find products that don't have genetically modified corn and/or soy in them, for one thing, and challenging to find products that use true *organic soy and organic corn.*

Monsanto, founded by a veteran of the pharmaceutical industry, was among the first companies to genetically modify a plant cell. In fact, it is estimated that now "Monsanto-patented genes are in 93% of the soybeans and 80% of the corn grown in the U.S" (Kaldveer, 2013; Organic Consumers Association, 2013).

Many ingredients are derivatives of corn as well, including ingredients you would not think are corn-based like sorbitol, MSG, xanthum gum *(I keep forgetting about this one, it sounds so innocuous)* monoglycerides and diglycerides, maltodextrin, dextrose, and many malt and sugar extracts.

The United States and Canada do not require GMOs to be labeled. In October 2013, Coca-Cola contributed more than $1.5 million to the Grocery Manufacturers Association (GMA) to campaign against the labeling of GMOs (again, check out legislation like the DARK Act).

The Washington state Attorney General says that the GMA violated the state's campaign disclosure laws when it bundled more than $11 million for the anti-labeling fight, while shielding the identities of the companies, led by Coca-Cola, who were donating that money. ~ Ocean Robbins

Here is a quote from Phil Angell, director of corporate communications at Monsanto, that pretty much speaks for itself:

Monsanto **should not have to vouchsafe the safety** of biotech food. ***Our interest is in selling as much as of it as possible.*** Assuring its safety is the FDA's job. (Pollan, 1998)

What are the environmental and health concerns? Well, there are environmental safety worries. GMOs are said to threaten biodiversity, partly because of genetic transfer. And then there is the impact on us:

> There are several types of potential health effects that could result from the insertion of a novel gene into an organism. Of primary concern ... are production of new allergens, increased toxicity, decreased nutrition, and antibiotic resistance. (Bernstein et al., 2003)

For someone like me who doesn't detoxify properly, it's challenging to process most things synthetic or altered. GMOs are really bad news for me. I have to be extra vigilant in my search for real, healthy food. As I've said elsewhere in this book, I thank god for stores like Whole Foods that evolved in the 60's from small health food stores into markets selling just about anything under the sun that meets your unique health needs. Without stores like Whole Foods and without companies that make the products I buy there and at other independent and chain stores whose proprietors carefully select what they offer, who knows where I would be today. I remember stories of how successful companies like Herb Pharm started with selling herbs out of the back of their truck. It is this type of passion to spread the word of natural health and natural medicines that has saved my life.

Here's a partial list of genetically modified crops.

Some Genetically Modified Crops in the U.S.*	
Soybeans	85%
Corn	45%
Cotton	76%

More than 170 million acres worldwide are planted with genetically modified crops, two-thirds of which are in the U.S., representing more than a fortyfold increase [from 2003 - 2013] The financial benefits to farmers - at least in the short run - are so great that more and more of them are embracing the genetically modified crops. (Phelan, 2013)

*percentages are not absolute

These photos compare standard and modified cornfields. *Thank you* goes to *imgarcade.com* for sharing the images.

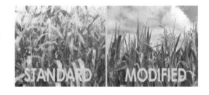

Cell Invasion Technology

There's more to the story.

Using the idea that bacteria and viruses, which are good at invading cells - *DNA naturally transfers across plants* - (Lederberg, 1986), can be introduced into plant cells to modify their resistance to certain chemicals or other forces around them, about half of the American soybean crops planted in the mid-90s carried a gene that made them resistant to the herbicide *Roundup*. Farmers liked this idea because they could *control weed growth without harming their soybeans*. Normally Roundup kills anything green. Round and Roundup we go.

With Roundup resistant bacteria and E. coli bacteria, the same soybean creators used cell invasion to bring forth modified corn which, like the soybean, could resist being killed off by Roundup.

Then an oxymoron was born: *insecticide corn*. Genetically modified corn is *registered as an insecticide* because every cell in it has been engineered to produce BT, a natural bacterial toxin. Bacillus thuringiensis (BT) is a bacterium that produces proteins which are toxic to insects. In fact, health researchers are studying the effect of BT on human cells after consumption of modified BT corn. There's a concept to ponder: *corn as insecticide*. What will they think of next? I am sure I do not wish to know.

Monsanto created Roundup as well as saccharin, aspartame, artificial vanilla flavoring, DDT, and produced, you guessed it, Agent Orange. *Their goal is sustainable agriculture.* While this is a noble goal, there are many other factors to consider: What about bio-diversity? What about bio-availability? How do GMOs affect the microbiome and absorption of vital nutrients? Proponents of sustainable agriculture (and, truly, who doesn't want that) also often claim that organics are no more nutritious than GMO and non-organic food. My body knows the difference between organic and GMO food, etc.

As far as DDT goes, it has a long, sad history. Thankfully, it was banned by Congress in 1972, due largely to environmentalists' efforts. DDT was challenged by Rachel Carson in her book *Silent Spring** which sought to inform the public of the side effects associated with the insecticide (it was nerve gas in WWII.)

As we think about the concepts of genetically modified organisms and cell invasion, there are three ideas, among others, to keep in mind:
(1) GMOs are living organisms. (2) You cannot control a plant once it is released into the ecosystem. (3) Everything is connected and behaves as such.
This groundbreaking book launched the Environmental Protection Agency...

Plant and Animal Extinction:
Violating the Species Barrier

Think about these facts:

It is estimated there are 8.7 million species living on our planet, excluding bacteria (Alford, 2014). However, it's estimated that between 200 and 100,000 species go extinct each year (Walsh, May 13, 2013). A joint research team of paleontologists at the universities of Brown and Duke recently concluded that the average pre-human extinction rate, or the natural background rate, was "0.1 extinction per million species per year" (DeVos et. al. 2015). The current extinction rate is approximately 100 extinctions per million species per year, or 1,000 times higher than the natural background rate. They predict future rates may be as much as 10,000 times higher. These are alarming statistics. We know species evolve over millions of years. Most last around one to ten million years if not disrupted. But we may be disrupting the natural order.

New Wave of Extinction
For the first time since the dinosaurs disappeared, humans are driving animals and plants to extinction faster than new species can evolve, a world expert on biodiversity has warned. Conservationists agree the rate of loss has increased. Dramatic predictions of experts like renowned Harvard biologist E. O. Wilson [indicate] that in two more decades the rate of loss could reach 10,000 times the background rate* (Jowit, 2010).   *the normal rate of extinction before humans became involved*

Scientists have produced comprehensive evidence that the diversity of butterflies, birds and plants is in decline. According to a study in the US journal *Science*, about 70% of all butterfly species in Britain have declined. About 28% of plant species and 54% of bird species also declined. Findings come from government-funded scientists using data amassed over 40 years by 20,000 naturalists (Radford, 2004).

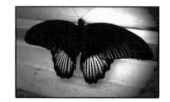

Manfred Bauer - publicdomainpictures.net

Are we to conclude that we are moving toward genetic uniformity? Trouble is, genetic uniformity can lead to disease. Additionally, GMOs contribute to the breakdown of the integrity of the *species barrier*, weakening the natural mechanisms that prevent disease from spreading from one species to another. And who knows what plants could have been used as medicine that now have become extinct?

Modern conditions like population growth, toxic pollution, habitat degradation, and global warming are factors which may contribute to the rapid increase in the extinction rate. Do you think we're messing with evolution? Outcomes thus far suggest *yes*. And, lest we forget, we *are* part of the ecosystem, vulnerable to evolutionary change. I do not believe we're protected from extinction, or separate from other species, just because we're conscious of our aliveness (and what is "consciousness"?). *We are only separate if we believe we are separate.* In fact, as humans, we're trying to survive just like any species tries to survive - we labor to produce food, etc. But because we're *aware,* we have more responsibility. We really are, or should be, *stewards of the earth.*

Of Bees and Butterflies

In a rural area of the beautiful Pacific Northwest, my brother and his family are home farmers and beekeepers - honeybees. In this six second silent video he is at work with the bees. Double click to open.

Pinterest.com

Beekeeper & Bees.AVI

Recently, a massive amount of honeybees died all at once in the Pacific Northwest. What a disheartening feeling this brings. Even more disheartening is one possible reason for their decline:

"So what's killing the honeybees? Pesticides - including a new class called neonicotinoids - seem to be harming bees even at what should be safe levels [of application]" (Walsh, Aug 19, 2013).

If the honeybee is vanishing at an alarming rate then what are we doing about it? The French, Germans, and Italians took action several years ago to control the use of *neonicotinoids* and protect pollinators. The U.S., in 2014, created a task force to study the situation. Let's hope they move swiftly (PANNA, 2011).

Neonicotinoid Pesticides
EPA's current review of neonics like clothianidin isn't due to conclude until 2018. Meanwhile, bee-harming pesticides continue to be widely used.
While pathogens and habitat loss* are also at play, a growing body of scientific evidence points to neonicotinoids - alone and in combination with other pesticides and pathogens - as a clear contributing factor to recent pollinator declines.
U.S. beekeepers reported record-breaking losses in recent years, with some losing 40-70% of their hives. Beekeepers, and the agricultural industries relying on their bees, are in trouble.
Bees need action before 2018. (PANNA, *2011*)

Bryan Walsh, in his *Time* cover story of August 9, 2013, <u>A World Without Bees</u>, goes on to discuss other reasons, in addition to pesticides, that threaten bee colonies.*

> Biological threats like the Varroa mite are killing off colonies directly and spreading deadly diseases. As our farms become monocultures of commodity crops like wheat and corn - plants that provide little pollen for foraging bees - honeybees are literally starving to death. If we don't do something, there may not be enough honeybees to meet the pollination demands for valuable crops. But more than that, in a world where [thousands] of species go extinct each year, the vanishing honeybee could be the herald of a permanently diminished planet. (Walsh, August 9, 2013)

According to Hannah Nordhous, author of *The Beekeepers Lament*, honeybees are the "glue that holds our agricultural system together" (as cited by Walsh, August 9, 2013).

What would we do without the honeybee?* What would you and your health do without the crops pollinated by bees - like blueberries, apples, pears, blackberries, raspberries, cherries, cucumbers, almonds, and spices like anise, cardamom, coriander, and nutmeg, and so on?

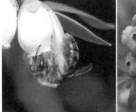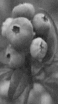

(Left photo by Rufus Isaac/AAAS) (Right photo courtesy of Daniel M. Turner)

(Both photos retrieved from npr.org)

*The bumblebee is disappearing too. See the **Resources** section ...

The monarch butterfly is in trouble too:

> A critical factor in the decline [of the monarch] is expansion of cropland and increased use of genetically modified crops that are resistant to herbicides, which in turn has led to more herbicide use against native plants that compete with crops. Crop expansion is happening in grassland ecosystems across the US, especially California, where western monarchs breed and feed. Because these herbicides are killing developing seedlings, as well as perennial plants, the only host plant for monarch caterpillars, milkweed, is disappearing along with the nectar plants used by adult monarchs. What are we to expect of these butterflies if we destroy their only form of food? (Argueta, 2014)

> Monarch butterflies are in crisis! What's at stake? One of the most extraordinary migrations on the planet. Each year, as they have for generations, North American monarchs take an epic journey, flitting upwards of 3,000 miles across the US and Canada to a few wintering grounds, including Mexico's Sierra Madre mountains. Less than 20 years ago, one billion monarchs migrated yearly. [In 2014,] a mere fraction of that - 33.5 million - made the journey - the ninth year in a row the migrating population fell below its long-term average.

> Why? In large part it's because industrial agriculture, using a new generation of herbicides, is killing native milkweed on which monarchs depend - the only place they lay their eggs.

> If the EPA placed limits on herbicides like glyphosate - marketed as Roundup - the EPA could increase the monarch's survival. But it may take hundreds of thousands of us to make the point heard! (Beinecke, personal communication, March 20th, 2014)

Our Energy Crisis

Perhaps the current state of the world's energy crisis mirrors the same disconnect that is currently going on in our war with our own bodies.

To see the world's disconnect, we only need to look at the disasters involving the Exxon Valdez oil spill in Prince William Sound, and British Petroleum's (BPs) oil rig explosion in the Gulf of Mexico.*

*I don't believe in pointing fingers. We are all responsible for our world's well-being.

Those millions of gallons of crude oil spilled into our pristine waters, and onto the surrounding beaches, may be symbolic of our ailing environment. In fact, we could go so far as to say that our environment is sick - as the acidification* of the oceans indicates- or, at the very least, is out of balance.

The world energy crisis is not a simple problem with a simple solution, I get it. But it is known that solar energy is abundant, and it could meet all of our energy needs, were it affordable. I hope for the day we can use it as a primary energy source.

Sustainable energy for our planet and mind-body balance is what we should be seeking both collectively and individually. On a global level isn't it time to move away from unsustainable power for our energy needs? On the individual level, so many of us struggle with stress, stuck in fight-or-flight, and struggle with unnecessary disruptions in our well-being. We must drop our addiction to fear, quick fixes like stimulants to boost energy, and drugs for imbalances in our bodies.

We have been given what we need to thrive on this planet if we truly look at what is all around us. The answer is never grand and rarely easy, but it is real and it is doable if we choose it.

But as long as the disconnect with our own bodies and our own lives continues, we will continue to see that mirrored back to us in our outer environments. Chronic fatigue and/or stress are the top reasons people go to the doctor. Our energy deficits on all levels have reached massive proportions. We are stuck in the fight or flight response.

Being stuck here is wreaking havoc on our collective well-being.

It is time to wake up. There is a better way to live that is sustainable, and that includes all of us, all of life … all living beings …

We can move out of living in fear and move into living in harmony with the whole universe. Life is meant to be savored and not survived.

*see **Resources** for link on *The Acid Sea* – the acidification of the oceans is a by-product of CO2 emissions and global warming.

Health is a commodity these days, and your body is the currency. The problem - or catch - with this system is that *health is deeply personal.* At the most basic level of our being we know that our health - our bodies and minds - belong to us, and are not for sale. Yet, as long as there is a for-profit healthcare system, your health will be a commodity. So much time, energy, and, of course, money goes into advertising and promoting prescription drugs, etc. Make no mistake about it. Your well-being is for sale in the current market.

Energy and health are precious. They are probably our most precious resources. Most of us don't realize just how important our health and energy really are until we lose them. The body is our vehicle to experience this amazing world and yet we only seem to want to take care of it when it is broken down on the side of the road.

Health is so unconsciously important to us that the first thing we ask one another is *How are you?* Although we usually are asking how the other person is doing emotionally, we are indirectly asking about the person's physical health as well because our emotions and the state of our health are inextricably linked. In fact, they are profoundly linked. Our inner environment, like the environment around us, is directly affected by our interaction with it.

The term that connects body and mind is now called *bodymind,* first coined by Ken Dychtwald (Dychtwald, 1977) and made popular by the neuroscientist and molecular biologist, Candace Pert. According to Pert's work with neurotransmitters and her book *Molecules of Emotion* (Pert, 1999*),* there is no differentiation between where your *mind* ends and your *body* begins. They are one and the same.

Dr. Pert also believed there's a causative connection between synthetic chemicals and chronic illness. Formerly, she did not used to think so, but then changed her mind. If we introduce synthetic chemicals, we may stimulate a causative internal environment resulting in chronic illness (Bland, on Candace Pert, October 25, 2013).

When a renowned scientist backs up what I have also experienced first-hand, I take note.

One of the oaths of medicine is to *do no harm*. While I believe most people who take this oath believe it when they take it, the continued practice of blindly prescribing of drugs as a first order of health care is quite possibly doing major harm to our well-being. In addition:

> According to a 1999 report by the Institute of Medicine, as many as 98,000 Americans were dying every year because of medical mistakes [including prescribing the wrong medication]. A reasonable estimate is that medical mistakes now kill around 200,000 Americans every year. That would make [medical mistakes] one of the leading causes of death in the United States. (Gupta, July 31, 2012)

> Medical errors are the eighth leading cause of death - higher than car accidents, breast cancer, and AIDS combined. Common medical errors are medication errors ... [which] occur when a patient is given the wrong drug, the wrong amount of the right drug, a drug known to cause allergy in the patient, or a drug known to interact poorly with a patient's other medicines. Errors also happen when medicines known to help a patient with a certain illness are not prescribed. About 7,000 people yearly are estimated to die from medication errors - more deaths each year than deaths due to work-related injuries. One study found about two out of every 100 people admitted to a hospital had a preventable adverse reaction - or unwanted effect - from medication. (National Partnership for Women & Families, 2009)

There were 484 deaths from the prescription drug Heparin since May, 2008, as reported by the FDA (US Department of Health & Human Services, 2009). With Heparin, side effects include nausea, vomiting, and breathing difficulties.

Yaz, a drug that kept me awake at night with severe cramps, was questioned for showing higher blood clotting risks. In an independent study of one million women, Yaz was 2-4 times more likely than other prescription birth control pills to cause blood clots, with some deaths associated, as well ("FDA to Review," 2011).

What is the message here? *Some prescription drugs are healing, and I know people whose health has been positively affected. But, let's not be naive. Drugs of any kind are extremely powerful, and drugs can and do kill.*

Fosamax, and other osteoporosis drugs, may have been associated with side effects such as femur breaks. Merck, maker of Fosamax, was cleared of charges, however the plaintiff claimed: "Merck knew Fosamax could trigger atypical femur fractures, but didn't alert regulators or doctors until after the drug lost market exclusivity" (as cited in Staton, 2013).

Another alarming statistic: U.S. citizens consume about 80% of all anti-depressants produced, such as opiates, which are some of the most dangerous prescription drugs available ("Americans Gulping Down," 2012).

I don't believe in demonizing people or companies. I believe most of us are doing the best we can. I choose to believe the best about people, regardless of the actions of certain individuals or companies. Yet, power and control is not given up easily, and, it doesn't mean we bury our heads in the sand when it comes to a glaringly obvious issue: **some prescription drugs are causing major harm to our health, and are gateway drugs to be sure.** Every day we see commercials funding the news that tout the latest pill that will cure us of our supposed ills. Yet, it is easy to find examples of prescription drugs which have been recalled for causing serious complications and/or death. Often we hear of yet another drug under investigation or pulled off the market due to people getting sick or dying.

Chronic conditions, for the most part, are preventable and/or treatable when addressed through nutrition and lifestyle. Yet some patients choose to self-medicate symptoms instead of addressing the underlying causes. Even worse, we are getting sicker: "By 2015, chronic diseases will be the most common cause of death even in the poorest countries [and] more than 75 percent of health care costs are due to chronic conditions" (NIH, 2009).

Why have pills become the norm? Why do we think a little white pill is the answer? These are simple questions with complex answers. It may be in our mythology to assume a magic pill will fix everything. It's normal that most people want an easy solution.

Yet your body is an intricate organism with multi-layered needs. It is like a plant or a garden more than anything else. Gardens need soil, water, sun, care and time to grow and flourish. The same things are true for your body to heal.

In Chapters Four and Five, we'll explore, in detail, suggestions for natural healing, ways to work in harmony with your body and the natural world, sans the quick fixes of the magic white pill.

One more observation: The little white pill is an enormous money-maker. In 2011, total sales for prescription drugs reached over $300 billion (Lindsley, 2012). That's a lot of investment in our health. But are we investing in our well-being the sustainable way?

Maybe not. And sometimes it takes a major shock to wake us up like when we witness the grave misuse of drugs resulting in untimely deaths. No one is immortal, except for maybe the jellyfish. But we should not be playing Russian Roulette with our health either.

Several celebrities such as Heath Ledger, Anna Nicole Smith, Michael Jackson, Brittany Murphy, Brad Renfro, Prince, etc. have died in recent years due, at least in part, to overdoses of prescription drugs.

Heath Ledger died from a lethal combination of six different drugs, prescribed by multiple doctors, which suppressed the breathing center of his brain: the painkillers oxycodone and hydrocodone, the anti-anxiety drugs alprazolam and diazepam, as well as the sleep aids doxyleamine and temazepam. The names alone scare me.

Anna Nicole Smith died from *acute combined drug intoxication* (Duke, 2009). Chloral Hydrate was one of the sleep aids she was prescribed.

Sleep aids can be temporarily usefu, but they are tricky. Some medications are used as sleep inducers because they cause tiredness, but often the fatigue can persist until the next day, or even longer.

Commonly Prescribed Sleep Drugs
• psychiatric drugs, especially antipsychotic drugs and tricyclic antidepressants
• benzodiazepines and other tranquilizers
• sleep aids you may recognize: Ambien, Intermezzo, Halcion, etc.
• anticonvulsants (epilepsy drugs)
• antihistamines
• muscle relaxants
• narcotic painkillers (opioids)

Each drug has a set of side effects. Here are *26 side effects* that come with various prescription drugs:

1. Drainage, crusting, or oozing of eyes* or eyelids
2. Swollen, black,* or "hairy" tongue
3. Changes in the shape or location of body fat*
4. Decrease in testicle size
5. Sores or swelling in rectal or genital area
6. Blue lips* or fingernails
7. Purple skin spots
8. White patches or sores inside mouth or on lips
9. Irregular back-and-forth movements of eyes
10. Enlarged breasts in males
11. Unusual risk-taking behavior,* no fear of danger
12. Extreme fear*
13. Hallucinations, fainting, coma

14. Fussiness, irritability, crying* for an hour or longer
15. Paralysis
16. Thoracic hematoma (bleeding into chest)
17. Blood clot in lung
18. Liver damage
19. Kidney damage
20. Breast lump*
21. Decreased bone marrow function
22. Congestive heart failure
23. Shingles
24. Nerve pain lasting for several weeks or months*
25. Bleeding that will not stop*
26. Coughing up blood or vomit that looks like coffee grounds
("The Terrifying Side Effects of Prescription Drugs," 2008)

*On the foregoing list, side-effects I experienced are *marked with an asterisk.*

Additionally, my symptoms during my illness included:

- chronic fatigue
- constant runny nose (a sign of Candida, or food sensitivities, and Body Burden - toxin overload)
- bloodshot eyes (continued to worsen over time)
- flu-like symptoms (constant in the beginning)
- nosebleeds
- hair loss
- mild headaches
- short term memory loss or trouble concentrating

- strong reactions to EMF's (electro-magnetic fields)
- strong reactions to chemical smells
- bad body odor
- teeth, hair, tongue turning black
- ringing in ears
- shaky nerves/trouble with motor control
- pain, tightness in chest
- feeling my body had been poisoned

I don't believe prescription drugs are "bad." I have taken bio-identical pregnenolone and progesterone, and still use a progesterone cream occasionally. I also tried Isocort (cortisol) when I was ill, and used Elavil, Xanax, and Ambien for sleeping (not recommended).

Even many vitamins are synthetic, including most of the *food-based* ones

 (except some of the *all raw* vitamins.) The notion that only *natural* is good for us is a misnomer. Most vitamins are *pharmaceutical grade*. In fact, before drug companies switched to money-making prescription drugs, they made many of the vitamins. Both prescription drugs and supplements have merit and can impact health and lives for the better.

But remember this: Drugs - prescription or street - have a seductive effect on the body. Prescription drugs* may suppress symptoms and push them deeper into the body, making it difficult for the body to regain balance and heal.

Symptoms are adaptations or defenses of the body to stress, infection, or toxic exposure. ~Dana Ullman, MPH (homeopathist)

Drugs also sedate the body and cause it to behave in ways that nature did not intend. For instance, when I took Benadryl, Elavil, Xanax, and Ambien for sleeplessness due to extreme anxiety, I would wake up with massive nervous system *hangovers*, at least at first.

With Xanax and Ambien, the intensity of my hangovers never really diminished. I just felt funny and off all day. Granted, part of the problem may have been my trouble detoxifying those particular drugs. However, not all of my symptoms can be traced to a liver disorder. Some of the blame is in the nature of the beast, i.e. the drugs.

With Elavil, my symptoms decreased a lot, but then I needed more Elavil to sleep as time went by. I started with about 10 mg/night and I was up to about 100 mg/night a few years into taking it.

Benadryl contains diphenhydramine known as a histamine-blocker that makes folks sleepy and is used in many over the counter sleep aids. The first time I took Benadryl, I woke up groggy and felt like I was swimming under water all day. But I ignored the feeling - a big mistake - as it was my nervous system crying for attention. I continued to take Benadryl for the next four years, starting with one per night, but soon that wasn't enough and I increased dosage to two per night.

*I am not condemning prescription drugs. I believe they can be life-savers for certain individuals. They don't work for me as I cannot detox them properly and I believe in taking the route with the least potential for side-effects. Natural, however, is not always better. Do your research and listen to your body!

However, I'm sad we don't think to look at what was naturally created for us to take when we are ill. **Herbs exist for a reason.** And 30-40% of prescription drugs are based, at least partially, on herbs. It's something to ponder, especially when it can break the bank to pay for a prescription drug that may end up causing more harm than good.

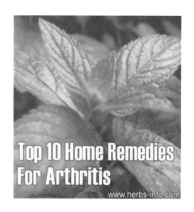

Yes, herbs are not regulated. No one can patent an herb. That is an

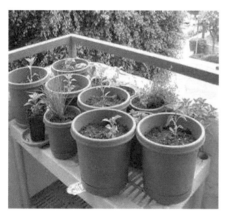

issue for some, although, in my opinion, I'm glad they aren't. But herbs and organic food are part of our *environment* as a whole that we have, in part, failed to notice. We have ignored the medicine given to us. Perhaps, no wonder we're not as vital as we could be.

Try growing your own herb garden!

Public-domain-image.com

Photo courtesy of ods.od.nih.gov

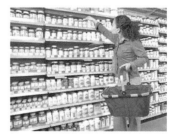

Be an informed, conscious consumer and a proactive, empowered patient!

For the majority of us, prescription drugs should be used for acute emergencies, or as a last resort, and not as a first line of defense, if used at all. Prescription drugs, in large part, suppress symptoms. And symptoms, my friend, are part of the solution to getting well again.

Chapter Three - Waking Up Tired

The Shadow of Fatigue

There is often in people to whom the worst has happened an almost transcendent freedom, for they have faced the worst and survived it.
~ Carol Pearson

The ideas, experiences, and theories in this chapter, or in any chapter of this book, are what I've found along my healing jourey and are for informational purposes only. They are not meant to diagnose, treat, or prescribe for any kind of condition or illness. I don't presume to be a doctor. Further, it is wise to seek the professional advice of a qualified health care practitioner before making any changes in your self-health care routine and practice.

First, let me say this: Chronic Fatigue Syndrome (CFS), or any other chronic disease, is *not* all in your head. This myth needs to die. There is good evidence that the *condition* of CFS is a physical disorder. Perhaps it is the fact that the majority of people who develop CFS are women that this disorder has been dismissed. Regardless, plenty of men, teens, and young adults are affected. Plus the variable symptoms are found across all racial, ethnic, and economic lines. CFS doesn't discriminate.

CFS is *not a psychiatric disturbance*, although it may indeed be neurally-mediated. The CDC has even stated that 29% of people with CFS have a *personality disorder*, compared with only 7% of a study-controlled, healthy population. I wish to note here that I'm not knocking the CDC. The CDC staff members have been very gracious to me.

Here's the thing: Generally, people tell you how they're feeling. So, if someone says *I'm not feeling well*, then newsflash, they aren't feeling well, and there *is* a reason.

Multiple Sclerosis (MS) was once thought to be caused by *hysteria* - I can't stand that word - or *alcoholism*. Ulcers were imagined to be the result of stress. We now know ulcers are caused by bacteria. With MS, we suspect that myelin, which is the protective coating around nerve fibers, may be affected by an auto-immune response or by neuronal loss, with the progressive type. By the way, CFS is now considered as serious a condition as MS. In the past, we believed many theories that have turned out not to be incorrect. Healing itself may be moving out of *groupthink* and into a more holistic way of seeing and being.

CFS is an illness caused by a system or systems that is/are out of balance, in my opinion. Speaking of systems, remember this: the mind and body are intrinsically, inevitably, and irrefutably linked.

Science is great, and necessary. Scientists conduct research and note patterns. But perhaps scientific research works best for longitudinal studies, to show probabilities. For instance, it is *probable* if one is obese when young to develop Type II Diabetes sooner or later. But research statistics may not work so well on the individual level, and *the personal level is where people heal.* In my humble opinion, scientific research, no matter how great - *although I wish we didn't test on animals* - only tells part of the story. For instance, as Deepak Chopra says, the more science understands about the brain, the less science understands about consciousness. This is why I'm fascinated with *systems biology* which notices patterns, watches for the surfacing of self-organizing models, and observes healing from a *holistic point of view.* The thing is, *nature is a dynamic system*, which learns, evolves, and grows. Our planet is a living being, a system, as the Gaia Principle would say, as well.

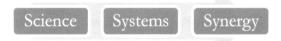

Studying systems leads one to notice *synergy* and *coherence.* Please see Chapter Five. The study of systems also teaches us that the whole is greater than the sum of its parts. The systems level is where healing happens: where we find synergy and possibly even coherence, as well as the energetics of holism - pleasure, engagement, resiliency, and connectedness - helping us discard the downward spiral of illness.

When we try to pick out anything by itself we find it hitched to everything else in the Universe. ~ *John Muir (Naturalist and Conservationist)*

CFS, and other conditions like it, is a prime learning opportunity for us to understand that the *mind* and the *body* are not only linked, *they are the same thing*. So let's stop differentiating them, because the differentiation doesn't truly exist. We also take note that mind and spirit can heal us, I believe. So in the end, *mindset* is hugely powerful in healing, as may be *spirituality*.

Consider this: CFS may be an *auto-immune condition*, much like MS or lupus, perhaps mediated by changes in the hypothalamic-pituitary-adrenal (HPA) axis, which in turn affects the immune system. It may affect women more as well, due to different genetic expression:

> The genes that switch on and off differently from person to person are more likely to be associated with autoimmune diseases. Another is that women and men use different switches to turn on many immune system genes... that difference in activity might explain the much higher incidence in women of autoimmune diseases such as scleroderma, lupus and rheumatoid arthritis. (Stanford, 2015)

Also, extremely important to note, is that a major component of CFS is chronic stress, as doctors have long suspected. All stressors affect the body the same way. In other words, your body does not know the difference between types of stressors, whether they are viral, social, emotional, physical, environmental, etc. However, the critical factor in whether or not a person may be susceptible to CFS is the way each person's body, spirit, and mind interprets stress. This is a very important point, since I believe the pathogenesis of CFS, as well as other chronic illness, can begin with a breakdown in the body at the systemic level, brought on by some kind of acute or unrelenting stressor, and played out, on an individual level, by genetic variability.

Waking Up Tired

Fatigue and/or stress are the two main reasons *by a landslide* people go to their doctor. **Twenty percent** of the population may face chronic fatigue in some capacity at any given time in their lives. According to alternative practitioners, about 80% of adults in the general population suffer unbearable fatigue at some point in their lives.

Fatigue is a big topic. I'm almost too tired to write this book, or at least I was in the beginning. The CDC along with DePaul University estimates CFS costs the US economy $30 billion annually in health care and lost productivity. *What is going on here?*

CFS (also known as ME/SEID) has been called by many names:

- ✓ A disorder of the HPA axis (hypothalamus-pituitary-adrenal axis) which may be in a state of chronic down-regulation, which means the genes are under-expressing
- ✓ CFIDS (chronic fatigue immune dysfunction syndrome)
- ✓ SEID (systemic exertion intolerance disorder) a name being tried on by the Institute of Medicine as of 2015
- ✓ ME (myalgic encephalopathy)
- ✓ Gulf War Syndrome
- ✓ EI (environmental illness)
- ✓ Autonomic dysregulation
- ✓ Neuroanasthenia
- ✓ Mitochondrial Disease
- ✓ A *women's disease*, (ouch) since two-thirds of all cases are *women of childbearing years;* one reason may be *estrogen dominance*, coming up in this chapter; it could be people who are HSP's (see page 204)

But the truth is men get this illness as well (see *Chemical Injury* later in this chapter where I discuss *Gulf War Syndrome*.) One male subject in a study said he became chronically fatigued after a stressful divorce. Men can be affected by estrogen dominance as well (*I am not suggesting this is the only cause*). As I stated earlier, CFS does not discriminate.

Trauma seems to be an indicator of future fatigue. Many report getting CFS or even FM* after going through a stressful life event such as personal illness or serious illness in the family, divorce, death of a loved one, car accident, etc. There is a describable pattern, or a set of patterns, associated with acute or chronic stress and the onset of CFS.

So, which name do we pick - A, B, C, or all of the above? If CFS has so many names, perhaps we need a new model to explain what it even means to be *sick with CFS*, or, at the very least, we need to explain how to get and stay well. *Finally*, the name *CFS* is a misnomer. It is only a *syndrome* if its causes are unknown. Are they?

*Fibromyalgia

Let's start with *fatigue* itself. There are many conditions that have fatigue as a symptom. Here are just some of them:

Addiction
Anemia
B-12 Deficiency
Cancer
Candida
Chemical Injury
Chemotherapy and/or Radiation Treatment
Chronic Fatigue Syndrome (CFS)
Diabetes
Diet - inadequate
Environmental Illness (EI)
Fibromyalgia (FM)

Heart Disease
Hypoglycemia
Hypothyroidism
Lupus
Medications like diuretics & beta-blockers
Mold
Multiple Chemical Sensitivity (MCS)
Multiple Sclerosis (MS)
Stress
Toxicity from modified or synthetic foods

What Causes CFS? ... The Million Dollar Question

The truth is, no really knows, or at least there's no general consensus on it. Race, gender, and socioeconomic status are factors as well (Jason, et al., 2009). There are many theories out there however.

> CFS is a debilitating and complex disorder characterized by profound fatigue that is not improved by bed rest and that may be worsened by physical or mental activity. Persons with CFS most often function at a substantially lower level of activity than they were capable of before the onset of illness.

> CFS ... is a diagnosis of exclusion...the cause or causes of CFS remain(s) unknown, despite a vigorous search. While a single cause for CFS may yet be identified, another possibility is that CFS represents a common endpoint of disease resulting from multiple sudden causes. Some of the possible causes ... might be due to infectious agents, immunological dysfunction, stress activating the HPA axis, neurally mediated hypotension, and/or nutritional deficiency. (CDC, 2015)

Some conclude CFS is caused by a virus like Epstein-Barr* or HHV-6A. Others say it is due to *burnout* from chronic stress *or* one stressful event that alters the way the body functions. Dr. Teitelbaum says CFS acts as a "circuit breaker" on the HPA axis to protect it from perceived, overwhelming stress (Teitelbaum, 2009). Still others focus on weak adrenals, hypothyroidism, or immune dysfunction.

CFS has been called a neuro-immune disease, as well as an auto-immune disease. Others ask: is it related to ATP depletion or loss of energy in the cells…mitochondrial dysfunction in the Krebs Cycle perhaps? Or maybe it is akin to a blood pressure regulation disorder called neurally -mediated hypotension, or perhaps vital exhaustion?

Some suspect CFS could be multiple and shifting combinations of the forgoing. *Perhaps being an HSP is a factor.** It's tough, unfortunately, for those suffering from CFS, since *fatigue itself is a marker of most disease states. Therefore, it's hard to pinpoint what CFS is, exactly.*

With all these theories floating around, we must ask: Is chronic fatigue or chronic illness simply about cause and effect? Is it about input and output, plusses and minuses, checks and balances…or lack thereof?

Because CFS, so far, has defied any attempts to being pigeon-holed, it is therefore categorized as a *non-specific illness*, which I think does us a great disservice. There is nothing non-specific about feeling awful most of the time, every day. I understand where the classification *non-specific* comes from, but I think applying it to CFS shows a lack of respect. Further, if it's true that fatigue is a marker of most disease states, *and it is*, then the fact that we have *unrelenting fatigue* should be a *huge red flag* to those who treat us, and to those who love us.

More than one million people in the U.S. have CFS, according to the Centers for Disease Control and Prevention. About 17 million deal with it worldwide. *At any given time, 1 in every 5 people feel unusually tired and 1 in 10 have prolonged fatigue* (Timms, 2012).

Chronic fatigue is most prevalent in what are known as neurological disorders including Multiple Sclerosis and CFS. Why is this? What is the common link? Is CFS a *mind-body illness*, but with symptoms that are primarily organic (*biological*) in origin?

*Please see "Highlights" at the end of this book for more information on HSP's & The Epstein-Barr Virus. I cover the definition of HSP's coming up later in Chapter Three, including coping techniques.

Yet this is not to say that there are not other sources of *chronic fatigue*. *Chronic fatigue* is actually classified into different types of fatigue including peripheral and central fatigue. For more information on different types of fatigue, see MS, CFS, and Chronic Fatigue coming up in this chapter.

I hope this book helps sheds more light. But to be clear, I'm just getting the conversation started. I'm the messenger, not the expert. That being said, I've lived with chronic fatigue and studied CFS and related chronic conditions for over twenty years. For example, I *do* believe some of the causes of CFS are most likely known, just not widely publicized. Then again, there is much we are still learning about how our amazing bodies truly work.

In my case, I'm not even sure I have or ever had CFS. *Chronic fatigue?* For sure, no doubt. *CFS?* What happened was that I was diagnosed with it, and *that label followed me like a black cloud for years.*

Actually, as I will describe and draw comparisons in this chapter, it's possible I had a mild case of *fibromyalgia (FM) as well*, at least the second time. FM is linked to auto-immunity. There are around 150 kinds of auto-immune conditions. They are not all the same nor do they respond the same to treatment. However, some of the symptoms in CFS, MS, and FM overlap, such as with the symptom of *chronic fatigue.*

I believed I had CFS after I was diagnosed with it, but I found, when I stated my diagnosis, people generally gave me *the raised eyebrow, or the blank stare, or the sigh.* Yet, why would you judge someone for the burden they bear? What about giving us the benefit of the doubt? I've never understood this trait in human nature.

~ I wish I could make my body do what I need it to do. I wish I was not judged for not being able to make my body do what I need it to do. ~

I think my doctor diagnosed me with CFS because he didn't know what else with which to diagnose me. What about sub-clinical hypothyroidism, or hypocortisolism or tertiary adrenal insufficiency, or an auto-immune condition, or a neuro-inflammatory disorder, or a mitochondrial disorder, or just a disruption of the microbiome?

The first time I dealt with chronic fatigue in my early twenties after my ski accident and subsequent surgery, I knew about CFS but never thought that's what I had. I could still exercise, for starters, even when I was tired, although an extra-long hike could knock me out for days. Low tolerance for exercise can be one of the main indicators of CFS.

In fact, since starting grad school, I've had two major crashes. I had made so much progress, I considered myself *healed*, whatever that really means. After weeks of studying while working out at the same time on my treadmill, practicing yoga, and training to teach yoga, my body crashed and demanded rest - lots of it. In the second crash, I was attempting three graduate courses in six weeks, not by choice. I worked my butt off and crashed again. It took a number of weeks to find balance. What was it that made me crash? Was it iron or B-12 deficiency? Was it mitochondrial meltdown or lack of oxygen in my muscles? What was or is this *thing* that haunts me like a ghost limb? I will not let it rule my life. It has no power here. My strategy now? Self-care. See Chapter Four for details.

The second time around when I experienced extreme fatigue, my symptoms were much worse overall, and I started to believe it myself. Did I have CFS? After my research findings, I would say *yes*. Does a label make a difference? In my experience, definitely *yes*, especially if the *label is inaccurate, and does not fully describe a condition.* Then again, even if a label does fully describe a condition or disorder, it can still be damaging. Today there is a growing movement to rename CFS. The name SEID (systemic exertion intolerance disorder) is being tried out.

It's not that I care if what I had was CFS or not. Whatever I had doesn't matter. It matters that I got better, that I feel better. But the stigma attached with the nebulous name, *CFS*, is notorious at best. For example, *I could not get regular, affordable health insurance.* I was denied health insurance coverage by all sources due to my *pre-existing condition.* They did not take into consideration that *I rarely used my health insurance. I most certainly didn't use it for chronic fatigue,* beyond the second time around when I was looking for answers, blood-work, etc. Even then I only used it a handful of times. I told them on my application forms that I used alternative medicine. I was trying to get off of my sky high. expensive portability health insurance that came to me as part of my divorce. It cost me $600/month for something I rarely used.

All I wanted was accident coverage and possibly some alternative, preventative coverage, if I could get it. Thankfully, I finally got health insurance through Providence Health. When they received my application, they called to ask me in person about my chronic fatigue. I told them how I managed it through diet and certain supplements, and with homeopathy. The staff at Providence Health took the time to connect with a potential customer on the personal level. I was able to explain my situation and how having *a chronic condition does not have to be a life sentence* if managed properly. I believe this may be why they gave me health insurance where other companies had not ... and Providence earned another customer. It benefited both of us. Also, I believe it is no accident the name of my health insurance is *Providence*. When you speak up for yourself, and yet also surrender to a greater energy, amazing things unfold. See Chapter Five.

The Shadow of Fatigue

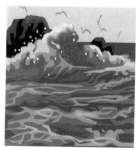

I breathe in every breath as if it were a shadow of air. Where is the substance of my breath and why does it not sustain me like it does others? Where is my original energy that supports all life without struggle? How do I recover what has seemingly dissolved forever? Where is my share of lifeforce and energy?

As I describe elsewhere in this book, chronic fatigue is feeling that you have no energy, like the main switch in your body has been turned off. It's like your car battery has mostly died, but somehow still sort of runs, by a miracle. You feel, literally, *too tired to breathe.*

I have experienced some chronic pain as well, and I also have heard from others that it is horrible to live with. Previously, I've described the young woman I met in group therapy whose back was in constant pain from injuries sustained when a car fall on her in her teens. She was hoping to deal with her pain on an emotional level. I'm not comparing chronic pain and chronic fatigue except to say both are physically and emotionally agonizing, although in different ways.

The body breaks down in different ways. There is temporary change or breaking down, called *acute illness*, and there is considerable breaking down called *chronic illness*. With chronic illnesses like CFS, Gulf War Syndrome, fibromyalgia, auto-immune illnesses, AIDS, or certain stages of cancer, the body feels like it has broken down to such a degree that what normally restores health to someone with acute illness seems to not work.

No matter how *broken* your body feels, I believe there is a way to feel well again. With CFS, perhaps the body's *protective mechanisms* for stress have failed or there is chronic inflammation. Yet my body is infinitely wise, and no matter my circumstances, I choose to inhabit well-being.

Chronic, severe, persistent stress - no matter what the source - may cause the body to kick into a state of hyper-vigilance in order to protect itself. The problem is, you can't maintain this state of being, i.e., chronic stress, without creating an imbalance of the *systems* of your body, possibly leading to chronic inflammation of the gut, brain, etc.

Is CFS an imbalance of a system or systems? And, if so, what is causing that intelligent system to break down? Chronic inflammation? Chronic, oxidative stress? Is the shadow of fatigue an indicator of protein or mitochondrial damage? Or, perhaps it is our overuse of antibiotics leading to loss of tight junctions, or genetic vulnerabilities?*

Regardless, I tried everything it seems to get rid of the shadow of my fatigue: eating well, eating "normally," eating extra super well, not caring at all what I put into my body, no stimulants, some stimulants, not worrying about how I was going to recover (just trusting that I would), extreme attention paid over every hour and day over how to recover, working full time and just hoping it would all go away by some miracle, and the list goes on and on.

I tried raw foods, sprouted foods, no sugar, etc. And, in my case, I *do* have to eat very well, although staying in The Relaxation Response helps a great deal and can greatly affect digestion and absorption.

But, even with all my attention and discipline, there was this *shadow of fatigue* that would not leave, no matter what I did. It haunted me like pain haunts a soldier who has lost her limb. It drove me crazy.

*See page 452 for more information on tight junctions.

To feel a constant pull of even slight fatigue is beyond frustrating. It marks your day. It's like a constant reminder that something is not right. You lose your *freedom*, in a sense.

I read somewhere once that dying is like realizing that you've dropped a backpack you weren't conscious of carrying around. It's pure freedom. Having chronic fatigue is like being super-conscious of that backpack, and it feels like it weighs a ton many days. *With chronic fatigue, there is no "unbearable lightness of being," there is only unbearable heaviness of being. Regardless, I have chosen to be "well in mind" (coming up).*

Some Theories of CFS*

*Note: While I have included many theories about what may cause CFS/chronic fatigue, I don't believe one shouldn't focus too much on the origins of chronic illness. Functional medicine would disagree with me and, of course, progress and research are key. But, more than anything, my body wishes is to be well, not subjected to endless tests and trials. While we have immune biomarkers now (Lipkin & Hornig, 2015), I found *focusing on my immediate symptoms helped me the most* to build the most synergy of health and well-being. Am I cold? Put a sweater on. Am I nervous or shaky? Do some gentle vinyasa yoga and/or take some type of supplement, etc. Am I hungry? Eat and eat well. Am I tired? Take it easy, practice self-care, and check within...

The Brain and ME/CFS: A Neurally-Mediated Condition?

When water travels down rock, it etches pathways, which shape the stone. This is how canyons are formed. Our experiences create similar pathways in our brains. The formative process can be a beautiful thing, because experiences are kept in mind to protect us, as well as to give shape and meaning to our lives. Yet, can these remembered pathways also keep us stuck in a state of chronic pain or fatigue?

Is on-going fatigue caused by ingrained neural pathways? Do chronic stressors become conditioned or programmed stimuli that keep our primitive brains stuck in a state of sympathetic (fight or flight) response? This may be what is known as limbic kindling.

Limbic kindling is the theory that the central nervous system develops facilitated pathways due to intermittent exposure to chemical, microbial, electrical or emotional factors. This intermittent exposure, in turn, "kindles" or programs the brain (through new, neural pathways) to stay stuck in a chronic stress resonse (N. Gratrix, personal communication, 2015), just like what happens in Posttraumatic Stress Disorder (PTSD). Is there a way to diminish these pathways? How does one move out of this chronic state of fear? Or is chronic fatigue the result of irreversible white matter damage?

I've come to wonder if chronic fatigue may not be completely healed due to already established brain pathways. More likely is that it is due to genetic tendencies, and how we turn on or turn off gene expression, or the condition of our microbial interactions system (our gut). It's also not my place to tell you what your body can or can't do. Your body is capable of renewing itself in many ways. It renews itself all the time, from three days (stomach lining) to six weeks (liver) to one year (98% of your atoms are renewed!). I wonder what it is, then, that lingers with chronic fatigue, that feels like a faded scar? Is it conditioned neural pathways? It is unexpressed genetic potential?*

Yet, still, I believe there are possible methods for facilitating new, positive, ingrained neural pathways. This is concept of neuroplasticity, which we will explore deeper. I believe what you focus on, takes focus, and that this intense concentration of energy can cause real, lasting change.

The Law of Facilitation

The Law of Facilitation states that:

"When an impulse has passed once through a certain set of neurons (known as the 'facilitated section') to the exclusion of others, it will tend to take the same course on future occasions. And, each time that impulse traverses this path, the resistance will be less" (source unknown).

What's also true is that negatively associated pathways can develop, and it can take much longer to break the negative hold. For example, if it takes 300-500 repetitions to facilitate (to make easy) a healthy pattern, it can take 3000-5000 times to diminish an unhealthy pattern.

Because the brain is affected by many things, like trauma which shrinks the hippocampus, it is also possible we can recondition the brain through restorative exercises such as yoga, Tai-Chi, Qi Gong, and walking. This powerful characteristic of the brain is known as brain plasticity. Exercise has been shown to help the hippocampus recover. We will explore *brain remodeling and brain plasticity* in Chapter Five.

*Whatever can or can't be healed, we all have potential to whole in some capacity: this is our unlimited potential, whether it's in mind, body, or even spirit, which is connected to the source of everything.

Focus on Multiple Sclerosis (MS)

I am honored and blessed to be part of the MS community through MS Station, run by the remarkable Ms. Rae Edwards. To listen to programs, visit http://multiplesclerosisradio.com/

I don't have MS and I'm not an expert on it, not by any stretch of the imagination. I'm presenting a bit about this auto-immune condition of the CNS so you know you're not alone.

One of the common symptoms of MS is fatigue. In 1997, Sheean and his team conducted an electrophysiological study of 21 MS patients.

"We postulate that central fatigue in multiple sclerosis is due to impaired drive to the primary motor cortex and several lines of evidence strongly suggest that this is not due to a lack of motivation" (Sheean, Murray, Rothwell, Miller, & Thompson, 1997).

There are two types of MS: progressive and relapsing-remitting. Many people report relief from relapsing-remitting MS by following lifestyle changes through diet and exercise, supplementation etc. Yet, the progressive type of MS may be due to neuronal loss, according to Dr. David Pleasure:

> For instance, without Charcot's discovery that MS affected axons – white matter – as well as myelin, for instance – we wouldn't have the important discovery that permanent disability that eventually develops in patients with progressive MS is chiefly due to axonal loss, rather than to demyelination. ("White Matter Matters," 2015)

However, here is a formal definition of MS:

> MS is a disease of the CNS characterized by destruction of the myelin sheath surrounding neurons, resulting in the formation of plaques. ... MS is progressive and fluctuating, with exacerbations, i.e., patients feeling worse, and remissions, i.e., patients feeling better, over many decades. ... The cause of MS is unknown. The most widely held hypothesis is that MS occurs in patients with a genetic susceptibility and is triggered by environmental factors. MS is three times more common in women ... with diagnoses usually made as young adults; however, it is estimated that 2%- 5% of cases begin before age 16. Since MS is not widely recognized as a childhood disorder, diagnosis is often missed or delayed. [Also,] many symptoms are similar to those of other pediatric neurological conditions, leukodystrophies, and metabolic disorders. (CDC, 2011)

Another reason for us to discuss MS is that myelin plays a big role in facilitation. *The law of facilitation locks in a neural message via the laying down of myelin sheath.* Is MS in any way affected by - or does it affect - the law of facilitation? Or, perhaps, this could this be why CFS is hard to shake? Is it a vicious cycle perpetuated by stress or the repeated interpretation of events as stressful? Is it just limbic kindling or is there more to it?

Myelin insulates your nerves, including your neurons in your brain and spinal cord, i.e., your central nervous system (CNS.) Myelin is made up of fatty substances and protein, and conducts impulses between your brain and the rest of your body.

I understand this to mean that *myelin communicates the electrical-chemical signals inside your nerves* to your CNS as well as to your muscles, and essentially *tells them what to do.* According to Catherine Spader, RN (2013): "Healthy myelin is vital to the normal, rapid movement of electrical impulses through the nerve pathways." To me, this translates as *energy.*

In facilitation, it is the *repetition of patterns* that speeds up production of myelin (made by little cells called oligodendrocytes) around axons that helps to improve neural conductivity. Thus, facilitation, or repetition of patterns, can lead to mastery, such as playing instruments or participating in sports, but it can also make it harder to break habits.

"Myelin makes movement mastery, and repetition of a movement makes myelin" (Moy, 2011).

In people with MS, the myelin can become damaged and affect motor control. But can myelin also be recovered through the Law of Facilitation? Research points to that possibility. Mary and Dick Bunge produced "the first unequivocal evidence that spontaneous myelin repair occurred in the mammalian CNS" (Bunge, Bunge, & Ris,1961; Scolding, 2001).

Also, research points to the immune system attacking and destroying the myelin sheath in MS - although the cause of MS is inconclusive. Remyelination does occur in people with MS, but happens less so over time. Nonetheless, teams are trying to find ways to encourage remyelination in the body when auto-immunity is involved.

Photo credit: A 3D rendering of microscopic human nerve cells showing axon dendrites and myelin sheath. 3Dme Creative Studio / Shutterstoc, via the courtesy of Caroline Reid at iflscience.com

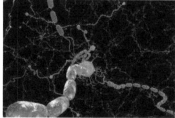

Remyelination occurs in MS lesions but becomes increasingly incomplete ... and eventually fails in the majority of ... patients. Efforts to understand the causes for failure ... have fueled research into the biology of remyelination and the complex, interdependent cellular and molecular factors that regulate the process. Examination of the mechanisms of repair of experimental lesions has [shown] that remyelination occurs in two major phases. Future challenges confronting therapeutic strategies to enhance remyelination will involve the translation of findings from basic science to clinical demyelinating disease. (Chan, 2007)

For most of the general population, when the myelin sheath is affected, say due to high cortisol levels, remyelination occurs on its own. The body can repair itself, although the new sheath may be thinner. **Does this thinner sheath affect the conduction of electrical impulses and therefore result in lower energy levels?** *Or is energy affected by inflamed white matter and/or neuronal loss leading to poor signal transmission* (Matute & Ransom, 2012)? Or is reduced energy due to an activated immune system and pro-inflammatory cytokines? What about other conditions that present chronic fatigue as a symptom? Does the propensity toward auto-immunity play a role?

My answer is *yes* - to one or more of these theories. Under stress, my body feels *shaky*, sensitive and raw. Is this due to demyelination and/or inflammation of white matter in my brain? Does inflamed white matter lead to a compromised blood-brain barrier? Your brain is powerful but sensitive. It's command central. If inflammation and reduced blood flow lead to a compromised center of control can you imagine what kind of implications this may have for your health and nervous system?

The question remains: *Is there a link between MS, CFS and neuronal loss or demyelination?* If they're classified as neurological conditions, and both bring crushing fatigue, is the fatigue from demyelination, white matter inflammation, or both? While the thickness of myelin is correlated with "conduction velocity of nerve fibres," it may be that *less* myelin is implicated in higher brain functions and may be dynamically involved in neuroplasticity (Costandi, 2014).

Research points to two types of fatigue: central and peripheral. Peripheral may be more due to neuromuscular fatigue, while central fatigue may be more due to metabolic and structural instability in the nervous system, precipitated by stress (Chaudhuri & Behan, 2004).

The HPA axis is affected by stress (including oxidative, inflammatory, and psychological) which results in dysregulation of the axis - either hyper or hypo activation of glucocorticoid (GC) receptors - also called *hypercortisolemia,* meaning there are *high cortisol levels* in the body.

The resulting condition can be either pathological or non-pathological. We will be discussing the effects of *too little cortisol*, and how this may be another biomarker of chronic fatigue (and, perhaps, a protective mechanism by the body so we slow down and heal). Cortisol targets so many areas in the body it's no wonder too much or too little can affect our health and well-being so greatly. It targets the liver, the immune system, the blood vessels, the kidneys, the muscles, our bones, and our brains. It also shares the same precursors as DHEA, which repairs cells, is made in times of low cortisol production, is the most common hormone in the body (Church, 2009).

And myelin? A great movie to watch is *Lorenzo's Oil*, to learn more about courage and perseverance from a true story about parents trying to help their son who had *adrenoleukodystrophy* or ALD.

"Myelin makes movement mastery, and repetition of a movement makes myelin" (Moy, 2011).

Is this phenomenon, pointed out by Moy, connected to brain plasticity? Is this why yoga helps? Also, does yoga affect the neuromuscular junction (where a nerve meets a muscle) in a positive way either in the reduction of and/or interpretation of fatigue?

Is the Law of Facilitation similar to the concept of neuroplasticity, and can we heal ourselves by rebuilding and strengthening our brains? Neuroplasticity is the ability of the brain to adapt and restructure. We will address neuroplasticity in further detail along our journey here.

Also, see *Focus on Your Neurotransmitter System* in this chapter for more information on the possible connections between MS and CFS.

Fatigue and Your Thyroid

Hypothyroidism/Sub-Clinical Hypothyroidism, Euthyroid Sick Syndrome (ESS)

Alternative practitioners talk about hypothyroidism and sub-clinical hypothyroidism and how they may be sources of chronic fatigue.

Hypothyroidism can make you feel very tired, cold, weak and nervous. It can cause your hair to fall out (mine did, for years – was it related?).
One sign of an underactive thyroid may be if you wake up well-rested but then rapidly develop fatigue after exertion such as exercise.

Hypothyroidism increases liver enzymes and can lower blood sugar. It may also increase allergies, promote digestive problems, cause you to swell up, and trigger sleep, pain, and weight fluctuation issues. Your cholesterol levels may be elevated as well.

Every cell in your body uses and needs thyroid hormones. So, if hypothyroidism is left unresolved, low thyroid levels can possibly lead to diabetes, high blood pressure, depression, arthritis, migraines, etc. to name a few conditions. Note the interconnectedness of all processes.

Actually, almost every cell in your body has its own circadian clock, too. See Chapter Five and *Riding the Wave of Health/Well-being* for more details on how keeping your body in balance affects your whole body.

It's no wonder people with chronic fatigue and even pain syndromes may feel they have hypothyroidism as well, or may be diagnosed with it. It could be that chronic fatigue is indeed from sub-clinical hypothyroidism or hypothyroidism. To find out, you would need to get your thyroid hormone levels checked.

Most conventional doctors treat hypothyroidism with synthetic thyroid hormones which you may take for life. There *have* been cases of spontaneous recovery in 5% of patients with chronic auto-immune thyroiditis. It seems conceivable, then, that some people recover without replacement therapy. This is something to keep in mind.

Sub-clinical hypothyroidism may be an early stage of hypothyroidism. It presents when tests come back within normal range (how many times has that happened before?) but the patient still has symptoms of possible hypothyroidism.

Sub-clinical hypothyroidism may stem from thyroid auto-immunity, radiation treatment of the neck, a pituitary or hypothalamic disorder, or ill-treated hypothyroidism among other causes.

LDL cholesterol levels may be elevated and there is a good chance sub-clinical hypothyroidism can progress to hypothyroidism. Yet, there is not a consensus to treat sub-clinical hypothyroidism with levothyroxine, a synthetic thyroid hormone (Wilson & Curry, 2005).

However, there's *an additional possibility that requires examination here.* That possibility is known as *Euthyroid Sick Syndrome (ESS.)* Many seriously ill people develop low thyroid levels (suppressed thyroid hormone/abnormal thyroid tests) and yet don't have sub-clinical hypothyroidism or hypothyroidism. Instead, they may have ESS - where levels of thyroid hormones are low yet patients do not require synthetic medication for life. Some practitioners are not sure whether it is a good idea to use synthetic hormones for ESS at all.

Research is needed to determine if ESS is due to an *adaptive response* that conserves energy, meaning ESS *may stem from another primary illness,* but one the patient may be able to readapt and recover from. Or is ESS due to a *maladaptive response* which could cause thyroid tissue damage? If an *adaptive response* is in progress, it may be a way to protect the body from oxidative stress and pro-inflammatory cytokines or other kinds of inflammatory conditions that could influence the HPA axis. Research at the Department of Biochemistry, Jawaharlal Institute of Postgraduate Medical Education and Research in India produced valuable results about oxidative stress and ESS (Selvaraj, Bobby, & Sridhar, 2008). Sections on oxidative stress, the HPA axis, inflammation, inflammatory conditions, and cytokines are coming up in this chapter.

Some of the illnesses and situations that may be connected with ESS include sepsis, having had surgery (heart or other kinds as well), having gone through serious trauma including a heart attack or a serious accident (car, ski, etc.), lupus, psychiatric depression, fasting, starvation, or certain kinds of malnutrition (lack of protein), cirrhosis, diabetic complications, anorexia nervosa, and acute and chronic illnesses, including which I would propose CFS, FM, etc.

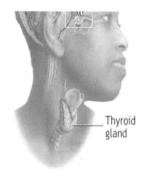

Thyroid
gland

seeker7.hubpages.com

Our thyroid gland absorbs iodine from what we eat and converts it to thyroid hormones which we call T3 and T4. Those seriously ill with other conditions caused by major trauma, for instance, may develop low thyroid hormones, including decreased T3 and T4 levels. However, they may show increased rT3 (reverse T3) and serum cortisol levels. Whereas, cortisol levels may be low in hypothyroidism.

Keep in mind the *Thyroid Stimulating Hormone (TSH)* produced by a small but significant organ called the pituitary gland. The pituitary is part of the HPA axis (discussed later in this chapter,) theorized to be a major player in CFS. To remind you, the pituitary, below our brain and behind our sinuses, helps keep T4 and T3 steady in our blood stream and controls the amount of energy we use.

One major distinction between people with ESS and those with true hypothyroidism is that *those with ESS have low, normal, or only minor elevated levels of TSH,* whereas those with true hypothyroidism have significant elevations of TSH.

And then there is Reverse T3 (rT3) which does the opposite of T3: it blocks your thyroid receptor. In situations such as chronic illnesses, infections, severe stress or trauma, etc, rT3 may be increased. The symptoms of rT3 include brain fog, difficulty losing weight, muscle aches, fatigue - basically the same symptoms as hypothyroidism, and many similarities with CFS, etc. Brain fog, muscle aches, and fatigue alone should ring the bell for those of us who have gone through it.

Basically what can happen in ESS is that people do not convert T4 to T3 very well. T3 is the active form of the thyroid hormone. In addition, T4 may be converted to rT3, resulting in high rT3 serum levels. Very few labs can accurately measure rT3. Plus patients with ESS may have elevated cortisol. Excess cortisol may interfere with thyroid hormones, possibly activated by pro-inflammatory cytokines, our chemical messengers.

This discussion might be giving you brain fog. Remember, ESS patients usually have low to normal TSH. That seems to be the main factor between *hypothyroidism* - which is elevated TSH levels and possibly requiring medication for life - and *ESS* which might allow your body to find its way back to normalcy, or at least a new normal.

Yes, it's complicated. You could ask yourself if your situation involves the conditions of ESS plus CFS and/or FM? Or might you have hypothyroidism or sub-clinical hypothyroidism and need medication? There are no easy answers. The only sensible solution is to become a health detective. Get tested, work with a knowledgable and open-minded health care practitioner and, most of all, *trust your gut, literally.*

Each individual is a unique case. For me, my LDL cholesterol was high and my cortisol was high, but then it dropped as I developed chronic inflammation - discussed later in this chapter. My TSH was low but within normal range and my T3 low, yet my reverse T3 was low. I also had yellowing of the skin and hair loss.

The facts that my TSH levels were within acceptable range and my reverse and total T3 levels were low, all suggest CFS/ESS. I could not tolerate glandular supplements which are often suggested for sub-clinical hypothyroidism. Yet I did well with homeopathic glandulars, but only the kind with real adrenal and thyroid.

Another major fact is that medication may not be required for people with ESS. This is good news. But first, hypothyroidism must be ruled out. If it seems you may have ESS, as we said, it means your underactive thyroid may be a secondary illness, due to a prolonged primary illness. It means there is great hope you can recover.

I call the thyroid my *second battery*. Some people call it the *check engine light, the idling speed of your engine, or the furnace of your body*, as it controls the metabolism of every cell. Metabolism is the basis of life. It's a set of chemical reactions that happen in each cell, converting oxygen and calories into, you guessed it, energy.

So if you're low on energy you may not be getting enough oxygen into your cells. Is this due to an underactive thyroid, or mitochondrial dysfunction, or both? We'll discuss the latter one later in this chapter. Either way, if your *check engine light* is flashing, find out if you have an underactive thyroid. Although I'm not a fan of medication, it may be necessary. You certainly don't want to go into a coma.

One possible cause of an underactive thyroid may be *hypothalamic dysfunction*. Your hypothalamus helps to control the pituitary, which in turn controls your thyroid (and adrenals). Thus, the hypothalamus has a close, strategic relationship with the thyroid.

There is no doubt in my mind that if the hypothalamus is up or down-regulated, it may affect thyroid function. See *hypocortisolism* toward the end of this chapter for discussion of *hypothalamic dysregulation*. Read the section in this chapter on *auto-immunity* for information on an activated hypothalamus, meaning whether or not it's up or down-regulated.

For all of us, nutrition may play a role in thyroid health, along with stress management, and strengthening the immune system, to control cortisol levels, inflammation, etc.

Kelp, selenium, manganese, and L-Tyrosine (thyroid cells combine iodine and the amino acid tyrosine to make T3 and T4) along with other nutrients and foods may all influence thyroid hormone levels.

Eggs* can be great for the adrenals, which in turn balances the thyroid (*they also contain lecithin – like soy, mustard, and sunflowers - which supply phosphatidyl choline, vital for healthy mitochondrial cells. Phosphatidyl choline may be used as part of lipid therapy to improve cell health and energy levels). T3 tells your body to use more oxygen. Low oxygen consumption may be yet another symptom of an under-active thyroid.

For your immune system, Vitamin D (from sunlight or D3 sources), exercise, and stress management are crucial. Natural *immune-modulators* include chamomile and plant sterols, such as the compounds found in olive oil. Immuno-modulators help your immune system up or down regulate. Natural *anti-inflammatories* include flax, fish oil, turmeric, olive oil, and ginger. Real Vitamin C from plant sources may help as well.

Even more than nutrition, exercise has the capacity to protect and even enhance the immune response by boosting antibody and natural killer responses (T cells). See Chapter Four for more about the power of movement and exercise, and this chapter for more on immunity.

Find out what works for you and consult your healthcare practitioner.

Iron-Deficient Anemia and Intrinsic B12 Factor

Many people who have hypothyroidsim are also anemic, although science is not clear whether this is due to low B12, low iron, or low folate levels. Iron is a crucial nutrient for your health. Iron facilitates production of crucial enzymes, strengthens your immune system, and helps with synthesis of DNA and synthesis of the neurotransmitters serotonin, dopamine, and norepinephrine in your brain. Also, we need B12 for nerve function, formation of red blood cells, and the creation of material like DNA, as well as proteins and hormones. We have trouble using the B12 we take in from the foods we eat. The reason we have trouble is related to a glycoprotein called *intrinsic factor.*

"Intrinsic factor is a glycoprotein released by parietal cells that line the internal surface of your stomach. Without intrinsic factor, your body can only absorb about 1 percent of the B-12 you ingest. With the help of intrinsic factor, this amount increases to 56% of a 1 microgram dosage of B-12" (Grey, 2011.)

To reiterate, lack of intrinsic factor can inhibit absorption of vitamin B12 which may affect the absorption of iron. When your doctor orders your labs, ask to have intrinsic factor absorption checked.

Richard Crookes, designer of my bookcover, may have had chronic fatigue due to lack of intrinsic factor. He now gets B-12 shots and is fine. Here is Richard's story in his own words:

I was walking with a stick and I was only about 35. I had been living in France for a few years and had just got back to the UK. Not sure whether I picked up a virus over there or maybe a liver problem from once drinking river water - anyway after lots of tests the doctors found the B12 was low. I wondered if it was because I'd been vegetarian* for nearly 20 years but they said no - it was nothing to do with that, which was a relief. (*Note: Richard is no longer vegetarian.)

I had to wait for it to get to a really low level before they put me on injections, but once they did I picked up within weeks. I have them every 3 months now for the rest of my life which is no hardship. A couple of years later I was walking the mountains and climbed almost 50 of the highest in England in a year with a friend. I'm 50 now and feel great - thankfully. Determinaton and positive thought are the way. ~ Richard Crookes, cover designer for The Memory of Health

Low Iron Saturation

There is new information on how important iron is for energy. Your body needs iron to help transport oxygen and to generate energy. As you will find out later in this chapter, having enough oxygen can be a big part of feeling energetic. For example, if your muscles are low in oxygen, you can feel tired.

Again, we know that anemia is caused by a deficiency in certain nutrients that make red blood cells like iron, B12, and folic acid. When you are tested for anemia, ask to have your *serum ferritin* levels checked. You are getting checked to see if your body is binding and transporting iron correctly. According to Dr. Oz, doctors may not know to check serum ferritin levels. If your transferrin saturation (TSAT) levels are low, as mine were, that is considered anemia/iron deficiency. This is also known as *low iron saturation*.

Symptoms include headaches, severe chronic fatigue, hair loss, and muscle fatigue. Remember, the red blood cells in iron carry oxygen to the muscles. If you have low TSAT levels, i.e., ferritin and transferrin saturation that predict your body's iron stores and serum iron levels, you may also experience pale skin, abdominal pain, sore tongue, low blood pressure, dizziness, headaches, irritabililty, weakness, light headedness, etc.

I still recall being at Herb Pharm for training, and one of the trainers told me I looked pale. She wondered if I could be anemic. I have been asked this throughout the years. I was tested, and my iron and transferrin sat levels were indeed low. My red blood cell (RBC) and white blood cell (WBC) counts were low as well, the different times I was tested. I have pale skin in general, but my tests proved that it was more than low melanin. Your RBCs are the vehicles that carry oxygen to your cells.

It generally takes 90 days to grow new red blood cells, but iron is easy to supplement and replace, thankfully, if this happens to be the cause. I like either Solgar Gentle Iron or Floradix. However, you may want to check with your doctor for supplementation guidelines, especially if you have an inflammatory condition. Iron supplementation alone may not work for everyone - the iron may not be turned into new RBCs - and it is recommended to be supervised by a healthcare practitioner.

As mentioned, many who have hypothyroidism are also anemic, which may be due to low intestinal motility and therefore poor absorption. Your body may also not be able to absorb iron very well due to Celiac disease or Crohn's disease, or because you are lacking in intrinsic factor. Prescription medications may also interfere with absorption.

Origins in the Digestive Tract

Are you aware you have a complex and intelligent brain in your gut which contains over 500 million neurons and is the equivalent size and complexity of something like a cat's brain? ~ Unknown Source

Yes, I *am* aware. And I believe it's very possible the breakdown of my health and subsequent onset of chronic fatigue stemmed from the large amounts ibuprofen I was taking which began to compromise my GI tract and perhaps even – or most very likely - my gut microbiome.

Don't get me wrong, I love ibuprofen. I'm glad it was invented. There are days when I need it. It's one of the best things I've found for cramps, although valerian is good, too. I recently figured out that valerian is effective because of the natural *gamma amniobutyric acid (GABA)* in it which calms down the HPA axis, which, in turn, modulates hormones. Actually eating well is the preventative for cramps, as well as the avoidance of refined sugar. ☺

Ibuprofen is thought to reduce inflammation in the body by inhibiting prostaglandin synthesis. Prostaglandins are created by inflammatory responses in your body. Of course, the better you eat with none to low amounts of simple sugars and a diet high in omega 3's and EPA, the less need to inhibit prostaglandin synthesis in the first place. In fact, *oleocanthol*, a substance in olive oil, works in the same fashion as ibuprofen to inhibit the inflammatory enzymes COX-1 and COX-2.

Again, you ask, why am I talking about ibuprofen? Because, as I said, I suspect my trouble with chronic fatigue originated during the time I was taking it. It often occurred to me that my difficulties may have started in my gut, after having surgery, and taking the prescription pain killers and/or having taken eight months-worth of anti-inflammatories (also known as non-steroidal anti-inflammatory drugs or NSAIDs.) Did I upset the balance of my digestive tract, which communicates, in turn, with my nervous, immune, and neuro-endocrine systems?

I was taking an unnatural amount of ibuprofen, considering my sensitivity to it, every day for eight months. I'm not even sure how well it helped my swelling. I gained 20 pounds. My skin turned yellow and I wondered if it could be due to myxedema or jaundice.

Ibuprofen stopped working to reduce inflammation in my knee, so doctors switched me to Naprosyn, now sold over the counter as Aleve. I did even worse with Naprosyn. After a week or two, I fell into deep depression. I remember lying in bed when I was supposed to be at school. I felt like I was falling into a dark, bottomless hole. If that was hell, I was surely in it, or on my way. The next day, I went to school to turn in a paper, but could not stay for class. After that experience, I took myself off Naprosyn. I never wanted to have that feeling of powerless despair again. That was when my life and the condition of my knee changed. I took action (self-directed and purposeful) to get my life and health back on course.

For years I thought my chronic fatigue came from trauma to my central nervous system (CNS) as a result of surgery and/or the subsequent eight-month rehab process, including pain-killers. In fact, it may be due to inflammation of the nervous system - coming up.

I still believe the stress of surgery and rehab, including subsequent oxidative stress - coming up - contributed greatly. Research has proven that early stress and/or trauma can change your stress response or set point. Cumulative effects of stress may trigger illness in vulnerable individuals (Broderick & Blewitt, p.471, 2010).

But I believe my taking something for so long that I was sensitive to, i.e., *ibuprofen*, may have started the *chain reaction*. Next, *leaky gut*, also called *intestinal permeability*, triggered further stages in the chain reaction, and caused my immune system to react to what would normally be non-threatening food particles, toxins, etc. As a result, I believe this is where my food sensitivities (or possible delayed onset allergies) originated, as well as subsequent immune and inflammation issues. The end result of the chain reaction, for me, was chronic fatigue.

Why do I believe that the type of a chain reaction I have described was possible? I believe it because, after much trial and error to figure out how to get well, the thing that has consistently worked for me is *diet*, and *healing my digestive tract*. It's black and white: eat not so well and my symptoms flare up; eat well and I feel pretty good or even great. I also have learned that enjoyment of food is crucial to efficient digestion.

Another thing I've learned is that the whole body and its systems are *inter-connected* and mediated/influenced by feedback loops. So, if we take the chain reaction model a step further, it's possible that my compromised immune/digestive system may have *affected* other systems and organs in my body, perhaps tripping their genetic predisposition to weaken, or even exacerbating how they become reactive of stress, etc.

In my case, the systems affected seem to have been my (1) central nervous system (CNS) including my HPA axis, vagus nerve, etc., (2) my thyroid, resulting in sub-clinical hypothyroidism, and ultimately (3) the mitochondria in my muscles. *All three systems are important sources of energy in the body* and all three, in *my* body, felt the effects of an injured digestive tract and/or a compromised immune system.

The gut is important for so many reasons: its how and where you absorb nutrients (hello iron and B Vitamins.) It is closely connected with your immune system, about 70% of which is in your gut - coming up in this chapter. It is intimately tied in with your brain, and is called your *second brain*. In fact, about 90% of your *serotonin* is produced - you guessed it - in your gut. *Feeling happy* takes on a whole new meaning, and may explain our obsession with refined carbohydrates too, even beyond the temporary rush they produce in the primary brain.

To review, *leaky gut* is named as such due to the increased permeability of the intestinal mucosa - or lining of your intestines - to food, toxins, macromolecules, and anitgens. In other words, the lining of your gut is supposed to keep out and differentiate the bad guys from the good guys.

What causes *leaky gut*, as it were, in the first place? There are many suspects, and several are listed here: NSAIDs are high on the list. In fact, they can cause the intestinal lining to bleed (Wolfe, Lichtenstein, & Gurkirpal, 2006) and can "disrupt intestinal integrity" (Bjarnason, Zanelli, Prouse, Williams, Gumpel, & Levi, 1986). Thus, it is possible that a person whose intestinal lining bleeds or is impaired may set off a chain reaction that puts that person in jeopardy of developing CFS or other chronic conditions?

NSAIDs may lead to a decrease in nutrient absorption - say from iron, for instance - and may contribute to *leaky gut*. Also, poor nutrient absorption *may retard energy* (ATP) production through the inhibition of glycolysis and oxidative phosphorylation. More on this topic shortly.

Other suspects causing *leaky gut* may include stress (go figure - it depletes nutrients in general, a big problem), allergies, celiac disease (one in every 133 people have it), gluten intolerance, alcohol (no surprise), poor diet (hello refined sugar, the original "anti-nutrient"), candida (yes, it's real), and gut dysbiosis.

Does intestinal permeability lead to auto-immunity? What other roles may it play? Some say that *leaky gut* may be responsible or contribute to auto-immunity, arthritis (some say RA too), CFS, food allergies, celiac disease, Crohn's, acne, eczema, psoriasis, malnutrition, anemia, etc.

NSAIDs can cause damage and inflammation to the small intestine in what is known as NSAID enteropathy. They can cause blood and protein loss, and even ulcers. On a positive note, as I have mentioned, NSAIDs also decrease prostaglandin synthesis which can be a very good thing, as anyone who has had cramps will tell you. But let's emphasize that NSAIDs *may* cause damage. I would say they *do cause inflammation* because I have experienced it after consuming some kind of nightshade. But I am wary of words such as *damage*. Words are powerful suggestions to our subconscious minds. Are we sick? Perhaps in the moment. Are we damaged? I certainly hope not.

Some say that L-Glutamine can help repair the walls of the intestine due to leaky gut. I am not sure I had much luck with this. But my body responded well to extra strength probiotics, eating whole foods, and avoiding foods that irritated my stomach and intestinal walls.

But I now know I am sensitive to nightshades. Ibuprofen and all NSAIDs are part of the nightshade family, believe it or not, and after long, intense exposure to NSAIDs, I found myself extra sensitive to foods I previously tolerated pretty well that are a part of that family such as potatoes. Now I only eat them without the skins such as mashed potatoes, and once in a blue moon, potato chips.

Other nightshades I've always been super sensitive to, or even repelled by include eggplants, peppers, and even the adaptogen ashwaganda and the popular gogi berries. I've always hated the smell of tomatoes which can make me almost puke. However, I pretty well with tomato sauce (cooked) and tomato soup. Well-being is about enjoying your food and life as well!

There is an on-going dance and balance between your immune system and inflammation levels (produced by your immune system, again 70% of which is in your gut.) Your body tries to mitigate chronic/excessive inflammation, but in return your immune response goes down. How does your immune system and/or gut achieve or maintain balance? How can you stack the scale* in your favor to heal in general? *The scale effect or the tipping poing of well-being may be trying multiple approaches at once until the scale is tipped in your favor. Try something, then keep it on the scale and add more techniques until you heal. Thanks to Niki Gratrix for this idea: nikigratrix.com

Science still understands very little about how the immune system operates. However, here is more information on your immune system and the role chronic inflammation plays in the progression of chronic illness. I am grateful to Linda Schmidl (personal communication, September 3, 2012) Administrative Assistant, from the Max Planck Institute of Immunobiology and Epigenetics in Freiburg, Germany for allowing me to use the following quote:

The intestine is the largest barrier surface of the body with the outside world. As such, it needs to be able to mount quick, efficient immune responses against possible pathogens. However, most of the intestinal antigens come from the food and the commensal flora, which need to be tolerated. Hence, the intestinal immune system combines a high number of inflammatory cells with a strong population of immune regulators that prevent detrimental reactions against harmless antigens. How the balance between inflammation and tolerance is achieved is still not well understood.

The complex intestinal flora is separated from the immune system by a single layer of epithelial cells. In the thymus, epithelial cells play a crucial role in T cell development through antigen presentation and provision of survival, apoptosis and differentiation signals. Intestinal epithelial cells can also produce signals that modulate lymphoid activity, however, the role of the epithelium in intestinal immune responses is not completely understood at the moment.

We are trying to identify in which way communication between epithelial cells and the immune system shapes inflammation and tolerance in the gut.

Thymic epithelial cells play a crucial role in T cell development through antigen presentation and provision of survival, apoptosis and differentiation signals. Intestinal epithelial cells can also produce signals that modulate lymphoid activity, for example IL-7 and TSLP. **On the other hand, the immune system produces cytokines that have an impact on epithelial cells. The outcome of immune responses depends on this crosstalk.** *We want to identify how intestinal epithelial cells interact with the immune system to establish and abrogate tolerance. By analysing systemic and intestinal immune populations and their activity, our lab aims to understand how tolerance is tailored to the different needs of each environment.*

~Ana Izcue, Group Leader, MPI of Immunobiology and Epigenetics

Microbes, DNA, and Your Health

There is an area of research in medicine that is gaining increasing significance, and it just may be one of the major players in chronic conditions such as ME/CFS/SEID as well as many other disorders.

I have been talking about systems. Well, the *ecosystem* of your body is more than just you. It is much, much more. According to *Dr. Simon Park (2014) you are made up more of bacterial cells than human cells.* The ratio is indeed 10:1 of bacterial cells to human cells. Perhaps these are the true aliens amidst us.

Bacteria are single cell microbes. The role microbes play in our health and even the onset or remission of chronic illness may be a major factor to consider. Microbes are even part of our our DNA. That's right: part of our DNA is non-human, at 8 million genes. That is a heck of a lot of DNA that is non-human. Also fascinating, not to mention probably super relevant, is that the two DNA systems of human DNA and microbial DNA evolved *together.* 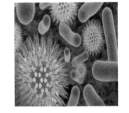 (Photo: Humans add millions of microbes to the air every hour. Photo credit: Forbes.com)

> There are 140 times more genes coming from microbes on and in our bodies than there are from our own cells. We have this relationship where they rely on us. We rely on them, a symbiotic relationship where life for both of us could not happen without one or the other. Perhaps we could gain a little bit more mutual respect. (Malterre, 2014)

Microbes help digest your food, fend off and help you recover from illness, help create vitamins, and may determine who responds well to a prescription drug and who doesn't.

In addition to the mysterious immune system, this brave new (well, kind of new to us) world of microbes is largely unknown. Is this why so much of our immune system is in our gut? Just like there is dark matter in space we are just beginning to explore and understand, there is the enigmatic world of bacteria that is still so new to us.

Already science is showing links between IBS and microbes, as well as acne and even enigmatic childhood fevers (Park, 2012).

It is possible that fending off conditions such as asthma, cancer and even obesity may be linked to microbes as well. How strong is the immune-based response that is informed by the world of friendly bacteria? What else will we find that is connected and affected by this world of bacteria? (See Highlights at end of book for more discussion.)

The great news is that good bacteria far outweigh bad bacteria (less than 1% are pathogenic.) But certain types of bacterial strains, when linked with milk fat, seem to promote inflammation. I personally love kefir, cheese, yogurt, etc. but is culturing the key to avoiding inflammation when it comes to dairy? We still have much to learn.

Also, if your digestive system, and therefore the ecosystem of your body, gets out of whack, can you imagine what ensues and unfolds? Disruption of the gut microbiome and chronic inflammation have already been linked to CFS/SEID (Lakhan & Kirchgessner, 2010).* The ecosystem of our body may be strong, but it is not inpenetrable.

Check out the movie *Origins* for more information on the microbiome and the importance of it in getting well and maintaining your well-being. http://origins.well.org/

Acidic Body and Candida

Candida is yeast (there are many strains) and is often downplayed, overlooked, or even scoffed at by medical professionals who practice modern medicine. But the thing is, candida does get out of control due to excessive antibiotic use, eating too many refined carbs or sugars, or because of a compromised immune system, as well as other reasons.

When the body is out of balance (*low HCI may allow candida to flourish, not to mention latent viruses*) it's more susceptible to candida, especially – *or because of - a chronic illness*. Again, keep in mind that if you eat an excessive amount of refined sugars or have on-going chronic stress, it may be that your candida levels will be higher than normal. If candida is out of control, it can become problematic. Look at your tongue. Is it coated in white? Candida - may be out of control in your body and it can cause a host of symptoms, including chronic fatigue. Excessive candida can *act as a stressor in the body*. Does candida affect and stress out the HPA axis as well? I can only surmise that is a possibility. Chronic stress does for sure, and it can affect fatigue and immunity.

*http://goo.gl/HILdMv

Normally, the Th1 mode of your immune system takes care of excessive yeast. If the Th2 mode of your immunity is activated (discussion coming up), your immune system may not properly rid the body of excessive yeast, possibly causing a multitude of problems.

Here's the thing: candida can cause or contribute to inflammatory conditions in the body. Overgrowth of candida can even lead to auto-immune and endocrine conditions if it is left unchecked for years on end. Sound familiar?

Symptoms of *systemic candida* include:

- severe fatigue
- white-coated tongue
- inability to concentrate
- mood swings
- blurred vision
- headaches (migraines too?)
- sensitivity to light
- digestive issues (related to IBS?)
- improper pH balance in digestive tract
- dark circles under eyes
- chronic runny nose
- chemical sensitivities (see **Chemical Injury** in this chapter)

Chronic fatigue and IBS obviously have other potential causes, but *systemic candida* is very important to address. The more I study and connect the dots, the more I think *systemic candida* plays a huge role, and develops when the body breaks down from illness, or perhaps it is part of the reason the body breaks down.

Systemic candida is often a first warning of other serious illnesses, such as diabetes and immune disorders, etc. It can also carry with it a host of symptoms, some of which seem to mimic CFS, such as chronic fatigue and brain fog – also, perhaps, caused by HPA axis dysregulation, etc.

We often crave the foods to which we are sensitive. In the case of candida, these cravings can cause serious imbalance in the system, and even be deadly in some cases. *Out of control candida is also a sign of an overly acidic system.* Candida thrives on acidic foods such as meats, dairy, refined sugar and grains. One of the most important things you can do is eat predominantly alkaline foods. *Here are some alkalilne foods.* Also, follow this link for great information on stress and well-being:
http://www.sarahbesthealth.com/why-stress-is-your-number-one-health-risk/

Alkaline Foods
most fruits, vegetables, greens (green super-foods and leafy greens) almonds, eggs, non-fat milk, buckwheat and millet, sprouted grains and beans (more alkaline, at least)

A fresh, alkaline diet may diminish candida. Certain supplements may work as well, like the *AquaFlora* line. This is homeopathic, and this along with functional medicine (personalized medicine) and may be the protocols of the 21st century. You can read more about homeopathy in Chapter Five's section titled, *Riding the Wave of Health/Well-Being.*

The best tactic I have found for an overgrowth of candida is apple cider vinegar. *I use Bragg's, and dilute a small amount in water. I add stevia to cut the taste. I also like Kevita's Lemon/Cayenne.* I use the approach of avoiding refined sugar as much as possible, eating raw, alkaline, and fresh foods and occasionally taking extra strength probiotics. I use Nature's Way Optima Max Bifido 90 Billion. I also love the Trader Joe's* brand for traveling. We are still learning how much protbiotics can help us, as our understanding of the microbiome is still in its infancy. I also suggest checking out *The Body Ecology Diet* by Donna Gates. She covers candida extensively in her book and reviews many options to rebuild and repopulate your body (Gates, 2011).

We're heading into the section about the mysterious immune system. A compromised immune system may lead to an overgrowth of candida. There are potentially many factors that affect the immune system. For example, did I develop food sensitivities due to a compromised immune system damaged by oxidative stress? Or how about the eight months I took six ibuprofen tablets a day for my knee rehab? What was going on? Perhaps we need to look at the immune system more closely for deepening clues.

The Mysterious Immune System

Our immune system is the system that not only keeps us well, but helps us communicate with the outside world (yes, really!). Yet immunologists are the first to admit that only abut 1-2% of the immune system is currently understood. As a matter of fact, they even have a new name for the immune system: *the microbial interaction system.*

*There are three different types of probiotics they offer, and you don't have to refrigerate them.

We cannot talk about the immune system anymore without factoring
in the microbiome which is our personal inner ecosystem.
When our microbiome is out of whack, we are in trouble
because, according to Summer Bock in the documentary
Origins, "A lack of biodiversity in the gut that can lead to
obesity, diabetes, arthritis and inflammation "(Shojai, 2014).

‘

Also, check out Science magazine's issue on the microbiome and gut health: *The Gut:
Inside Out, The Inner Tube of Life* (Simpson, Ash, Pennisi, & Travis, 2005).

There are many complexities involved, including different cell types
and thousands upon thousands of genes, which may or may not be
affected by lifestyle, age, etc. This phenomenon is also known as
epigenetics. In fact, 50-80% of your genetic potential is turned on or off
by what you eat, how you move, and what you think (Gottfried, 2014).

In other words, your immune system is - you may have sensed it - a
system that affects other systems in your body as well. See the section
in this chapter on *psychoneuroimmunology.* This is why medicine is now
using systems biology to study the immune system: touch the web, and
see what is affected, see what creates more vitality, or disturbs or
reduces health. I think this is what is beautiful about health and your
body: it doesn't just give you one option to be well. It gives you many
options and backups too. Your body wishes to be well. Not only that,
it desires to vibrate with wellbeing like a finely tuned instrument.

But, back to *epigenetics.* Epigenetics is potentially so crucial to health
that I am posting my musings on it both here and in Chapter Five.
Again, epigenetics means *above and beyond the cell.* In addition to your
genetic makeup, *mindset* is fundamental to well-being. Therefore, what
you *energetically* bring to the table, i.e. *your energetics,* may play a bigger or
as big a role as *your genetics* with respect to your health and well-being.

              Energetics vs. Genetics

When your belief systems intersect with your biology, the landscape of
your body can literally change. Results of research in the field of
epigenetics help to explain how this phenomenon can occur. In a
nutshell, the choices you make and your environment have the
potential to influence your genetic code. This is a major breakthrough.

Similarly, in the book *The Biology of Belief*, Bruce Lipton (2008) describes how our thoughts, whether positive or negative, have *the most influence* on gene expression. In other words, the *energetics* of our thoughts may influence our genetic potential more than our genetics.

Also, *daily practice* of the Relaxation Response (Benson, 1975) – around 20 minutes - *turns off* gene expression of cells that produce inflammation and improves mitochondrial function (Bhasin et al., 2013).

Why is this big news? First, it points to the powerful connection between the mind and the body. Secondly, it indicates that what we think and our behavior can affect immune function, just like the field of *psychoneuroimmunology* states. Please see *Story of Your Body* later in this chapter for further discussion of psychoneuroimmunology, and Chapters Four and Five for more on The Relaxation Response (RR). I also suspect that this is how placeboes work: they work because they give you peace of mind. Consequently, *peace of mind gives you peace of body*, and invokes The Relaxation Response. It's a domino effect.

Perhaps the laws of Nature really do work all the time, it's just that we're out of touch with them and the natural cycles of our bodies. Any way you look at it, the *power of the mind* is undeniable. This is critical, as we can harness the power of our mind to help with such issues as **chronic inflammation**, which is an enormous problem these days, and can lead to chronic conditions such as heart disease, MS, and possibley even CFS, etc. Remember, chronic inflammation is one of the main biomarkers of chronic disease.

Self-Regulation is Key

Meta-research on stress shows that chronic stress may influence white blood cells to downregulate cortisol receptors, which in turn "allows cytokine-mediated inflammatory processes to flourish" (Segerstrom & Miller, 2004). Acute stress (or rather, probably acute eustress, as acute stress can be implicated in CFS, PTSD, etc.) may enhance immunity (at least in vivo) but chronic stress may suppress it (Segerstrom & Miller, 2004).

Likewise, and this may be very relevant for people with M.E./CFS/SEID, "increased antibody production to [a] latent virus, particularly Epstein-Barr virus...is also consistent with suppression of cellular immunity" (Segerstrom & Miller, 2004). What does this mean in plain English? Remember when we talked about Th1- Th2 shift? This phenomenon is seen in people with CFS. Chronic stress may play a role in shifting the immune system to Th2 dominance, whereas it should ideally be balanced between Th1 and Th2. The body's ability to self-regulate stressors is key, and may influence optimal immune function.

How do we strengthen our immune systems and self-regulate? By using all of our tools which include some daily form of practice such as yoga or meditation, eating real food, cultivating healthy social connection, finding balance between up and down time, and cultivating The Relaxation Response. I believe the immune system is like a matrix. We can influence it both physically as well as mentally, emotionally, and even spiritually.

Between all of our choices in what we do, eat, and think, we have way more control than we realize. This is the study and field of epigenetics.

For every action in the universe there is an equal and opposite reaction. This can be a beautiful, comforting law but an extremely frustrating one as well. When you're sick it seems as if the law doesn't apply to you. There are ways the body breaks down that seem to go against the design of nature, as with cancer, CFS, and AIDS.

Then again, what is the design of Nature? She seems to be built on both order and chaos. Scientists talk about *entropy* and the nature of all things to tend toward disorder. Yet nature also is clearly organized and works on an *order of patterns*. See *Riding the Wave of Health*, Chapter Five.

But there are also ways the body recovers that seem to defy the laws of nature. Perhaps spontaneous healing owes it trick to the deck of cards it uses: quantum healing.

Just as there seem to be at least two decks of cards that explain the laws of Nature – the *theory of relativity* to explain how gravity and large objects behave, and *quantum mechanics* to explain how the sub-atomic universe behaves – perhaps there is more than one way to heal. Just as there are a million ways to be happy, there must be a million ways people can heal.

There is much to be discovered about the immune system and I believe people who deal with chronic and life-threatening illnesses are brave pioneers in the field of medicine. Regardless of what the future holds in healing or medicine, the point is to realize the power of your thoughts and your energetic nature. You have more power than you realize, and even much more than you currently use.

What does this potentially mean for you? I encourage you to make the best use of the energy that inhabits your body at any given point in time. I also encourage you to believe in the *potential* of your body and combine it with the powerful forces of your mind and spirit. When you become self-aware great things can and do happen.

Th1 to Th2 Shift

Scientists and practitioners are noticing that many people who have CFS, FM, AIDS, etc. have immune systems that have shifted from Th1 to Th2 activation. Let's break down what this means.

Th means *T helper*, and there are two classes of T cells: Th1 and Th2. Normally, your immune system swings back and forth from Th1 to Th2, depending on what your body needs.

Th1 goes after viruses, cancer, pathogens, and yeast (very important) that are *inside the cell*. This is called cell-mediated immunity. On the other hand, when your immune system is in Th2 mode, you are fighting invaders *outside of your cells*, like toxins, allergens, parasites, etc.

When your immune system has shifted to operating more from Th2 activation, you tend to over-respond to toxins and allergens, while under-responding to viruses, yeast, etc. **Your immune system can actually produce these symptoms: fever, pain, or fatigue that never seem to go away. These may be some of the clues that your immune system is not working as it should.**

So, your body can be out of balance in either direction. If your Th1 overexpresses, this situation is called *hyper-immunity*, and can lead to auto-immunity. If your Th2 overexpresses, this is condition is called *hypo-immunity*. This may lead to out of control infections, and also where candida may get out of control (sound familiar?). This also may be why CFS has been implicated in being connected to viruses, and not being able to shake them as it were.

With fibromyalgia, where a shift to Th2 has been noted, perhaps auto-immunity is not what's happening. At the same time, fibromyalgia has been already suggested as possibly being an auto-immune condition, and it is part of the rheumatic family (just like rheumatoid arthritis).

Here's a further complication. *Both Th1 and Th2 can be implicated in* **auto-immune conditions.** There are at least two examples. First, there is evidence that Type I diabetes, which is cell-mediated, may elicit a Th1 type immune response.

Conversely, Lupus, which is anti-body mediated, may call forth a Th2 type immune response. In either system, what may be crucial is the ***balance of cytokines***. Cytokines are chemical messengers secreted by immune cells as proteins which act on other cells to mediate immune responses. Also, other immune factors such as *Th1/Th2 CD4 T cells* play a role in the balancing act.

Th1 cells activate pro-inflammatory cytokines, and Th1 is associated with *acute inflammation*. Conversely, Th2 cells activate anti-inflammatory cytokines. What does this all mean for CFS sufferers? Previously, we said people with CFS may have shifted to Th2 activation. Is chronic inflammation in people with CFS, at least in part, due to **low cortisol levels**, as opposed to inflammation stimulated by autoimmunity, as that may indicate Th1 dominance? It's confusing, for sure. That is the mystery of the immune system.

Also worthy of note is the fact that allergic diseases may shift to Th2 dominance. Vaccines also stimulate your Th2 immune system. Is it possible that too many vaccines could send one's immune system into overactivation either direction? (*I am not saying don't use vaccines.)

Also *people who cannot sleep* due to the prevalence of pro-inflammatory cytokines, seem also to not make the **usual shift to Th1 at night, *which greatly enhances immune function.***

On a positive note, it has been suggested that *probiotics* can help the immune system normalize its swing between Th1 and Th2.

There is so much we do not understand yet. The immune system may be influenced by many factors, including physical, mental, emotional, spiritual, and environmental.

The bottom line is: **get your vitals tested (including thyroid, etc.**). Try a practitioner trained in functional medicine, so they can test for small ranges of abnormalities - even small abnormalities can create big symptoms - and customize (personalize) and tailor your treatment to you. This can make all the difference.

We've been talking about inflammation. But what exactly is it, and why does it matter?

Inflammation

What is inflammation, and what role does it play in such diseases as CFS, FM, and others? These conditions, we have said, have many alternative names, but in the field of health psychology, they are now called *chronic inflammatory diseases*. So it may be that what has been labeled as *CFS is really a chronic or neruo-inflammatory disorder*.

More about this topic in a bit, but first, what is inflammation, and specifically what is *chronic or systemic inflammation*? What role does it play in chronic conditions? And what role may it play in auto-immunity and delayed onset allergies?* (*coming up later in this chapter)

Inflammation protects us from toxins, trauma, bacteria, and so on. Histamine and prostaglandins are released and the body swells to further protect us. I have dealt with excess swelling for years, so it's hard to think of it as a protective mechanism. But I believe in my body's infinite wisdom as well.

Your body is designed to keep excess inflammation in check, yet the process can dampen your immune response. Even just a short amount of *stress* can affect natural killer (NK) cell activity. What happens to the NK cells is they shut down their vigilant watch against invaders. Of all the types of cells in our immune system, NK cells are the most sensitive to stress. (Image: ninds.nih.gov)

Excessive or blunted amounts of cortisol can also affect your immune response. If your cortisol levels become really low, you may develop chronic inflammation, chronic fatigue, hypothyroidism, etc.

Inflammation was designed to protect us. But, what happens when inflammation runs unchecked? *This may contribute to fatigue.* Also, what about when inflammation turns against the body, as it does in auto-immunity, which is considered an inappropriate *inflammatory response?*

It could also be that CFS is the result of an inflamed nervous system, although I personally believe it also involves reduced vagal tone, and perhaps even insufficient ATP production or energy recycling.

But, nonetheless, chronic inflammation is implicated in nearly all chronic conditions, and may indeed be the underlying factor or cause. Personally, I've often felt that inflammation - whether cause or effect - plays a role in CFS. I reached the point where I could feel when my brain and/or body were inflamed. My symptoms invariably flared up at the same time, including fatigue, loss of motor control, etc. Does inflammation caulse chronic fatigue, and if so, how?

I have noticed inflammation in my body due to eating refined sugar or exposure to chemicals (excess sugar or stress raises insulin levels, which can cause inflammation). For example, its summer as I'm writing and I love this time of year, but excess air conditioning bothers me. My inflammation levels go up, and I feel *out of sorts*. Does inflammation contribute to dysregulation of the HPA axis?

Inflammation promotes free radical production, yet isn't the reverse true as well? Doesn't free radical production, caused by on-going stress that turns into oxidative stress, promote inflammation? I believe the answer is *yes*. It goes both ways and establishes a vicious cycle.

Keep in mind signs of inflammation: *body heat, redness, pain, swelling, the release of histamine*. What do these symptoms tell us about CFS? I can say what they meant for me: I had bloodshot eyes (*redness*). I had systemic inflammation - *interpret this as swelling in my face and body, for instance* - for a number of years and still struggle with it to a degree. I thought it was due to low cortisol levels, but when I was tested at one point, my cortisol levels were high. I wasn't healing properly either - for example scarring from shaving my legs. However, my cortisol levels dropped after having laser surgery. This is when my experience with chronic inflammation started to develop.

Surgery is clearly stressful to my body, for whatever reason (due to the production of pro-inflammatory cytokines?) Most of my inflammation was due to low cortisol levels. I also think **part of my low grade inflammation was due to an *over-active* immune system/brain's immune system**. I tested negative for C-Reactive Protein, and certain auto-immune conditions, but my Vitamin D levels were super low and my *histamine levels* were high. My cortisol levels did rise over time, and, although my inflammation got better, it remained at a low flame like a smoldering fire I couldn't put out.

But, here's something significant that works just about every time with my inflammation: sunlight. Now I know why I always felt better when I traveled. I was getting more sunlight. After nine days in California with my mom – or when I lived in San Jose for work - my fatigue levels dropped. I wasn't doing anything differently, besides getting more sunlight which allowed my body to produce more Vitamin D and all of the other body processes Vitamin D regulates like serotonin production, etc. (Rutberg, 2015).

Back in the Pacific Northwest, my body couldn't get well. Yes, the region is notorious for low sunlight – many people look pale up here. Fall and winter can have an UV index of 0; a UV index of 3 or higher is recommended to raise Vitamin D levels.

As I mentioned in the introduction, Vitamin D regulates "about 1,000 different types of genes in the body, about 5 percent of the entire human genome" (Rutberg, 2015). Vitamin D may also greatly enhance serotonin production, which may have far-reaching implications for people with autism (Medical Xpress, 2014).

According to Mark R. Haussler, "[Vitamin D enhances] the ability of the brain cells to produce serotonin by anywhere from double to 30 times as much" (as cited in Rutberg, 2015). What does this mean for you? While I believe sunlight is the best source of Vitamin D for synthesis, Vitamin D3 supplementation is recommended by practitioners to combat inflammation, enhance the immune system, and now, perhaps, to enhance serotonin production. Ask questions, do your research, and see what works for you.

Chronic Inflammatory Disorders and Chronic Systemic Inflammation

Systemic inflammation is linked to many auto-immune conditions such as lupus, rheumatoid arthritis, and even fibromyalgia. However, not all chronic inflammation is linked to auto-immunity. Some instances where it is not linked include cancer and heart disease. It is linked with most degenerative diseases, however. What causes systemic inflammation?

Remember The Zone Diet? The premise is that proper nutritional ratios can control hormonal response and damaging inflammation in the body. The Zone Diet balances proteins, fats, and carbs, and is a proponent of balancing the proper ratio of Omega 6 to Omega 3's, which tame prostaglandins that lead to an over active immune system.

Some of the culprits in chronic inflammation are what are known as **pro-inflammatory cytokines and eicosanoids**. Let's take a closer look. "Cytokines are signaling proteins that help cells communicate with one another" (UC Davis, 2014). Cytokines are short chains of amino acids and are **messengers** which signal there is inflammation in your body. They are referred to as *communication molecules*. They are secreted by the immune system and can be pro or anti-inflammatory.

Cytokines can be created by stress, i.e., anything your body interprets as stress, by injury, and by illness. Cytokines may also play a role in brain cell death.

Eicosanoids (signaling molecules that affect inflammation and immunity) are hormonal messengers that communicate between the brain and the immune system. *Emotions, stress, and diet can all influence inflammation levels, as well as whether or not inflammatory genes express themselves or not.*

You'd be amazed at what is considered *stress* to your body. One that surprised me was when I had laser surgery for my veins. That stressed my body and increased my inflammation - even started it. *I had never noticed chronic inflammation before those surgeries.*

Cytokines are also involved in modulating neurotransmitters, as a well as influencing the hypothalamic-pituitary-adrenal (HPA) axis. I'll be talking more about the HPA axis as this chapter progresses. I believe these are significant points.

How much of a role do cytokines play in the way the HPA axis can up or down regulate and stay stuck, as it were, in the on or off position? In other words, how much *does chronic inflammation influence the endocrine and central nervous systems? And do diet and a healthy environment (i.e. the ecosystem of your digestive tract) keep inflammation, and therefore cytokines, in check?*

Important note: Since so much of our immune system is mysterious and is again a *system*, perhaps we need to look a bit deeper into the roles our emotions, thoughts, and even our spirits play in whether we secrete pro or anti- inflammatory cytokines.

Psychoneuroimmunology will be discussed in this chapter, addressing part of this mystery. Also, I delve into the role spirit may play in influencing the immune system in Chapter Five.

Is getting chronic inflammation under control the way to reverse how the HPA axis seems to stay stuck in either *up-regulation* (overly activated) as it does with depression and possibly fibromyalgia (FM) or *down-regulation* (inhibited) as it seems to do with CFS?

Or is it by **regulating and strengthening the vagus nerve** through yoga, and other forms of restorative exercise? Or are these both important and even interconnected? In my experience, they are both work to control inflammation. Also, diet creates a healthy inner ecosystem. Moreover, it's essential to stay in the relaxation response which is, indeed, the relaxed, infinite, indefinite, and dynamic present moment.

Pro-inflammatory cytokines are implicated in systemic inflammation and chronic inflammatory disorders. *In fact, they seem to be one of the main bio-markers of these conditions.* They can affect depression, allergies, sleep, (more on all three of these coming up) immune function (positively or negatively,) and they are implicated in numerous other conditions such as heart disease and chronic pain.

Eicosanoids are produced from essential fatty acids (EFAs) and are less inflammatory when made from Omega 3 fatty acids. When they are out of balance, say from too much Omega 6 consumption, they can affect heart health, cholesterol, high blood pressure, arthritis, and inflammation levels. *They can also cross the blood-brain barrier to stimulate the production of pro-inflammatory cytokines in your brain. High levels are implicated in depression.* The ideal ratio is 2:1 of Omega 6 to Omega 3 EFAs.

Let's talk about Omega 3 EFA's. There are many kinds of Omega 3 EFAs derived from food and from supplements. Two of those types of Omega 3 EFAs are *eicosapentaenoic acid* (EPA) and *docosahexaenoic acid* (DHA.) You can find EPA and DHA in fatty, cold-water fish such as tuna, salmon, and halibut. EPA and DHA reduce pro-inflammatory cytokines and pro-inflammatory eicosanoids. You might also try flax oil, fish oil, walnut oil, evening primrose oil, borage oil, hemp seeds and/ or hemp oil. Hemp oil is *a perfect ratio of Omega 6 to Omega 3, and a complete vegetable protein.* Along with the sources just mentioned, olive oil is great for Omega 3s and/or gamma linoleic acid (GLA) which is possibly helpful for inflammation and auto-immune conditions.

Mono-unsaturated fats, low in Omega 6 EFAs, are recommended over saturated fats. However, coconut oil is an exception since it contains medium-chain triglycerides (MCTs) making it a great form of saturated fat for easily accessible energy. Do consider reducing or avoiding animal fats which can have excessive Omega 6 EFAs and arachidonic acid (AA) - a possible cause of inflammation.

Clearly, diet is crucial to immunity, as we shall investigate further in a bit. A really great book is *Fats that Heal, Fats that Kill* (Erasmus, 1993).

In the next box set, I list foods, herbs, and supplements that may reduce inflammation. Some are also known as immune-modulators.

Reduce Inflammation, Modulate Immunity
Foods, Herbs, and Supplements

Adaptogens like Siberian Ginseng ~ may strengthen immunity

Aloe Vera

Antihistamines ~ Vitamin C and the bioflavonoid *hesperidin* are natural antihistamines

Antioxidants and micronutrients like zinc

Boswellic Acid

Chamomile ~ also an immune-modulator

EGCG ~ stands for *epigallocatechin gallate*, found in green tea

Fruits & Veggies ~ high in plant sterols and/or bioflavonoids - think bright colors, but they are all great for you: plant-based nutrition

Ginger

Lemon

Olive Oil ~ immune modulator

Omega 3 Oils ~ borage oil, flax oil, and fish; avoid hydrogenated fats, trans-fats, polyunsaturated fats, margarine and fried foods; only consume expeller-pressed/cold-pressed oils; I recommend Nordic Naturals* (vegetarian option, too.) *Nordic Naturals Omega 3 Oils have been tested in double-blind studies. https://www.nordicnaturals.com/en/Pro/Education_and_Events/1075

Oregano

Plant sterols ~ found in walnuts, seeds, vegetables and fruits

Resveratrol ~ found in red wine

Spirulina, Wheat Grass and Chlorella

Turmeric ~ also raises glutathione and serotonin/dopamine levels

Vitamin D ~ from sun, from food such as eggs and certain seafoods, and perhaps from Vitamin D3 supplementation as well

Exercise is a powerful tonic for the immune system. It also reduces inflammation by raising your cortisol levels. See Chapter Four on *Exercise* for more information.

Of course, the loophole for people with CFS and possibly fibromyalgia as well, is that too much stimulation through traditional exercise can put your body into fight or flight mode - the sympathetic state - and where you most definitely don't want to be.

Instead of traditional exercise, consider the beauty of restorative exercise like yoga, gentle walking, Tai Chi, and Qi Gong. You can still raise or modulate your cortisol levels, reduce inflammation, and strengthen not only your immune system, but your nervous system as well. These types of mind-body fitness keep your body in the parasympathetic state, which is where healing takes place, and this can be a game changer. For more information, please see Chapter Five.

Focus on the Vagus Nerve

What may be most important in all of this **is the role your vague nerve plays in relation to the calming of your stress response system**, of which your hypothalamus plays a key role.

The vagus nerve is one of the main components of the parasympathetic nervous system (PNS.) It travels from your brainstem all the way down to your stomach and into other organs such as your heart, lungs, GI tract, and pancreas. If you look closely at that last sentence, you can see how chronic stress may affect all these different organs and systems in your body. Also, the vagus nerve communicates with your immune system, and plays a role in decreasing inflammation by affecting the HPA axis and the release of anti-inflammatory cortisol.

There are many reasons to activate and heal your vagus nerve and restore vagal tone.* I believe it is key in recovering energy.

Your PNS is activated by deep breathing. When you activate your vagus nerve with deep breathing, you calm your hypothalamus as well as your entire stress response system. The vagus nerve releases the neurotransmitter *acetylcholine* which tells the body to relax. You want this amazing phenomenon to happen so you can move from fight or flight (sympathetic response) to rest, relax and digest (parasympathetic response.) "Vagus" means wanderer. Read more here: http://goo.gl/8MBf5Q

 Some of the best ways I know to activate the vagus nerve are: yoga, deep breathing, quiet meditation such as sitting or gazing at a candle, or active meditation such as music
Riaan Badenhorst walking, making love, passion - anything that gets and keeps you deeply in the present moment. Actually, one of the most popular activities is looking at baby animal pictures on the web!

*Vagal tone is best measured by heart rate variability (HRV), which should be, ideally, slow and variable (Heathers, 2011).

Seeking transformative moments by methods such as those just described can get you to the physiology and states of body and mind which can help you to heal. Collectively, these states are also known as The Relaxation Response.

Both the sympathetic nervous system (SNS) and the parasympathetic nervous system (PNS) are part of the autonomic nervous system (automatic - beyond conscious control.) Your SNS is activated during times of stress (even positive stress, known as *eustress*.) The SNS then in turn increases your heart rate and blood pressure and can even halt the peristaltic action in your digestive tract. Ring any bells?

When your PNS is activated, you move into rest and relaxation, your appetite returns, your heart rate and blood pressure go down, and your immune system has a better chance of reaching homeostasis which can be due to reduction and regulation of inflammation by the vagus nerve.

Your SNS and PNS have opposite functions, yet work in synergy together. This is the point of recovery: to achieve balance and synergy between the two opposing forces. It may also be your tipping point.*

Something to consider is what is called the *polyvagal theory*, a term coined by Stephen Porges:

> Polyvagal theory considers the evolution of the autonomic nervous system and its organization; but it also emphasizes that the vagal system is not a single unit, as we have long thought. There are two vagal systems, an old one and a new one. That's where the name polyvagal comes from. The final, or newest, stage which is unique to mammals, is characterized by a vagus having myelinated pathways. The vagus is the major nerve of the parasympathetic nervous system. There are two major branches. The most recent is myelinated and is linked to the cranial nerves that control facial expression and vocalization . (as cited by Dykema, 2006)

Focus on Rheumatoid Arthritis (RA)

Rheumatoid arthritis (RA) is an inflammatory disease and an auto-immune condition affecting about 1% of the adult population. It is characterized by inflammation that leads to progressive destruction of cartilage and bone. Much like MS, ME, FM, and CFS, its origins are unknown.

*The tipping poing of well-being may be trying multiple approaches until the scale is tipped in your favor. Try something, then keep it on the scale and add more techniques until you heal.

HPA axis dysregulation (down-regulated in particular) may play a role in auto-immune and chronic inflammatory diseases, including RA and CFS. Moreover, an imbalanced autonomic nervous system, with reduced parasympathetic and increased sympathetic tone, has been a consistent finding in RA patients. This is similar to what happens with someone with CFS, if not nearly identical.

It has been shown that toning the **vagus nerve** may help regulate the immune system which is known in the field of *psychoneuroimmunology* (*coming up*) to be **connected to the nervous system** and affected by cytokines, hormones, and neurotransmitters (Tracey, 2009).

According to Dr. Frieda Koopman, a rheumatologist in Amsterdam, and her colleagues:

> The autonomic dysfunction in RA patients is characterized by an increased overall sympathetic tone and decreased activity of the vagus nerve. This indicates that the normal equilibrium, where the SNS and PNS act oppositely and have contrary effects, is in imbalance. When immune homeostasis is disturbed, both the SNS and HPA axis are activated to restore this [in a normal response.] In RA patients, however, inadequately low levels of cortisol were seen in relation to inflammation and controlled physiological stress [this is what happens in CFS as well.] An imbalanced autonomic nervous system, with a reduced parasympathetic and increased sympathetic tone, has been a consistent finding in RA patients. Our findings support and extend the pioneering work by KJ Tracey, suggesting tonic activity of the vagus nerve is essential to maintain immune homeostasis. (Koopman et al., 2011)

Blog on RA, Auto-Immunity, and the Microbiome:

Cort Johnson is a huge advocate and researcher in the field of ME/CFS: <u>Study Suggests Gut Bacteria May Be Able to Trigger Autoimmune Disorders</u> (Johnson, 2013). See References for the link if you have the physical copy of this book.

Auto-Immunity

There may be 100 different kinds of auto-immunity, with two of the biomarkers being *fatigue* and *cyclical symptoms*. Is CFS an auto-immune condition? It's not my place to answer that for you. But I wouldn't be surprised if it were, and also I suspect immunity is deeply connected to gut health. But I hope, and believe, one can move out of an auto-immune condition. Please see Chapter Five for support.

Someone once suggested that perhaps auto-immune responses in the body are not a sign of malfunction. Perhaps they are the body's way of being hyper-vigilant until a threat has passed. This idea makes sense to me, in that I believe the body is infinitely wise. Moreover, the wisdom and intelligence of the body are dynamic, ever changing, ever growing.

But the trick of course, with any kind of chronic illness, is how to unlock this intelligence. I believe much of that has to do with learning to speak your body's language, which many of us ignore or aren't fluent in as yet. Another part of the puzzle may be in cultivating and practicing *self-awareness*. See Chapters Four and Five for more details.

Your nervous system (brain and spinal cord) are linked with your immune system. This is an important piece of the giant puzzle to understand. Even more so, as I will discuss in greater detail, around 70% of your immune system is in your digestive tract. When you grasp these connections on a physical level, the mechanisms of how to feel better become more obvious. Chronic illness can seem like a mystery, but I believe the laws of Nature - both physical and spiritual - can help pull you out of it.

But first, stress plays a huge role as well. Here's the story, according to scientific research. The stress response affects the immune system which then can *increase* the stress response. Likewise, deviations in the immune system can also affect mind and behavior as well. It is a two-way street, a feedback loop. One of the concerns is that alterations in this two-way street may lead to *auto-immunity*.

I was tested for auto-immune conditions, i.e., rheumatoid and thyroid, and my tests were negative. Even if I had an auto-immune condition, the conventional solution is life-long prescription drugs, which I can't take because of my liver disorder, meaning I don't methylate properly. I've always had to find natural means to heal myself.

My Vitamin D levels were tested and the naturopath nearly fell off her chair. My D3 level, which is based on supplementation or sunlight exposure, was 14. My D2 level, which is derived from diet or supplementation, was 9. Thus, my total was 23 near the bottom of the reference range of *20-100*. Optimal levels are between 50-70 ng/mL. Vitamin D level should never be below 35 ng/mL. Whoops.

We know Vitamin D is a powerful anti-inflammatory. *No wonder I had chronic inflammation.* However, some of my chronic inflammation was also possible due to having very low cortisol levels.

Vitamin D also helps with the immune function and assists wound healing. My wounds weren't healing correctly and/or taking a long time to heal. I have many scars now from simple things like shaving that I never used to have. It is also possible I was not getting enough natural Vitamin C from plant sources. I now use a real food Vitamin C powder and I notice my body heals more quickly. I also get plenty of sunshine which is a powerful medicine, avoid refined sugar in my diet, and watch my stress levels.

What does this all mean in a nutshell? Is stress the big elephant in the room? And what do *down-regulated* and *up-regulated* mean?

Yes, it is critical to understand your stress response. *Down-regulated* essentially means your stress response system may have *adjusted,* or is *inhibited,* or is not easily responsive to stressors, resulting in a chronic under-release of cortisol. This, in turn, can potentially affect immunity and inflammation. To give a bit more scientific answer, *down-regulated* means there is a decrease in the number of receptors on cell surfaces. It means there is a decrease in gene expression. This is often due to overexposure to stress. *Up-regulation,* on the other hand, means an increase in the expression of a gene. For example, it can refer to an increase in the expression of inflammatory genes. Could it also mean a constant release of too much cortisol?

Up-regulation of the HPA axis is connected to melancholic depression. You can read more about depression later in this chapter under *Fatigue and Depression.*

Here are some clues to the nature of an auto-immune condition:

In people with auto-immune conditions, the cortisol response may be compromised. What this means is that inflammation may run unchecked. For other people, their stress response may still be responsive, but there may be irregularities in their immune cells/cortisol receptors. *This is relevant, because cortisol is released both in response to stress, but also in response to inflammatory triggers.*

Low/High Cortisol or Abnormal Cortisol Receptor Scenarios (based on the work by Esther Stermberg):

Cortisol - a powerful anti-inflammatory hormone and the main GC, glucocorticoid - in blunted and/or excess amounts can impair immune function. Cortisol is released in response to stress and after inflammatory triggers. Its main role is to help maintain energy to cope with stress. [Usually] it modulates the inflammatory process as well. But there are two ways cortisol expresses abnormally:

***Your stress response is abnormal**, resulting in an either elevated or lower release of cortisol than normal. Elevated cortisol impairs immune function, leading to slow wound healing and more intense viral infections. Low cortisol affects blood sugar, blood pressure, and immune function. It can show up as depression, nausea, vomiting, diarrhea, dehydration, irritability and fatigue.*

***Your stress response is normal**, but the cortisol receptor (in your immune cells) is abnormal (inflammation can cause cells to die.)*

*These two scenarios can **result in auto-immunity** according to Esther Sternberg (Sternberg & Gold, 2002). Also please review the research report of Jeanette Webster, Leonardo Tonelli, and Esther Sternberg (2002).*

Auto-immune means activated immune system. If we look to the field of *psychoneuroimmunology*, we find *the immune system is activated by stress.* In fact, this is where psychoneuroimmunology may shed light. The study of psychoneuroimmunology points to a relationship between your stress response system, HPA axis reactivity (more later in this chapter), and the development of auto-immunity. This field also points to the fact that health may depend on free flow of communication in the body. *~I'm indebted to Saul McLeod, Simplypsychology.org for a schematic of The Hypothalamic Pituitary-Adrenal (HPA) System.*

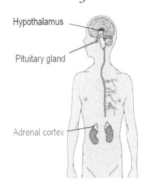

Hypothalamus

Pituitary gland

Adrenal cortex

Why is health dependent on free flow of communication? The central nervous system (brain and spinal cord) is how the body communicates messages. When we factor in that the hypothalamus is the place in the brain where emotions are turned into physical response along with what we know about how neuropeptides link the communication of our thoughts and emotions to all parts of the body, then we can see a *pattern.* We observe how the body and mind are not only intricately linked, but how they depend on the *free-flow of signals, information, and energy* between each other to function, to heal, and to thrive.

The Story of Your Body – Psychoneuroimmunology

The interconnection of all life is a profound and beautiful web. The fabric of being, and non-being, is all interwoven and inextricably linked. We rise with the sun, and feel the inexorable pull of the moon. What if we were to approach health and well-being from this perspective?

Psychoneuroimmunology is the study of interactions between the psyche, the neuroendocrine system, and the immune system. It is the study of how your brain and body are inter-connected and **communicate** through feedback loops, and can influence whether you stay well or get sick. Even more so, *your emotions play a role in the health of both your body and your immune system.* Expressing your true emotions is critical to staying well.

Likewise, keeping your body strong through diet, exercise, and mindset tip the odds in your favor of keeping your body, brain, and immune systems strong. As I've mentioned, this is what the famous book, *Molecules of Emotion by Candace Pert* is about: your mind and body are actually the same thing, part of the same field (the web of being), and they communicate with one another through **neuropeptides**.

Neuropeptides link the communication of thoughts and emotions with all parts of our body. Did you know 90% of your serotonin and a good deal of dopamine are found in your digestive tract? We also have receptor sites for serotonin and dopamine in our brain as well as other sites throughout the body. Our "mind" and our "body" are constantly communicating with one another through these neuropeptides.

Our digestive tract is often called our *second brain*, and it even looks a like a brain. One is more rational, and one is more visceral (our gut and "intuition"). But, the point is, our brain is communicating with our body, and vice versa.

Our *mind* and our *body* are part of the same unit: the *mind-body* field. Our thoughts and emotions are so powerful they can switch on or off gene expression, **including inflammatory genes**. This is one of the premises of the book, *The Biology of Belief,* by Bruce Lipton (2008).

I am so grateful to *David R. Hamilton* for permission to use his quote:

The entire body is actually hardwired to feel every emotion. Neuroplasticity is how your thoughts and emotions impact the physical structure of your brain. ~David R. Hamilton, Ph.D.

Because everything is interconnected, it is essential to feel and express your emotions. To keep them bottled up and unexpressed creates stress, and may even lead to chronic illness. We will explore this concept further in *Mind, Body, and Spirit* toward the end of this chapter as well as in several sections in Chapter Five.

But, here's the critical part, maybe even in terms of auto-immunity: Again, about 70% of your immune system is in your digestive tract - *your small intestine* to be more specific. According to Dr. Donald Kirby, your gut is "your biggest immune system organ" (McMillen, 2015). What does this mean? I believe it means that diet and lifestyle may significantly impact your immune system, and may determine whether or not you develop auto-immunity or move out of it if you have symptoms.

It's hard to know what comes first: stress - which can compromise your gut - or lifestyle or genetic vulnerability - that can compromise your gut and immune system. But, as researchers of systems theory and even psychoneuroimmunology point out, maybe it doesn't matter because our systems are all connected anyway.

Are you starting to see a bigger picture here? **This is why lifestyle is implicated as so fundamental in mitigating the onset of chronic illness *and helping one to heal from chronic illness*.** Its how you eat, think, feel, and behave that all add up overtime. As Sara Gottfried, from the movie *Origins* says:

> One of the most exciting scientific discoveries is that the way you eat and move turns on and off certain genes. It's empowering, because 50% to 80% of your genes and how they're expressed is determined by the way that you eat, move, and think." (Shojai, 2014, Section 43:11-45:23)

You do have the choice to be an empowered, proactive patient and and an informed, conscious consumer. Your lifestyle choices can make a huge difference in how you heal or how you get or stay well.

Lifestyle and Chronic Illness

There are many instances of how the interplay between the systems in our body can affect our health. For example, even small changes in your hormone levels can affect the quality of your well-being greatly. Very small changes in cortisol can make you feel truly awful. It can affect your energy levels, and even create inflammation. The same is true for small changes in your thyroid levels that can affect you greatly.

This is why it is important to be proactive and seek out healthcare practitioners who not only **A.** listen to you **B.** have the foresight and capacity to test you, even if your results thus far have been "normal." I recommend seeking a practitioner who has training in Functional Medicine, who can not only test your hormone levels, etc. but treat you with personalized medicine. This is how medicine should be: personal

Of course, what you know about and how how feel in your own body is the most important. This is why lifestyle is so crucial in preventing and healing from chronic conditions. You have to know and take responsibility for your own well-being. Know yourself and your body.

Know the rhythms of your own body. Know what energizes you and what short-circuits your vitality. Be honest, but kind, with yourself and have the courage to make change. Subtle changes add up.

Take small, actionable steps toward revamping your diet and lifestyle until you notice a difference in your well-being. This is mindful living. This is well-being. Have faith and courage in yourself and your body's ability to achieve a dynamic homeostasis, a living balance of sustainable well-being, where you can *feel* all systems living in harmony.

You feel awake. You start to feel subtle, ecstatic *joy* ... You feel the healing energy of sunshine, feel the pull of the moon and stand in awe of the stars (where you can see them). You feel hopeful, peaceful, grateful and, most importantly, dynamically and vitally ALIVE.

If I could send a love letter to you and your body about the importance of lifestyle, this would be it. What you do everyday - what you think, what you eat, how you move, how you interact with your environment - both with yourself and socially – all make up how you *feel* ... and how you experience your precious, irreplaceable life.

We have been talking about immunity, systems, and the interplay of these systems in your body that may contribute to well-being. We have also delved into specifics of how certain conditions, illnesses, and symptoms may play out in the body.

For instance, your immune system is made up primarily of proteins. If those proteins are damaged, it can be an uphill battle since the immune system perceives altered proteins differently.

What role do diet and lifestyle play? Can ancient, single-celled organisms such as spirulina and chlorella that are high in the building blocks of life help?

What about stress? Remember, stress and low energy are the primary reasons people go to see their healthcare practitioner. What can can we do to mitigate stress and what happens in the body in the presence of severe, on-going stress?

How are the proteins in your immune damaged in the first place? Through **oxidative stress** and an action called glycation, i.e., when a sugar molecule attaches to protein (Arora, 2008).

Oxidative Stress, Baby

We've all heard of oxidative stress by now. It's when free radicals attack healthy cells and cause them to "rust" like a nail, or how skin can get that leathery look.

Free radicals are a byproduct of metabolism in your body for instance. They can also be produced by environmental toxins, when sun and air pollution mix, or by your liver due to poor detoxification.

> If free radicals overwhelm the body's ability to regulate them, a condition known as oxidative stress ensues. Free radicals thus adversely alter lipids, proteins, and DNA and trigger a number of human diseases. Oxidative stress is now thought to make a significant contribution to all inflammatory diseases. (Lobo, Patil, Phatak, & Chandra, 2010)

You might be wondering what exactly is a free radical anyway? A free radical is a molecule with an unpaired electron. What does that mean?

Remember high school chemistry where you learned cells are made of molecules? Molecules, in turn have one or more atoms of one or more elements joined in chemical bond. You may recall (or may not ☺) images of an atom as a circle with a nucleus holding protons.

Electrons circulate in the shells (or circles) around the atom. Atoms like to have a paired number of electrons in their outer shell for stability. So atoms get together and share electrons, forming stable molecules. To share they must split their bonds.

Here is how free radicals are made: when a weak bond splits and leaves a molecule with an unpaired electron, a free radical is formed. A free radical is smart and unstable. It quickly attacks a stable molecule to steal an electron. If the attack is successful, the molecule that gives up an electron then becomes a free radical itself. You can see where this is going. The end result is the disruption, oxidation, and death of healthy cells. Oxidative stress. Stressful enough?

What you may not know is that **oxidative stress may play a role in auto-immune conditions.** How? Oxidative stress can create ***pro-inflammatory cytokines.*** Excessive toxins may cause your white blood cells to down-regulate. This inhibition of your immune system may lead to more infections, thyroid dsyregulation, hair loss, premature menopause, constipation, and, yes, fatigue.

This is the one main **reason I'm big on good nutrition and stress management.** Self-care and practicing a healthy lifestyle can make a huge difference in the quality of your health and well-being.

You want to **protect your cells from losing their structure over time due to free radicals and oxidative stress.** You can help protect your health by eating super dense foods which are high in anti-oxidants. Also, by managing stress levels, you may be able to minimize free radical damage.

Both of these strategies can go a long way toward protecting your cells.

Oxidative stress can affect not only your immune system and organs, but also your nervous system. Additionally, oxidative stress may damage the mitochondria, **the energy factories in cells**, affecting what is known as mitochondrial energy. This may play a huge role, and be a big reason why people with chronic fatigue in general are so exhausted.

I use CoQ10 (in water-soluble ubiquinone form) to support mitochondrial health and support my cells against oxidative stress (Bergamini, Moruzzi, Sblendido, Lenaz, & Fato, 2012). **What happens when you have created too many free radicals in your body? You can deplete your glutathione levels, your master anti-oxidant.** This scenario may lead to chronic illness.

Glutathione

Glutathione is present in every cell in the body and is **low in almost every chronic condition (about 80%)** including diabetes, cancer, heart disease, etc. Normally it soaks up free radicals. But if you don't make enough and/or create oxidative stress in your body, you are probably low in this most important anti-oxidant.

Glutathione may also strongly affect mitochondrial performance, which is what produces energy at the cellular level in your body. Low glutathione levels are implicated in several neurodegenerative conditions such as Parkinson's and Alzheimer's. Since CFS is strongly linked to dysregulation in the hypothalamus, there is speculation that low glutathione levels might be a culprit in this condition. Low glutathione levels have also been linked to autism (see the section on Autism in this chapter). Low glutathione is related to inflammation in lupus and arthritis. Also, it is implicated in MS. Low levels can affect the immune system and may lead to Th2 predominance (see the earlier section on Th1 and Th2). Are you seeing the connection yet?

In people who reach 100 years of age, there is a strong correlation between long life and high glutathione levels, some centarians even having levels as high as people in their 30s and 40s. How do you protect yourself? Your body makes glutathione, but if you are low, or don't produce enough, you want to eat foods that are glutathione precursors, like fruits and vegetables high in bioflavoinoids. Other great sources are raw foods like avocadoes, peanut butter, and whey protein. See the section on Autism for a full list (pg.186).

Free radicals can also be produced by the liver, if one doesn't detox properly (due to poor methylation, for example). Free radicals are produced anyway, but your body can make too many of them as well. There are actually two phases of liver detoxification: Phase I and Phase II. In Phase I, your liver needs anti-oxidant power (such as glutathione) to *regulate* the free radical production in your liver, and also everything that travels through your liver. You get this anti-oxidant power from that which is produced naturally inside of your body, and also from that which comes from antioxidants found in food.

Phase II is where your liver hopefully moves out unwanted toxins, compounds, etc. In some people, this phase does not work as well as it should, which can lead to a build-up of even more toxins and subsequent free radicals, i.e. oxidative damage in your liver, and send out free radicals into your bloodstream, causing oxidative stress due to excessive free radicals in your body. You can read more about the process of methylation coming up here in **Chronic Fatigue & Poor Methylation**.

One of best things I found for gentle, natural liver detoxification is eating leafy greens. I know it can seem hard to eat salad or leafy greens on a regular basis, but it can make a huge difference in your ability to detox and also raise your magnesium levels. What I have found that works, is to make organic greens the base of my meals, and then add whatever else I love on top. The point isn't to "detox," it's to aid in your liver moving out toxins. I will address this topic more soon here.

Some people use therapeutic grade *wild orange or lemon* essential oils **(check with your doctor first).** I find this works for me, via a few drops in yogurt or smoothies. One of the active ingredients in lemon and wild orange is d-Limonene, which *may* help with Phase II liver detoxification and *may* assist in building up glutathione levels (Brudnak, 2000; Sun, 2007). MSM and turmeric help me with liver health as well.

If your body produces excessive free radicals in Phase I, you may deplete your glutathione levels. You need glutathione for Phase II detoxification as well. If you don't have enough in Phase II, you may be susceptible to oxidative stress. You can't take a pill for glutathione - you can take *precursors* in pill form, but you *make* glutathione, you don't *take* it - but you can eat foods and that increase natural glutathione production and take supplements like MSM, etc. (Mercola, 2013).

Glutathione Deficiency and Oxidative Stress

As we have been saying, glutathione is one of the major anti-oxidants and the master detoxifier. It is a major component of your immune system, key to controlling inflammation, and a primary preventer of aging. If you are not as vital as you'd like to be, you may be low in glutathione – and possibly CoQ10 (Bergamini, et al., 2012).

Many of us do not produce enough glutathione, especially those with chronic conditions who may have some impairment of the genes involved in glutathione metabolism. How do you know if you are low in glutathione? Get a genetic test (try an alternative practitioner). There are other liver enzymes to consider being tested for as well, including the very important family of *Cytochrome P450 enzymes*. See Chapter Four for details.

Without glutathione, or without enough of it, your body cannot rid itself of environmental toxins, processed foods, efficiently detox hormones, heavy metals, prescription drugs, etc. How can you protect yourself? Eat more raw foods and more super-foods like wheat grass and spirulina. These foods naturally contain high levels of glutathione precursors. Increase your intake of peanut butter, sweet potatoes and turmeric. Try natural whey protein. Exercise increases glutathione levels and detoxifies your liver. The time is now to start down a new path toward health.

CFS and Oxidative Stress

It may be that people with Chronic Fatigue Syndrome or even other chronic conditions have impaired immune function due to low glutathione levels. This, in turn, may lead to muscle fatigue (myalgia – read fibromyalgia) and other symptoms associated with CFS.

Glutathione is essential to aerobic muscular contractions. Is there competition between your immune system and muscular system for glutathione? Testing does point to this (Bounous & Molson, 1999).

As Dr. Rich Van Konynenburg pointed out:

> As a result of the shift to Th2…the immune system responds [and] further drains the body's supply of cysteine to make glutathione, robbing the skeletal muscles of their supply, as Bounous and Molson hypothesized. The muscles thus go low in glutathione and the oxidizing free radicals there (including peroxynitrite) rise in concentration, blocking their metabolism and producing fatigue. Even though the HPA axis becomes down- regulated, there is still not an effective Th1 response to attack the viral infections, because of the **glutathione depletion** at this point. (Van Konynenburg, 2003)

You can read Dr. Van Konynenburg's full theory on ME/CFS at the end of this chapter.

MTHFR Mutation and Reduced Glutathione Production

As I mentioned, a major common factor in most people who have chronic conditions is reduced glutathione production. *Dr. Mark Hyman* describes it best in this classic article: *Glutathione: The Mother of All Antioxidants* (Hyman, 2011*).*

What's also relevant is what happens when you have a gene defect known as the **Methylenetetrahydrofolate Reductase** (MTHFR) mutation:

> When you have the MTHFR mutation, the pathway for glutathione production is partially blocked and you have much lower levels than normal. Glutathione is the key antioxidant and detoxifier in our body, so when its production is hindered one is more susceptible to stress and less tolerant to toxins.
>
> … accumulation of heavy metals and toxins may lead to a multitude of symptoms including disease, memory loss, rashes, premature greying hair, hair loss, social deficits, migraines, depression, anxiety, nausea, diarrhea, cancers, and more.
>
> [With children] who are autistic, 98% have a form of this MTHFR mutation. A lack of methylfolate hinders the multi-step process that converts the amino acid homocysteine, to another amino acid called methionine. As a result, homocysteine builds up in the bloodstream and the amount of methionine is reduced. The body needs methionine to make proteins and many other important compounds. It also aids processes in the body from breaking down histamine, serotonin, and dopamine. Thus, this defective methylation pathway is associated with psychiatric illnesses such as schizophrenia, *depression and bipolar, as well as auto-immunity disorders, ADD, autism.* ("MTHRF: Since an estimated 60% of the population has this condition," 2013)

To find out much more about the MTHFR gene mutation, visit the website created by Dr. Ben Lynch where he reports on research studies: http://mthfr.net/ (Lynch, 2015).

Estrogen Dominance:
ME/CFS, Cancer, Obesity, Diabetes, Endometriosis

Women may be more affected by ME/CFS for several reasons, including differences in immune system genes (Stanford, 2015) as we stated earlier in this chapter. But, estrogen dominance may play a factor (for men too), and the prevalence of synthetic estrogens is alarming (TEDX Endocrine Disruption Exchange, 2015).

Some argue that our exposure to synthetic estrogens is small and does not present cause for worry. They calculate we have one million times less exposure to synthetics than we have to natural estrogens we ingest from ordinary foods such as cabbage and legumes (Bast, 2000).

Yet, it may the inability to detox synthetic estrogens, such as those found in PCBs that is the issue, and not the exposure itself, at least for up to one-third of us.

Endocrine disruption in wildlife was proven in 1999 by the National Academy of Sciences (as cited by Bast, 2000). Have you seen the pictures of the frogs with extra legs and intersex genitals?

> Apprehension is growing among many scientists that the cause of all this may be a class of chemicals called endocrine disruptors. They are widely used in agriculture, industry and consumer products. These endocrine disruptors have complex effects on the human body, particularly during fetal development of males.
>
> "A lot of these compounds act as weak estrogen, so that's why developing males - whether smallmouth bass or humans - tend to be more sensitive," said Robert Lawrence, professor of environmental health sciences at the Johns Hopkins Bloomberg School of Public Health. "It's scary."
>
> The scientific case is still far from proven, as chemical companies emphasize, and the uncertainties for humans are vast. But there is accumulating evidence that male sperm count is dropping and genital abnormalities in newborn boys are increasing. Some studies show correlations between these abnormalities and mothers who have greater exposure to these chemicals during pregnancy, through everything from hair spray to the water they drink.
>
> Endocrine disruptors also affect females. DES, a synthetic estrogen given to many women to prevent miscarriages, caused abnormalities in children. They seemed fine at birth, but girls born to those women have been more likely to develop misshaped sexual organs and cancer.

There is also evidence from both humans and monkeys that endometriosis, a gynecological disorder, is linked to exposure to endocrine disruptors. Researchers also suspect that the disruptors can cause early puberty in girls.

A rush of new research has also tied endocrine disruptors to obesity, insulin resistance and diabetes, in both animals and humans. For example, mice exposed in utero even to low doses of endocrine disruptors appear normal at first but develop excess abdominal body fat as adults. (Kristof, 2009)

DES is a synthetic estrogen administered to millions of pregnant women from 1938 to 1971. The health effects are many (American Cancer Society, 2014).

Yes, we're talking about hormones in this section, but we're also talking about toxins and carcinogens. One thing we can do is improve how we detoxify our bodies. As noted, some people use therapeutic grade d-Limonene essential oil internally to detox **(note: check with your practitioner first)**.* It may help support liver health and detoxify excess estrogen out of the liver (ANP, 2001). While most essential oils are phytoestrogenic, citrus oils are not.

In fact, there is research that d-Limonene may not only help with both Phase I and Phase II liver detoxification, but also with Glutathione S-Transferase (GST) as reported by Mark Brudnak, PhD, ND (Brudnak, 2000). GST is a system that may eliminate some carcinogens. D-Limonene has been shown to dissolve cholesterol-bearing gallstones, and in patients with heartburn/GERD, d-Limonene may give relief because it provides a gastric acid neutralizing action and improves, in some cases, peristalsis (Sun, 2007). D-Limonene has also been shown to help modulate oxidative stress, and *may* affect certain types of cancer, including breast cancer (Kapoor, 2013). Using essential oils aromatically *may* directly affect your neurotransmitter system positively and **s-Limonene has been shown to improve moods.** Limonene seems to reduce serotonin, reduce glutamate (see page 209), and increase GABA (Zhou, Yoshioka, & Yokogoshi, 2009). It may also

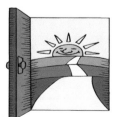

reduce dopamine (Yun, 2014). While I believe in integrative medicine, it is imperative we take charge of our own self-care and open the door to a brand new day. *Use caution when ingesting GRAS therapeutic grade essential oils, and check with your main practitioner or a qualified aromatherapist. Use extreme caution with kids/pregnancy. Other tactics to support liver health may include eating leafy greens, apple cider vinegar, green superfoods, and supplements like Liverite, milk thistle (as part of a liver formula), artichoke, dandelion, & warm, organic lemon juice. Exercise and deep breathing are ideal.

Although cancer-related fatigue is not associated with CFS or mainly what we are talking about here, it is certainly worth mentioning.

Again, chronic fatigue has many origins, and one of the goals of this book is to help you trace the origin of your fatigue. Of course, in many instances, that is not possible. In this case, one may be better off managing symptoms to find relief.

However, it is also very crucial that one rule out other origins of fatigue before coming to the diagnosis of CFS. This is important for several reasons, the most important being that you may be exhausted because you have MS, anemia, diabetes, or even cancer, to name just a few conditions.

Cancer fatigue is normally associated with exhaustion after having been diagnosed and given conventional treatments such as surgery, radiation and/or chemotherapy. I've known a few people who've received modern cancer treatments, my father included.

He was indeed worn out during treatments and afterwards. However, I can report that despite his fatigue, he made an effort to walk with a friend or a loved one outside as regularly as possible and did other exercises indoors. He followed a balanced diet full of nutrients, even when it had to be liquefied.

Another helpful trick was that he was mentally engaged every day with his project to finish writing his textbook. To gain comfort, he listened to music and especially loved performances by *Sarah Brightman*. He also listened to recordings of old radio dramas and comedies. My dad did what he could to endure and mitigate his relentless fatigue.

Finally, are the same mechanisms at work with cancer fatigue as are found in other cases of chronic fatigue? For example, is it the extreme stress of radiation or chemotherapy that leads to oxidative stress, which then leads to poor mitochondrial function? Is there one cause, a few, or many different causes of chronic fatigue?

Four Allergy Classifications

Type 1: Anaphylactic Hypersensitivity
Type 2: Anti-Body Dependent Cytotoxic Hypersensitivity
Type 3: Immune Complex-Mediated Hypersensitivity
(delayed onset, *auto-immune condition*)
Type 4: Cell-Mediated Hypersensitivity (vs. anti-body)

Does an activated immune system cause us to react differently to foods we once tolerated? I've always been sensitive to alcohol and caffeine. My tolerance for chocolate fluctuates up and down. At certain points I've been sensitive to dairy and eggs, and I'm still sensitive to GMO corn, corn syrup (although none of these may be allergic sensitivities). I sometimes sneeze when first exposed to bright sunlight, just like my dad. My mom is allergic to cats. Too bad for her! At any rate, allergies are influenced by both genetics and the environment.

Some of the signs of food allergies and/or various kinds of sensitivities are: runny nose, sneezing, digestive disturbances, dark circles under the eyes, bloodshot eyes, and *fatigue*. Some of the other reactions - which may be entirely or somewhat attributed to allergies - might be low blood pressure, rapid heartbeat, bloating, constipation, diarrhea, asthma, scratchy eyes, itching, nosebleeds, puffy face, flushing of the cheeks, coughing, hay fever, swelling, vomiting, hives, arthritis, headache, stomachache, irritability, hyperactivity, depression, ADD, trouble breathing, anaphylaxis, etc. Bleh.

Did I have what are called delayed onset allergies? My histamine levels were abnormally high. I had a constant runny nose, severe fatigue, bloodshot eyes, rapid heartbeat, and low blood pressure, to name a few symptoms. Delayed onset allergies (Type 3) are deemed auto-immune.

Most practitioners think that true food allergies are few and far between and that the storyline of a real allergic reaction to food is usually extreme and can include death. However, I must point out that, like most things in life, there must be a range - a spectrum - of reactions to things we ingest. And the digestive tract has the highest amount of immune cells. You do the math.

There is a school of thought that recommends waiting three to six months after ingesting a suspect food to give the immune system a chance to reboot and replace all of its IgG antibodies. Does this really work? For me, I do my best to avoid what I am sensitive to, and to strengthen my body at the same time. My tolerance for caffeine goes up and down. But is that because of changes in sensitivity or is it due to a stronger vagus nerve and/or HPA axis?

Something to keep in mind is that an overactive thyroid (hyperthyroidism) or an underactive thyroid (hypothyroidism) can result in increased *allergies,* skin problems, fatigue, nervousness, gastrointestinal problems, sleeping too much or too little, gaining or losing weight, swelling, and various types of pain. In an earlier section of this chapter under *Fatigue and Your Thyroid,* you can read about sub-clinical hypothyroidism and how your endocrine system is affected.

Chronic Fatigue and Poor Methylation
Mitochondrial Meltdown

That's one mouthful of a subtitle.

These are two huge subjects, and I am by no means an expert on this topic. Please take everything you read here with a grain of salt, and just consider it a subject matter to peak your interest to explore more about as you continue your own health journey. I am just giving the outline of how the subject of the methylation cycle may play a role in your storyline.

One of the main experts in these fields was the CFS advocate *Richard Van Konynenburg, Ph.D.,* who passed away suddenly in 2012. People in the CFS community showered Rich with praise for his expertise, research, and knowledge, and for the compassion he showed those who suffer. He will be greatly missed.

We will we explore some of Rich's theories coming up at the end of this chapter. Another CFS and mitochondrial expert is Dr. Sarah Myhill, whose theories we will explore in the section on Fibromyalgia.

According to Tom Malterre, "It happens to be that the mitochondrial DNA is extremely susceptible to damage. Out of the 87,000 plus industrial chemicals that are on the marketplace today - those that are researched for safety analysis - the vast majority are found to be mitochondrial disruptors" (Shojai, 2014, Sections 45:51-46.04).

Also, please read Tom's extensive review of research on environmental toxins and how **nutrition can help us process them** (Malterre, 2013).

Methylation helps us to detox and break down toxins and lipotropics (like estrogen and synthetic estrogens). It happens when chemicals known as *methyl groups* are combined with molecules in our bodies, like DNA, so that the molecules can do their assigned jobs (Matthews, 2008).

Methylation makes foreign substances more water soluble and easier to "wash" out of the body. Methyl donors like SAME, CoQ10 (a vital nutrient for those with CFS in my opinion), methylated B12 (methylcobalamin), curcumin, and 5-MTHF (a type of folic acid) all help to enhance detoxification (Kane, 2015).

Additionally, methylation is cyclical and the cycle is described as a *biochemical pathway* by Dr. Amy Yasco (2015) who works with autistic children. Processes of methylation that happen along the pathway are part of a host of essential functions: keeping mood on even-keel, helping immunity work, boosting energy, monitoring inflammation in the body, and perhaps most importantly, regulating detoxification. According to Dr. Yasco, "All these processes help the body respond to environmental stressors, to detoxify, and to adapt and rebuild" (Yasco, 2015).

The methylation cycle affects the immune system, detoxification system, and your glutathione/anti-oxidant system. It may affect anxiety levels as it synthesizes neurotransmitters.*

*__Note:__ enzymes, immune factors, hormones, and neurotransmitters are made up of proteins. Protein may be the most important macro-nutrient. For me, the more high quality protein I consume - like **raw, organic plant proteins**, greens superfoods like spirulina, organic whey protein, seafood, and organic, cage-free eggs, etc. - the better I feel.* Eggs and seafood are useful in other ways as they're high in sulphur and eggs provide **crucial cholesterol,** a precursor to vital hormones.

*I use Ester-C with Cranberry (by American Health) to help my liver detox properly among other tactics.

The crucial point, as far as the methylation cycle goes, in a nutshell, is that the **inability to detox properly** may lead to glutathione depletion, and/or oxidative stress. According to mitochondrial expert Dr. Jon Kaiser, **mitochondrial dysfunction** or even toxicity may occur, leading to *cell die off* and *DNA damage,* and leading to such conditions as CFS and cancer (2015). He recommends nutrient and drug therapy.

Poor detoxification, as in my case, may be due partly to genetic factors. I found out about my genetic vulnerabilities by getting a genetic test. If you decide to request such a test, you might also look for Cytochrome P450 enzymes that are involved in Phase I detoxification. In my case, I was low in Phase II enzymes, as well as natural glutathione levels.

It is interesting to note that two family trees of genetics may involve at least CFS and autism, if not more chronic conditions. Please see the next section *Focus: The Epidemic of Autism.*

The methylation cycle also produces CoQ-10 and carnitine. During the cycle, the rate of *glutathione production and recycling* as well as *sulphur metabolism* are controlled, both of which are involved in the detox process. Glutathione is a sulfur enzyme and sulphur helps eliminate heavy metals and *transport oxygen* - look for it in eggs and garlic. Vegans and vegetarians may be at risk for sulphur deficiency. **Low glutathione levels may also switch one's immune system from Th1 to Th2 dominance.** Please review the earlier section titled *Th1 to Th2 Shift* in this chapter.

If you are not detoxing properly, it could affect the rest of your body on many levels, as your body is an ecosystem. For people with MS, you might be interested to know that **the methylation cycle can produce myelin** for your brain, i.e. your nervous system.

Some people are proponents of restarting the methylation cycle using supplements. I personally am not a fan of this practice although I'm sure supplements can and do help. However, this process may, in fact, lead to major *die-off* symptoms. Such symptoms can be painful. They occur when the body rids itself of infectious colonies of bacteria and other organisms that have died off. If the body struggles to eliminate the dead material and toxins, then headaches, diarrhea, etc., may occur.

The first rule you learn in holistic health is to support and strengthen before *detoxing*, if you ever do detox. I'm not a big fan of forcing the body to detox. **Detoxing stresses the body, a big no-no in CFS**, as well as in other chronic conditions. Always remember to reduce or eliminate stressors, and not intentionally add them. Find that sweet spot where you are not bored or stressed out. Be present **in the zone**, cultivating eustress, in the flow of life (Mihaly Cziksentmihalyi, 1990).

I believe the body primarily detoxes naturally. If you give your body what it needs - what it is truly asking for - it will naturally find balance again. For instance, I prefer to eat well, avoid refined sugar or other foods that irritate or deplete my body, and use green superfoods. One such superfood is *pH Quintessence* that may help Phase II liver detoxification. It works very well and is gentler and more effective on my system than *plain milk thistle*. I don't notice any *detox* symptoms, just cleaner, better energy. I do use milk thistle in formulas, however.

Green, clean, serene energy is my favorite kind of energy from green superfoods. *I have found that some supplements work too, and I love apple cider vinegar. Any supplement I mention is what has worked for me.* I only refer to them as what may aide, support, or promote well-being. Since supplements are not regulated, brands can make a difference. As always, experiment with and find what works for you. Consult with your practitioner, and always do what's intuitively best for you.

Folate, B6, and B12 are said to be some of the important nutrients for methylation. Some practitioners recommend taking the active forms of folate, B6 and B12. However, I'm not a strong proponent of this tactic. **It's kind of a vicious cycle: if you don't naturally detox properly, why take synthetic forms of supplements or prescription drugs to help you detox?** I stick to the natural route, including deep nutrition, no prescription drugs (what works for me), self-care, stress management, and mind-body fitness. Also, deep breathing cleanses and alkalizes you. I have to use these methods, and they make a world of difference for me.

~ Go natural - to detox or find balance naturally ~

BalanceBeam Courtesy of www.Clker.com

Apples and cruciferous vegetables like brussel sprouts can help, as can citrus juices and green superfoods. You may want to try foods that are precursors to glutathione like raw foods and peanut butter. See a more comprehensive list coming up here in *Focus: The Epidemic of Autism.*

I believe in eating properly and doing exercise like yoga and jogging/brisk walking to help keep my liver functioning well.

Here is a recap to help with detox:

Many people drink warm water with organic lemon first thing in the morning on an empty stomach. My mother and grandmother used this practice for years. Lemon is also the most alkalizing food – it is great to help balance your pH levels! Citrus fruits help with Phase I detox.

As mentioned, I try to eat a lot of green leafy salads and use certified therapeutic grade lemon and wild orange essential oils to up my glutathione levels. These steps help my body to stay in balance easily.

Of course, as we know now, improper detoxification or an overload of free radical production leads to *oxidative stress*, a player in many chronic conditions. And what does oxidative stress do? It can cause *mitochondria meltdown*, i.e., damage to the mitochondria in your muscles. Remember we said your mitochondria are, in a word, **energy**.

They are cell structures that process oxygen and convert food into energy. When the mitochondria in your muscles are damaged, your energy levels may be reduced. Perhaps the damage occurs when glutathione levels are low due to competition between your immune system and your muscles (both need it.) Another point is that, believe it or not, loss of glutathione in your brain - which is where FM and CFS may start - may affect energy production in the rest of the body.

Energy loss may be the result of what is known as a slow recycle rate as *adenosine diphosphate* (ADP) moves to become *adenosine triphosphate* (ATP) - again, ATP is your energy. If this happens, not only do you not make enough energy, but you may also go into what is known as anaerobic metabolism to compensate. *Also, if your liver is congested, you may not carry as much oxygen and produce as much energy in your body.*

What does this mean? It means you may be creating too much lactic acid in your muscles, which leads to, you guessed it again, pain and/or fatigue. This could be a factor in CFS and Fibromyalgia (FM). Pain associated with FM may be caused, at least in part, by production of too much lactic acid (Myhill, 2014).* Lactic acid can be produced in excess in the body when the body is under a constant state of stress. Look for more on *Fibromyalgia* coming soon in this chapter.

What can you do? A few things: Request an ATP profile, but first you must locate a health practitioner who will order one. You can also visit our own Facebook page *Chronic Fatigue Support* to see a comprehensive list of practitioners who specialize in CFS, Fibromyalgia, etc:

https://www.facebook.com/ChronicFatigueSupport

Another thing to try is restorative exercise like yoga, gentle walking, Qi Gong or Tai Chi instead of traditional exercise which can keep you more in anaerobic mode (if you push yourself.) Yoga can be both aerobic (if you're doing vinyasa yoga) and anaerobic, but it doesn't tax your body the same way as other forms of anaerobic exercise often do. If you do develop any post-exercise fatigue, consider trying organic bananas, Dave's Kombucha Tea (it has added electrolytes), COQ10, green superfoods, magnesium malate, or green smoothies to replace electrolytes. Finally, try to avoid things that stress you. Also, consider **learning to re-interpret stressors as opportunities to grow**. I practice self-care, listen to mellow music, and take supplements support a calm state of being like *Milky Oats, Deep Stress (WishGarden), Seriphos, Mood UpStress Down (WellRoots),* and *lavender oil (like **CalmAid**).*

Remember: Practice self-care because prevention is the best medicine.

Focus: The Epidemic of Autism - A Few Natural Treatments

Autism is now considered an epidemic by many because rates have risen dramatically in recent decades. In the 1970's, autism occurred in 1 out of every 10,000 children. Today in the US, that number is *1 in 150* and UK numbers are even more shocking. In a recent study, Cambridge University scientists reported that 1 in 60 children were diagnosed with autism. For boys, it was 1 in 38. Predictions are that the worldwide ratio for boys and girls may be 1:2 by 2025.

*MSM supplementation may help with Fibromyalgia pain.

What are we doing about such alarming statistics? The National Institutes of Health (NIH) released funding of $60 million for autism research in 2009. In 2012, NIH awarded $100 million in federal grants for research at nine Autism Centers of Excellence (ACE.) But federal efforts remain scattered with disproportionate funds devoted to *causes* of autism, a situation perhaps prompted by practitioners who continue to claim there is lack of evidence as to how autism onsets. Yet our children may be getting sicker more often and at younger ages.

Jenny McCarthy (McCarthy & Kartzinel, 2009), in a book on her son's battle with autism, *Healing and Preventing Autism: A Complete Guide*, addresses the issue. She calls autistic children the new **canaries in the coalmine** because of their possible reactions to environmental toxins.

According to Dr. Jerry Kartzinel who co-authored the book with McCarthy, her son, Evan, is now healed from autism. **Not cured, but healed.** The authors examine differences between healing and curing as they describe natural steps that may be helpful to manage, reduce, or even eliminate many conditions that accompany autism. These conditions may include: immune system dysfunction, rashes, frequent ear infections, allergies, digestive disturbances, anxiety, seizures, obsessions, aggression, and candida. Kartzinel hypothesizes that these conditions may **coexist** as part of the same disease state as autism, and may, in fact, not be distinguished from autism.

Further, Kartzinel theorizes that massive **toxic insult** brought on by exposure to environmental toxins may be one of the main catalysts that triggers onset of autism. He tells how his adopted son's health rapidly deteriorated after a series of routine childhood vaccines administered by Kartzinel himself.

We have many concerns to weigh about each child's individual protection and the protection of the general population.

○ Should we vaccinate most of our children? *Yes.*
○ Are the systems of some children overwhelmed by too many vaccines given at once? *Possibly. It may activate their brain's immune system.*
○ Regardless of cost, must we search for and use safe preservatives in vaccines? *Yes.*
○ Is timing critical when vaccinating children? *Possibly…*

*See page 249 for information on Autism, vaccines, and microglia: the brain's immune system

Kartzinel's theory of *toxic insult* is similar to the theory of Body Burden as coined by The Environmental Working Group. *Body Burden is essentially toxin overload and is considered a potential cause of many disease states.* Whether or not toxins are the sole cause for the onset of autism, there may be a window of opportunity to arrest symptoms before a child reaches the *tipping point* in terms of toxin overload. According to Kartzinel, *once the immune system reaches the tipping point of exposure, there is a potentially rapid descent into autism.* To avoid reaching the *tipping point*, it is vital to be aware of environmental toxin exposure from the moment of pregnancy conception, and even before, and certainly after the birth of your child. Consider sources like paint, carpeting, and upholstered furniture, as well as childhood vaccines and food additives. Early awareness of potential toxic burdens may be nothing short of critical in halting and even reversing this disease.

In addition, many parents are on waiting lists of six months to a year for an autism specialist to see their child. Since timing is crucial, McCarthy and Kartzinel lay out a step by step protocol of how to reduce or even eliminate symptoms of the autism spectrum disorder, in addition to other conditions such as ADD, ADHD, OCD, personality disorders, even allergies and asthma. Some of these protocols include a *gluten and casein free diet,* and using a variety of supplements such as B6, zinc, Vitamin C, magnesium, caprylic acid, and probiotics to name a few. Other suggestions include fighting *candida,* addressing *food allergies,* detoxing heavy metals, and *keeping the methylation pathway open* which is a key component in moving all types of toxins out of the body.

Genetic vulnerability may play a roll in whether a child develops autism or not, according to Kartzinel, but *only if the child is exposed to environmental toxins as well.* Otherwise genetic influence is less than 1%. There are two family trees of genetics linked to autism. The first tree is the *Common Auto Immune Tree,* meaning family members exhibit common auto-immune diseases such as inflammatory bowel disease, **chronic fatigue,** fibromyalgia, lupus, and celiac disease among other auto-immune disorders. The second tree is the *Methylation Tree,* meaning family members had a *history of methylation problems.* On this tree are such conditions as **autism,** depression, alcoholism, ADD, ADHD, and schizophrenia, among other conditions. *All autistic children belong to at least one tree, if not both.* Knowing genetic background may help in selection of which natural treatments to pursue.

The methylation pathway in particular may be key to understanding why certain people become sick after exposure to toxins and others don't. Genetic vulnerability determines if methylation pathways are working properly in the body. If they are, then the methylation process produces glutathione. *Glutathione is the most powerful antioxidant and detoxifier in the body and is responsible for detoxing vaccines, environmental toxins, prescription drugs, food additives, etc.* If glutathione is not produced, toxins may not be eliminated, and they may be recirculated in the body and become even more toxic.

Individuals who are genetically predisposed to not produce enough glutathione may be prone to methylation diseases, including autism. This is one reason why *diet and supplementation are so crucial in raising glutathione levels in the body*, enabling it to move out toxins. Effective ways to raise glutathione levels include ***methyl donors*** such as: supplementing with methyl B12, trimethylglycine (TMG) or dimethylglycine (DMG) (found in brown rice), folic acid, SAME (in bubble packs only), or by eating glutathione rich/sulfur rich foods such as peanut butter (if your child is not allergic.) Milk thistle and raw foods contain high levels of glutathione as well, but may not be safe for children. Glutathione IV's, nebulizers, or transdermal crèmes are also options. Kartzinel says that about two-thirds of children are poor methylators and may respond to raising glutathione levels. Also, "Adequate levels of vitamin D may be required to produce serotonin in the brain where it shapes the structure and wiring of the brain, acts as a neurotransmitter, and affects social behavior" (Medical Xpress, 2014). I highly recommend the full article.

McCarthy emphasizes that *positive thinking* may be the most important step. She advises there are many biomedical treatments to try, and if one doesn't work, move on. Try another and another until you find what works. Not every child may heal totally and healing does not mean being *cured*, McCarthy and Kartzinel say. Much like being in a car accident, the child may heal from the wounds, but the original scars of toxic exposure may remain. However, they are cautiously optimistic that recovery is possible if toxin exposure is reduced or eliminated, toxins are removed from the body, and homeostasis in the body is restored. Kartzinel says about 20% recover but still must be *managed* with diet and supplements. Another 30% will end up with milder autism, and another 20% will have moderate persisting symptoms. He says 20-25% may still have ADD, but their neurological tests will show up as negative for autism. He says about 5% will recover entirely.

A note on mercury: symptoms of autism in children are identical to symptoms of mercury poisoning in children: loss of speech, social withdrawal, less eye contact, repetitive behaviors, hand flapping, toe walking, temper tantrums, sleep disturbances, and seizures (McCarthy & Kartzinel, 2009). Also, see the section on *The Sickness Response.*

Is this the cause or only cause of autism? Unlikely, and polyvagal theory and the social nervous system may play a role (Porges, 2001). However, contrary to reports, mercury has not been removed in vaccines. As of 1999, it only has been reduced. In its place, more aluminum has been added. The underlying issue of using toxins as cheap preservatives in vaccines remains.

Last, but not least, here is a synopsis composed by *Nick Meyer* on the work of *Dr. Stephanie Seneff*, senior research scientist at MIT, concerning rising rates of autism and the widespread use of glyphosate (and Roundup) in agriculture. You decide what's important.

Stephanie Seneff

Courtesy of YouTube,
Wellesley League of Women

Rising Rates of Autism

At today's rate, by 2025, one in two children will be autistic.

Children with; autism have many biomarkers indicating excessive glyphosate in their systems including key mineral deficiencies, seizures and mitochondrial (the cell's power center) disorders.

Monsanto claims Roundup weed killer, with glyphosate, is harmless because humans don't have a shikimate pathway. But our gut bacteria *do* have this pathway, and that's crucial because these bacteria supply our body with needed amino acids. Our gut is not only for digestion but also for our immune system. When glyposate gets in our gut it impedes our immune system.

Most studies are too short to show Roundup's effects as a cumulative toxin, one that builds up both in the environment and in our bodies over time.

Roundup has the following side effects: kills beneficial gut bacteria, allowing pathogens to grow; interferes with synthesis of amino acids and methionine which leads to shortages in critical neurotransmitters and folate; chelates (removes) important minerals like iron, cobalt and manganese, and much more.

(Meyer, 2014; Seneff et al., 2013; Seneff, 2014)

Fibromyalgia - The Story Continues - CNS/Nervous System Overload

They call fibromyalgia (FM) a neurological disease, or a neurologically mediated/neuro-immune disease. Many are now saying the same thing about CFS, i.e., that it is a neurological/neuro-degenerative disease. Some are also saying FM and CFS have *the same origins,* but they each play out in their own way depending on individual chemistry and genetics. The central nervous system (CNS) is how the body communicates messages. How may this system of communication lead to signals of pain and fatigue, if that is, indeed, a causal factor?

A related possibility is what chiropractors who treat FM and CFS identify as *deafferentation. Deafferentation* is when compressed nerves can interfere with signals so your brain and body can't communicate well, exacerbating the *facilitated* pathways brought on by severe stress or trauma. *Facilitation* is where repetition of pain or fatigue can create worn, neural pathways, as discussed earlier under *The Law of Facilitation.*

Or, is it possible people with FM and CFS are low in serotonin, both in the brain as well as digestive tract? Is there a correlation between FM pain points and neurotransmitter (neuropeptides) receptor sites?

Traumatic and/or extreme stress may be starting points of CFS or FM. For example, consider the incidents experienced by Laura Hillenbrand.

One evening in 1987, Ms. Hillenbrand was riding in a car which narrowly missed hitting a deer. Simultaneously, she spotted a meteor in the night sky and subsequently felt intense waves of nausea and wracking chills. After many months, she was diagnosed with CFS, a condition that has since kept her primarily house-bound (Hillenbrand, 2003). You know Ms. Hillenbrand as the talented author of *Seabiscuit: An American Legend (2002)* about the racehorse with crooked legs, and *Unbroken (2014)* about Louis Zamparini, a competitive runner in the 1930s, then a World War II bombardier and prisoner of war. Zamparini so admired the disabled author that he sent her one of his purple hearts.

Whatever the causes, there seem to be some potential links and possible commonalities between FM and CFS, whether the causal origins are in the brain, digestive tract, etc.

I will now explore some of these potential links between MS and CFS or even other auto-immune conditions such as rheumatoid arthritis (RA) and irritable bowel syndrome (IBS) from the perspective that conditions may be influenced by chronic stress that deeply impacts the stress response system.

Some Common Links

There is definitely a vicious cycle that seems to play out across some *chronic inflammatory conditions.*

For example, could it be that the pro-inflammatory cytokines that can keep one up at night do so by influencing cortisol levels? Many people who are exhausted have reverse cortisol patterns: low levels during the day (cortisol reduces inflammation and low levels can cause fatigue) and high levels at night, which means it competes with melatonin production. If you would like to know more about your own cortisol levels, you can ask for an adrenal stress index (ASI) test, to find out what your body is doing. I found *5-HTP* to help when you want to get much needed rest. It produces more serotonin in your body that leads to higher melatonin levels (up to 200% higher.)

Let's compare CFS and FM side-by-side (not a comprehensive chart). They seem similar in ways and certainly have chronic fatigue and/or pain in common. But CFS may be more implicated in viruses - read immune-deficiency - and FM is more implicated in auto-immunity.

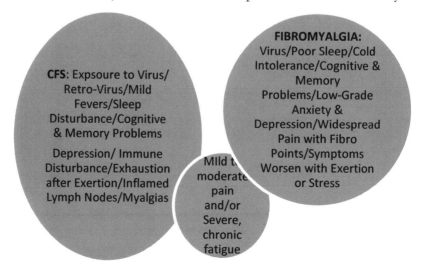

After looking at the chart comparing FM and CFS, I have two questions: Is FM the extended version of CFS after prolonged stress has migrated into auto-immune territory? Or are these two separate conditions with similar origins (acute and/or prolonged stressors) that play out differently depending on genetic predisposition?

I've had some experience with pain associated with CFS, but not the type of pain I understand others have with FM. And I've had an inflamed lymph node on my neck for years, like others with CFS. It showed up on an MRI, plus I feel it. Yet, overall, my symptoms more closely match FM, beyond the fact that my main symptom is fatigue.

What Causes Fibromyalgia?

FM is considered an *inflammatory myopathy*, meaning the immune system can attack certain parts of the muscle. FM has been called a *rheumatic disorder* and it often occurs along with other rheumatic conditions such as RA and lupus. It is also believed to be, or classified as, an *auto-immune condition* by many practitioners.

According to the Center for Disease Control, "Rheumatic conditions are characterized by pain and stiffness in and around one or more joints. The symptoms can develop gradually or suddenly. Certain rheumatic conditions can also involve the immune system and various internal organs of the body" (CDC, 2014). But FM has many symptoms associated with it beyond joint and muscle pain: dizziness, which is also known as *fibro fog*, headaches, depression, sleep and mood disturbances, IBS, and, of course, atypical *exhaustion* (not normal exhaustion after a long day).

But the truth is, just like CFS, we don't really know what *causes* FM. In general, research suggests FM, which affects primarily women, may be the result of various factors:

- Trauma: especially whiplash injuries, e.g., from a car accident
- Hypothalamus-pituitary-adrenal axis (HPA) activation
- Acute or chronic, non-specific stress
- Low thyroid function (see *Fatigue and Your Thyroid* earlier in this chapter)
- Low serotonin states
- Endocrine disorders
- Sleep disorders

As far as trauma is concerned, in addition to whiplash, we also note that in both FM and CFS cases, there are higher incidences of childhood trauma and/or post-traumatic stress disorder (PTSD). See *Trauma* later in this chapter.

Regarding the hypothalamus-pituitary-adrenal (HPA) axis, I have seen FM described as both an *up-regulation* and a *down-regulation* of the HPA axis. *Up-regulation* might implicate clinical depression, triggered by the secretion of too much cortisol (Pitcho, Herrera, & Ansseau, 2001). Up-regulation may also be the catalyst for chronic pain along with, perhaps, the build up of excess lactic acid in the muscles. *Down-regulation* of the HPA axis, as with CFS, would mean too little of the stress hormones are present which is how deep fatigue may originate, as well as pain. So which is it? Both? If FM is an auto-immune condition, that may suggest the HPA axis is *down-regulated*, yet pain is the pre-dominant symptom and is associated with *up-regulation*.

According to Peter A. Levine, FM is a coiled, tightened stress response that results in chronic pain. He calls this scenario "undischarged

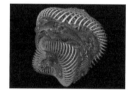

traumatic stress" (Levine, 1997). CFS would be the opposite: a flattened out stress response resulting in chronic fatigue. In either scenario, the *HPA axis is activated or inhibited*. The goal is to soothe the stress response, and *let it coil or uncoil to normalcy, like a slinky*. There's much more about *Peter Levine's* work and the notion of *traumatic stress* coming up in this chapter.

At this point, we can further refine our discussion because *FM is divided into two categories:*

- Primary FM (idiopathic: causes unknown)
- Secondary FM (causes known - such as surgery, injury, etc.)

Primary FM is idiopathic in the sense that the condition appears spontaneously and the *exact cause(s) are not identified*. However, even though primary FM may be idiopathic there is plenty to talk about in terms of *possible cause*. As we have said, like CFS, primary FM may be brought on by some kind of severe stress, such as trauma or a virus which upsets the balance of the HPA axis, and changes the way the brain, and therefore the body, responds to stress - and even the way pain signals are interpreted.

Primary FM may be, in part, *over-reactivity in the section of the CNS that processes pain, called the nociceptive system.* There may also be up to three times the amount of a neurotransmitter called *substance P* in patients, causing increased pain perception. This pain perception could also be interpreted as *hypervigilance.* In my opinion, *the notion of hypervigilance can play a role in FM, CFS, PTSD, and trauma victims, and may be one of the reasons it's so hard to turn off the stress response.* We shift into automatic gear, fueled by a primitive part of the brain, the amygdala. There is more on trauma and PTSD coming up in this chapter.

Secondary FM is thought to be caused by injuries such as *neck injuries* (in as much as 20% of people with this kind of FM), repetitive stress injuries, surgery, Lyme Disease, Hepatitis C, and endometriosis. In fact, an estimated 31% of women who have had endometriosis go on to develop either FM or CFS.

I've heard that *cranio-sacral therapy* can help at least the second type of FM and *myofascial massage* may be good for FM in general. *Water therapy* has been shown to be therapeutic.

Stef Miller, a yoga teacher, experienced an amazing reversal of FM. Diagnosed at age 35 as having FM, CFS, and RA, Stef set out a program to help restore her health. Utilizing alternative and complementary medicine modalities along with water therapy, restorative *hatha and yin yoga,* and tai chi, she managed her immobilizing pain and cognitive impairment and eventually came to a place of whole health.

It's not hard to connect the dots between CFS and FM, although they may play out differently in the body due to genetics. We're each unique, so of course we manifest symptoms accordingly.

Is it possible that fibromyalgia is an over-production of *lactic acid* produced by a system that can't turn itself off due to extreme stress? Is FM an *overload* of the body's detox pathways? Does the overload manifest primarily as pain as opposed to fatigue? Or is it all about mixed or misinterpreted pain signals due, perhaps, to low serotonin in the brain? Low serotonin levels may indeed lower one's pain threshold, as serotonin is known as the *feel-good* neurotransmitter. What causes such severe, rheumatic pain in the muscles and body?

Journal Entry

I had an environmental doctor test fibro points on my body, and he found a significant amount to be tender to the touch - in fact most of them. Does this mean I had FM and not CFS? He didn't officially diagnose me with FM. He did test my thyroid levels though, in addition to many other tests, and told me I had sub-clinical hypothyroidism.

I've only had a few fibro moments that I really felt, and that really stuck out for me - like the sunscreen incident [see Chapter Two]. But, just a few days ago on July 4ᵗʰ, the kids on the street behind me set off fireworks from 8:30 pm until at least 4 am. Smoke filled my room and I had no windows open. I could feel my body reacting to the smoke.

*My body was not doing a good job at detoxing the smoke. I got spacey almost immediately. My lungs ached. My body was overwhelmed. I slept with extra plants in my room and ventilated it but I still woke up with a **sore** body, especially in my hips. I was so sore it felt like I had hiked 10 miles. **Detox overload, clear as daylight**, at least to me.*

And, actually, when I was able to start exercising again after my injury, I would have severe lactic acid buildup after just walking. This doesn't happen any more, but I also do yoga now, which keeps my body in the parasympathetic state, and not sympathetic - fight or flight - like a lot of traditional exercise does.

Lactic acid is caused by oxygen debt, which leads to a buildup of lactic acid. There is a connection between excessive stress on the body and the buildup of lactic acid, whether that stress is from too many stimulants, toxins, or exercise, etc. This did not happen to me when I was well. I do think there is a connection between lack of enough oxygen in the body for whatever reason, and these conditions. Is this mitochondrial damage?

Build-up of Lactic Acid?

According to Dr. Sarah Myhill (2014), CFS may be "mitochondrial failure," and fibromyalgia may be an "inappropriate switch from aerobic mitochondrial production of energy [which uses oxygen] to glycolysis, [a] very inefficient anaerobic production of energy, not requiring oxygen, but with a large build up of lactic acid."

> All athletes recognise the moment when they switch from aerobic metabolism (requiring oxygen) via mitochondria to anaerobic metabolism (glycolysis) resulting in a build up of lactic acid. It is this build up of lactic acid that causes the pain, heaviness, feeling of exhaustion, deadened muscles, and 'muscles will not work or go any faster' sensation. (Myhill, 2014)

Do you recognize this feeling of "deadened muscles?" I sure do.

It is a lack of key nutrients such as potassium and magnesium that lead to oxidative stress and mitochondrial damage?

According to Dr. Emily Deans (2012), "Mineral deficiencies are known to predispose folks to oxidative stress … [and] low magnesium [can] cause problems with muscle cells turning fuel into energy, thus fatigue, weakness, and pain."

Magnesium, CFS, & Fibromyalgia

In fact, Dr. Deans refers to two studies on fibromyalgia and magnesium: one study showed how "300-600 mg of magnesium malate daily improved the symptoms of fibromyalgia" and another study showed how low serum and red blood cell levels of magnesium of fibromyalgia patients were lower than control groups, and [that] there is a correlation between magnesium, tender points, fatigue, sleep, etc. (Deans, 2012). Another study shows patients with CFS have low red blood cell magnesium and that magnesium treatment would improve their wellbeing (Cox, Campbell, & Dowson, 1991). In fact, "magnesium seems to act on many levels in the hormonal axis and regulation of the stress response" (Deans, 2011).

Chemical Injury:
Veterans, Environmental Injury, and MCS

Although CFS affects more women than men, there seems to be sub-group* that shows high incidence of CFS and fibromyalgia: **Gulf War Veterans (which, of course, includes women),** according to study done of a U.S. cohort (Eisen et al., 2005).

Not only is there the severe stress of being in war, but was the undue **exposure to chemicals** another type of severe stress that potentially led to CFS, fibromyalgia and even to **chemical injury? Gulf War Syndrome, chemical and environmental injury, and multiple chemical sensitivity are enormous topics.** *I can't do them justice here.* Please see a review of them, framed within the concept of the Gulf War Syndrome, as presented by The Environmental Illness Resource group (Gulf War Syndrome, 2015).

In addition to some veterans developing CFS and fibromyalgia after the Gulf War, some veterans may face a double whammy: **chemical injury** (possible tied in with CFS and/or fibromyalgia) and **post-traumatic stress disorder** *(PTSD).* PTSD and CFS may share a potential biomarker: **hypocortisolism.** This concept is discussed in the section coming up: *Adrenal Fatigue…Or?* Later in this chapter, I also discuss effects of *traumatic stress on the mind-body system,* as well as *PTSD and Memory* and *Post-traumatic recovery.*

*Race and socioeconomic status also play a role (Jason et al., 2009)

Gulf War Veterans who develop fibromyalgia do not have to prove a connection between their illnesses and service to be eligible to receive VA disability compensation (U.S. Department of Veterans Affairs, 2015): http://www.publichealth.va.gov/exposures/gulfwar/fibromyalgia.asp#sthash.7hnGHi5P.dpuf

Last, but not least, I want to make a point about the relationship of toxic chemicals to **allergies**: Any exposure to occupational chemicals, whether it be during military service, or as a member of the general public, can put the body at risk for developing **hypersensitivity** of the immune system, i.e. developing allergies, again due to limbic h:

> The limbic kindling model explains how multiple types of stressors (psychological, electrical or chemical) all result in the same outcome: chronic sympathetic nervous system activation that reduces the body's ability to "rest, digest and detoxify," and often results in allergies and hypersensitivities. (Gratrix, 2014)

The Stress of Immunotoxicity - Chemical Injury and Damage to the Immune System

They destroy the very enzymes whose function is to protect the body from harm, they block the oxidation process from which the body receives its energy.
~Rachel Carson on insecticides, Silent Spring, Chapter Three (Carson, 1992)*

Synthetic chemicals may downgrade the immune system and interfere with the body's ability to synthesize vitamins, just as glyphosate does by inhibiting the activation of Viamin D in the liver as well as inhibiting the cytochrome P450 enzymes in the liver, and amino acid synthesis in the gut microbiome (Samsel & Seneff, 2013).

Why is this alarming? Vitamin D regulates the expression of over 900 genes (Kongsback, Levring, Geisler, & Essen, 2013), and "the disruption of homeostasis by environmental toxins" may be linked to many of our modern, chronic conditions like autism, depression, obesity, heart disease, and cancer, etc. (Samsel & Seneff, 2013).

According to Seneff, "Glyphosate disrupts the liver's ability to activate vitamin D and that is a very simple explanation for the vitamin D deficiency" (as cited by Benson, 2015). As we mentioned before, Seneff also believes glycosphate (found in Roundup) may be responsible for the rising rates of autism (Samsel & Seneff, 2013).

*Originally published in 1962

In addition to immunity down-regulation, other issues related to MCS, chemical injury, EI, and/or **Body Burden** might include premature menopause or even andropause, thyroid function abnormalities, and, of course, fatigue.

At least 70 prescription drugs have been implicated in the onset of auto-immune conditions. Some of the drugs involved may include beta-blockers and anti-convulsants. Mercury, pesticides and other environmental agents may also be associated with immune system imbalances.

Dysregulation of the immune system may result in such conditions as auto-antibody production, inflammation, neurotoxicity, allergic-like reactions, hypothalamic dysfunction, and an imbalance of the Th1 and Th2 immune systems. Synthetic chemicals can alter nutritional levels by activating other enzymes in the body, leading to Vitamin D deficiency, crucial for immunity (T. Malterre, personal communication, 2015).

The Clinical Ecology Patient

The scientific study of how synthetic chemicals may adversely impact the immune system is known as **environmental medicine or clinical ecology**. From the latter, there has been spawned a whole new class of patient: *the clinical ecology patient.*

The term *clinical ecology* was first coined by *Dr. Theron Randolph*, physician and allergist. However, clinical ecology is not yet generally accepted by mainstream practitioners as a legitimate field of medicine. Yet, as usual, there are many people who have symptoms and feel unwell, quite possibly as a result of undue exposure to synthetic chemicals such as environmental toxins at their workplace or home, or foods they are eating, or other things they ingest.

From childhood into her twenties, my mom was diagnosed with allergies and sensitivities to toxins. As a result, there was no carpeting in her bedroom or curtains to trap dust, she used non-wool blankets and protective covers for mattress and pillows, her room was cleaned daily, and she had to avoid smokers. Thus, her environment was controlled, as were her medications and diet. She was a clinical ecology patient in the 1940s and 1950s!

Again, scientists understand little of the immune system. Is it so hard to believe that synthetic substances could be misinterpreted by our bodies, especially if we don't detox or assimilate properly, or are nutrient deficient?

As we have discussed, many people are experiencing a new kind of illness that seems to be *environmentally induced*. They are experiencing unusual and even severe reactions to their everyday, routine surroundings, including rashes, breathing difficulties, flu-like symptoms, fatigue, headaches, and depression.

These responses may be due to off-gassing from paint, furniture, carpeting, copy machines, mold, car fumes, pesticides, deodorant, perfumes, or tobacco smoke (which often has at least 100 different toxic chemicals in it if the tobacco has been grown near nuclear plants.) Other offenders are paper mills, chlorinated water, cleaning products like laundry detergents, **chemical warfare**, oil well fire smoke, biological weapons, and CARC (Gulf War Syndrome, 2015).

Other symptoms include headaches and even developing multiple chemical sensitivity (MCS). Multiple Chemical Sensitivity is a condition where someone has developed a severe, on-going sensitivity and/or sensitivities to even minute amounts of everyday chemicals. They have reached Body Burden, the tipping point. I developed primarily CFS with some multiple chemical sensitivity (MCS) symptoms after having surgery.

Note: **The Environmental Illness Resource** website, http://www.ei-resource.org/ which is a source of social support and information on environmental illness and conditions like MCS, CI, CFS, and FM.

I developed severe MCS during my second round with CFS in my thirties. Even a whiff of perfume placed strategically on an advertisement sent to me in the mail could wipe me out (another example of limbic kindling?). I remember seeing the Sundance film *Safe* (Haynes, 1995) where Carol White (Julianne Moore) goes to a remote place to heal because she developed MCS after she had the interior of her home painted. She wears a mask to take a walk outside because she can't tolerate the exhaust from even one car passing by her. For me, her masked face is a surreal image to this day. Even back then, I knew Moore's dramatic portrayal was about something very real … and then it happened to me too.

In my case, I found out the hard way to be mindful of materials treated with fire retardant. Fire retardants are even worse now than they used to be, in terms of chemical makeup. One of the main chemicals that brought me down was the latest fire retardant that has *polybrominated diphenyl ethers (PBDE)* in it. Brominated fire retardants made me more ill than almost anything else alone in my second round with CFS. I felt so sick, I literally could barely stay in my body. I was dizzy with the neurotoxic effect on my brain. Was my liver unable to break down the chemicals, or was it a lack of biodiversity in my gut and nutrient deficiency that caused my symptoms? As I mentioned in Chapter One, I had to leave my house and stay in a motel until I could get my new *chair and a half* removed because it was treated with PBDE retardant.

What is happening here? David S. Buscher, MD, immunologist, allergist, and founder of the Northwest Center for Environmental Medicine, states that while the mechanisms are unclear, it could be some kind of immune dysfunction and overreaction. Or, it could be a lack of biodiversity in the microbiome (T. Malterre, personal communication, 2015). Many of these modern chemicals are also *neurotoxins*, affecting the brain in many ways, including the *hypothalamus*, which essentially governs much of the body, and can affect behavior, the endocrine system, and the autonomic nervous system.

PDBEs are also implicated in thyroid hormone dysfunction (with which I definitely have had trouble), decreased sperm count, and possibly even cancer. According to the Environmental Working Group (EWG), thyroid disruption can happen in fourteen days or less after exposure to PDBEs. This is a real concern, as PDBEs are everywhere. When you identify that familiar smell of new clothes or a new mattress, or the smell of new furniture or new dinnerware, you may be inhaling, in large part, PBDEs. *Fire retardants are used on everything these days.*

Electro-magnetic field (EMF) pollution may also be implicated in contributing to MCS or other conditions. This may seem silly, yet some people do experience symptoms when living near power grids, power lines, etc. I could not buy a particular duplex I liked because heavy power lines outside the bedroom area bothered me. I could tell I wouldn't be able to rest well in that room, and rest is essential to staying well.

According to Scott Forsgren, a.k.a. The Better Health Guy, in a report authored with Neil Nathan, MD and Wayne Anderson, ND:

> Molds are multicellular fungi and grow in ... long threadlike branches. They produce airborne spores and are often quite colorful. In nature, molds are the recyclers of organic waste. While they are closer to plants than animals, they cannot undergo photosynthesis and thus rely on organic matter for nutrition. (Forsgren, 2014)

We've talked a lot about toxins in this book. Now we come to the concept of *mycotoxins*. First consider the word *biotoxins*. *Biotoxins* are toxins created by living organisms. *Mycotoxins are a subset of biotoxins* and are produced by fungal organisms. Ah, but back to mold.

So what do mycotixins do for the fungi? Again Scott Forsgren:

> They are believed to be used by fungal organisms as a protective mechanism, as a way to stake out their territory, and to allow for further proliferation of the fungi. Also, within a host, they may be used by the fungi to weaken host defenses in support of persistence of the fungal organisms. (Forsgren, 2014)

So we are caught in a kind of war, it seems, if fungi are busy in our bodies producing mycotoxins to protect themselves. Evidentally, if the fungi feel under attack, they go into heavy production of mycotoxins.

Not only do **we play host to mycotoxins** through the courtesy of fungal organisms that colonize within us, but mycotoxins may also take up residence in us as a result of our external exposure to molds. I have several friends who became extremely ill from mold exposure. Mold exposure may lead to EI, MCS, ME, CFS and/or mycotoxin illness.

In fact, it could be that mold was an issue when I lived in the last condo and descended rapidly into illness. I *do* know for a fact the condo below me had high mold levels. I could smell the mold when I was in the unit several different times. One of those times was because we had it inspected for possible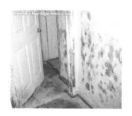
purchase. The inspection report confirmed mold problems in that lower unit. If your walls have black mold like this, get out a.s.a.p. and get your landlord to fix the very serious health issue.

For me, I had to use natural means to improve my condition, whatever the causes (mold, stress, surgery, etc.), because I can't tolerate prescription drugs. Either way, the point is to keep trying things. You never know what will work.

And then there's *Joey's* story about his battle with the disorder *myalgic encephalomyelitis (ME)* and how mold and mycotoxins affected him. He has reported improvements from his ME symptoms as a result of living in a mold-resistant trailer (Joey, personal communication, December 30, 2013).

Joey's Story

I figured since I started talking about my ability to exercise, I think it's only fair to paint an accurate picture of what that entails. For one, I've been hesitant to talk about how I got here, so that leaves the end result and if someone is reading just the end result, I might appear super healthy, like I never had ME at all.

But when I read this by Dave Asprey, a silicon valley executive I really admire, http://www.bulletproofexec.com/how-your-house-c... I realized this topic is going mainstream, and perhaps my story can help patients that have tried every drug and supplement prescribed for their illness, and only got worse in the process.

In 2010, I serendipitously ended up at my friend's house in Santa Cruz. While there, I was able to go off my sleep meds (including benzos) and my gut issues improved dramatically. Nothing changed but location. After that, I realized that @lisapetrison was onto something about the effects of mold on ME patients and I made the extreme decision to build a mold-resistant trailer made of foam and metal, following Erik Johnson's recommendations. I knew that it would be helpful, but I still thought I needed ampligen to get back my life.

In 2010, I moved into the trailer permanently during the depths of winter in Utah, when I was approved for Ampligen with Dr. Bateman. Within a few weeks I was able to do things I wasn't able to do in years: stand up and hang-dry all my laundry, use my computer for 6 hours straight. I was again able to go off benzos. I realized if I started Ampligen now, I'd never know what was responsible for what, and I needed to give <u>avoidance</u> a real shot. Plus, I would've needed to take out a loan to try Ampligen for six months and most patients regress after the drug is stopped. If <u>avoidance</u> worked, it would be a more financially-sustainable option.

When it got warmer, I headed to the desert to completely eliminate mycotoxins and brought none of my old possessions along. Soon I rolled the dice and went for a 40-minute walk. I expected to crash because I was laboring. My stamina was shot but I didn't crash. That was the first time I'd attempted to walk more than 10 minutes in years. One year ago, I could only travel that distance by wheelchair or bicycle. Soon, as my story goes, I was doing five-mile hikes, lifting weights again, playing basketball.

But the reality isn't black and white. I'm extremely sensitive to mold to this day, and that hasn't really waned to a significant degree. If I spend any time in a moldy house, I'm right back to my old ME self. I can't use my brain for the rest of the day, my muscles feel flu-like malaise, and I'm basically a vegetable until it passes. I lose all motivation. It's a pronounced neurological and physical letdown. But this is how I used to be, when I was exposed to this stuff in my old house.

When I say I can exercise now, it's only in 10% of the available buildings (maybe?) that I can do that, and that's while living in a dry city. In a good building I can play full-court basketball. In a bad one, I experience both short-term changes (breathing hurts, lactic acid builds up much faster, my coordination is off) and I crash as soon as I get home. This is a reaction no anti-inflammatory or anti-histamine drug has been able to block.

Many of you will say that you don't have what I have. But if you knew me three years ago, you would absolutely believe I have ME. I've been vetted by the top ME doctors in the world including Peterson. I believe this disease is auto-immune (why else would ampligen work better than valcyte, rituximab and chemo drugs clear PEM?) and our reaction to mycotoxins is by far the most underrated and understudied immune irregularity in ME patients.

Joey referred to ME as an auto-immune disorder. CFS/SEID may also be a *neuro-immune* or *auto-immune condition*. Whatever the label, we have to wonder how involved the *immune system* is in these conditions that have the word *immune* as part of their classification. I suspect the immune system operates on many levels simultaneously. As we learn more about the complex area of immunity, perhaps some of the mysteries of these disorders will be solved. The immune system – the microbial interaction system - is one of the true frontiers of medicine.

HSPs - Highly Sensitive Persons

"HSP's have an innate trait of high Sensory Processing Sensitivity (SPS) – or innate sensitiveness (Jung's term) - and include about 20% of the population, including animals. *It's also found in as many men as women"* ("The Highly Sensitive Person (HSP) Explained," 2015).

I believe HSP's may be more affected by many of mind-body conditions such as ME, MCS, CFS, FM, depression, pain states, etc. The book *The Highly Sensitive Person* (Aron, 1996) was written by Dr. Elaine N. Aron.

What does it mean to be highly sensitive? In terms of energy, it means that we may give a lot, but we then need time to reboot. I am an HSP, and when I give, I give of my whole self. This is great and can have great rewards, but I also need a lot of down-time to recharge and that's perfectly okay. ☺

Are HSP's more at risk because of sensitive nervous systems? According to Sarah Best (2016), "What all HSPs have in common is a hyper-responsive amygdala – the part of the brain that governs both fear responses and pleasure."

While being extra sensitive may not be a cause of M.E/CFS/SE.I.D, it may be a significant contributing factor. Giving yourself lots of downtime, eating for a sensitive system, and practicing boundaries and mind-body fitness may help you significantly, as they do for me:
http://www.sarahbesthealth.com/are-you-a-highly-sensitive-person/

Other effective strategies may include stress management and rewiring your brain utilizing new knowledge about brain resilience. See Superflex vs. Rock Brain.

https://bookofresearch.wordpress.com/2015/02/28/the-highly-sensitive-person-hsp/

Finally, if you feel you might be a highly sensitive person, do what you can to minimize your exposure to toxic chemicals and being overstimulated in general, i.e. toxins, toxic thoughts, people, etc. To read about one of my biggest reactions to a chemical sunscreen I used at the height of my illness, please see *In My Shoes, Journal Entry* in Chapter Two under *Cosmetics*. I think a big takeaway is that having a hyper-responsive amygdala may *lead to reversed cortisol levels*, and may also leave the body vulnerable to latent viruses, etc. *See Highlights for details.*

The Healing Crisis

In a nutshell, the *healing crisis* means the body may feel worse before it feels better. The healing crisis is called a "crisis" because your body feels almost like it's getting sick again as you begin to heal. I am not a big fan of this feeling, and I try to always support my body, instead of trying to officially detox, which may send it into this phase.

Instead of practicing official detoxing methods, I *first always try to support my body* by methods I've been discussing (diet, exercise, supplements, relaxation, self-care including stress management, cultivating a positive attitude, etc.) as my primary approaches to healing. Using chemically-induced detox methods may send the body into a crisis phase.

The body may go into this phase anyway, naturally, but the symptoms can be less intense if you just naturally adopt a healthier lifestyle.

It's easy to get discouraged during the healing crisis phase. God knows I have. It has freaked me out because the symptoms can be so intense. It is human nature to want to be comfortable and not in pain. The healing crisis seems in direct opposition to this requisite. But if you can listen and pay attention to your body's deeper need - the need to be well - it makes it easier to get through the healing crisis phase.

The so-called *healing crisis* is also the turning point for many, ironically. When you hit the creek bed - rock bottom - the only way to go next is back up again. Your healing symptoms may be excruciating, but they have awakened you and pulled you back into your body. The night is always darkest before the dawn. As you awake and are more and more present to your pain and/or exhaustion - as terrible as you may feel - you are *feeling*, and *feeling is the silver lining*.

You can heal whatever it is that you feel. (Dr. John Gray)

For every problem, I believe, the *solution is somewhere in the problem*. If CFS is really a *homeostatic imbalance in the hypothalamus and/or microbiome*, then the *solution is balance* again: eat well, de-stress, practice faith …

Yet, why does the healing crisis happen? And why does it feel so damn beyond awful? Here's one reason: When we ingest or are subjected to toxins our bodies will initially compensate. For example, if we take a new prescription drug, we may have side effects like fatigue congestion, etc., but our bodies adapt and symptoms seem to go away. However, the truth may be that the body has never really adapted. It has made a record of the toxin and the initial reactions are still there, just buried deeper in the body, i.e., perhaps dwelling on a cellular level as opposed to a causing a runny nose. The body's healing mechanism is to protect you as long as possible, but it still has to self-correct over time to toxic exposure. In other words: what goes in must come out.

A Day in The Life...

In the past, a day like this would have taken me down pretty low emotionally. I probably would have gotten psyched out and thought that this is just how it is for me. But this time, even though this was one of my worst reactions to a chemical yet, I didn't really think about it all that much. I knew the symptoms would eventually pass if I just kept up with my routine of diet and exercise, and positive thinking. I wasn't going to let this episode detract from my forward momentum. I was stronger than these stupid chemicals. Just keep moving forward, I told myself, and I'll find balance again.

All of this talk of synthetic chemicals and imbalance reminds me, yet again, of the importance of keeping it simple and natural, as much as possible, to stay or get well. I have to remind myself of this over and over again. If I start to eat not so naturally, my body sends me signals right away: fatigue, inflammation, anxiety, etc. Our gut knows so much. It is our primal, visceral brain (well, our amygdala is technically considered part of our primitive brain, but the gut feels primal to me as well. It's where you store your feelings, and where the story of your health and its journey begins to play out in your body.

Your Second Brain
The Enteric Nervous System

Know the feeling of butterflies in your *gut?* Those are the chemicals of the stress response being released. This release can be the result of negative stress or positive stress, also known as eustress.

In addition to butterflies, there's a lot more than fluttering going on in your gut, which includes your esophagus, stomach, intestines, and colon. Whether you realize it or not, your gut, is exceedingly perceptive and active. **In fact, it is an intelligent, fully operating, almost self-contained second brain, housing over 500 million neurons**. Wow! Even more astounding is that around 90% of your serotonin receptors are in your digestive tract.

Your *gut feelings* are literally that: feelings you feel in your gut. So much of what we feel, we mistake as being something we think. Thoughts are not emotions. You feel emotions in your gut, your body. When we follow our gut - listen to our emotions - and eat healthy foods (raw, cultured, sprouted, fresh, organic, alkaline, non-GMO) our bodies are inclined to naturally find their way back to balance.

Almost everything you'd find in your brain is also located in your gut, including dopamine, GABA, and serotonin, as mentioned. And there is an intimate connection between your *two brains*. Just like the axis of the hypothalamus, pituitary and adrenals, i.e., the HPA axis, there is a profound connection between your primary brain and your second brain, which is known as the enteric nervous system. That solid connection is called the *gut-brain axis*. Your gut and brain *talk* to one another and *influence* one another. They communicate back and forth. This is why diet, thoughts, and emotions all play strategic roles in health and healing, and fully manifested, dynamic well-being.

Focus on Your Neurotransmitter System

Before we head in any deeper, it's important to understand the role neurotransmitters play in your life and health. Essentially, deficiencies in neurotransmitters or receptors (weak links) may put certain people at a disadvantage to being more vulnerable to the effects of stress. In a nutshell, you need great nutrition as raw material (amino acids, antioxidants) in order to create/protect your neurotransmitter system.

Neurotransmitters act as messengers, with *neuro* meaning nerves or neurons and *transmitter* meaning the signaler. Your neurotransmitter system is super critical for the functioning of your brain and body and is necessary for the healthy functioning and operation of your central nervous system (CNS). This is very important for those of us who not only have potential disorders of the CNS, but for those battling anxiety, depression, addiction, etc.

Scientists are not sure how many neurotransmitters there are, but there are a few major players and some interact intimately with one another as well. Examples of the big players include: norepinephrine, GABA, acetycholine, serotonin, dopamine, endorphins, and glutamate.

> These neurotransmitters help orchestrate the smooth operation of various functions in you brain and body such as motor function, perception, cognition, attention, emotion, etc. (Maxmen, Ward, & Kilgus 2009)

An example of how your neurotransmitters interact would be how GABA modulates dopamine in the reward pathway. The reward pathway is heavily implicated in addiction. Another way would be how serotonin down-regulates dopamine.

Since the smooth operation of all of these neurotransmitters working in harmony is so key, is there a connection say between inflamed white matter and MS or CFS? With inflamed white matter, "the blood-brain barrier becomes partially ineffective, and peripheral immune cells and antibodies can enter the central nervous system" ("White Matter Matters," 2015). White matter is "full of myelin" ("White Matter Matters," 2015) and the myelin sheath acts as a conductor of electrical energy of the neurotransmitters for your 60,000 nerves. Demyelination can occur due to various conditions such as too much cortisol, inflammation, heavy metals, chemicals, or due to auto-immunity, e.g., when the myelin sheath is attacked as with MS.

Yet, it could also be that glutamate excitocicity (glutamate is an excitatory neurotransmitter) could lead to mitochondrial depolarization, increased production of radical oxygen species, disturbance in axon functioning, and multiple sclerosis pathology:

> Oligodendrocytes are particularly sensitive to alterations of glutamate and ATP homoeostasis, which may kill these cells by excitotoxicity ... White matter (WM) damage implies primary or secondary disruption of axon function causing disturbance of signal transmission and altered neurological functions that can [include] devastating loss of motor function. (Matute & Ransom, 2012)

Remyelination can and does occur naturally, and even in people with MS. However, as people age, it seems remyelination can become harder, and this may be when can lesions appear. When nerve impulses cannot travel efficiently, symptoms appear, such as fatigue. See *Focus on Multiple Sclerosis* earlier in this chapter for more discussion.

Also, deficiencies in neurotransmitters or receptors (weak links) may put certain people at a disadvantage by making them more vulnerable to the effects of stress. Over time, **repeated activation of the stress response** (perhaps kindling as well) takes a toll on the body. Research suggests that prolonged stress contributes to high blood pressure, promotes the formation of artery-clogging deposits, and causes brain changes that may promote anxiety, depression, and *addiction.*

Remember, you need great nutrition as raw material to support your neurotransmitter system and balance the levels. And, addressing neurotransmitter levels is a big part of how synthetic drugs work. Here are some examples of supplementation and support:

GABA - for your brain-gut axis; powerful in stabilizing the hypothalamus; GLA may work to calm your brain too, and counter-act inflammatory cytokines
L-Theanine - calms your brain down without making you feel tired; precursor to GABA, serotonin and dopamine
Spirulina - high in complete protein; improves norepinephrine which raises energy levels
L-Tyrosine - can support positive moods and even thyroid function

Why or How Does Provigil Work?

Provigil, also known as *Modafinil*, is widely prescribed, it seems, for ME/CFS and even MS. For some people it seems to provide more energy and is known for improving mood, memory, and alertness.

As I have said, I am not a fan of using prescription drugs when there are natural alternatives available. However, some people swear by this drug (and other prescription drugs for that matter), although it is not yet really understood how Provigil works in the brain and body.

Does Provigil work as an anti-oxidant, reducing reactive oxygen species (ROS) and therefore improving muscle contraction and energy metabolism, i.e., enhancing *mitochondrial performance?*

Is Provigil helping with general liver detoxification - **particularly those of the cytochrome P450 system, which is responsible for drug metabolism in the liver (Gerrard & Malcolm, 2007)** - that seems to be such an issue for so many people with chronic conditions? Is improved detoxification the reason people then have more energy?

Or do patients seem to have more energy because Provigil reduces *adenosine*, a natural organic compound in our system which helps regulate sleep, among other things? Consequently, with reduced adenosine, is alertness increased?

On the other side of the coin, let's look at potential side effects of Provigil: Some people have reported a rash. Others found excessive sleepiness continued even when taking Provigil. Psychiatric symptoms have been noted. Certain adverse cardiovascular events were recorded. However, in a controlled clinical study, the most common reaction to Provigil was that 34 out of 934 subjects developed a headache.

Please review some of the research. A place to start might be with the analyses offered by Paul Gerrard and Robert Malcolm in *Mechanisms of Modafinil: A Review of Current Research* (Gerrard & Malcolm, 2007). Of course, you can peruse more current research on the web. As with any drug, you must weigh the pros and cons and then decide if it could be a potential aid for you. As always, do what works for you. Whatever works, synthetic or natural, the goal is to feel better!

Serotonin and the Communication Connection
IBS, CFS, FM, and Depression

Science is searching for links between chronic conditions. Chronic stress and inflammation are common factors. What about Vitamin D, and the role it may play in the **production of serotonin,** and, therefore, immunity (Medical Xpress, 2014)? Why are we so low in Vitamin D? Is it exposure to glyphosate and inhibition of cytochrome P450 enzymes (Samsel & Seneff, 2013)? Or, is it lack of adequate sun exposure? How important are essential amino acids that form our crucial neurotransmitter system, including serotonin, and what role does serotonin play?

Serotonin* is a nervous system chemical messenger, and **its role is to communicate.** It plays a crucial role in nearly all of your brain cells functions, as well as other bodily functions. **Chronic stress can also create low levels of serotonin.**

Serotonin is low in people with fibromyalgia. It is low in many with depression. It is dysregulated in the digestive tracts of people with IBS, being either too high or too low. Likewise, it is low in some people with CFS and high in others. Low levels been linked to patients with migraines. Finally, **tryptophan (an essential amino acid) is the precursor to serotonin.** When tryptophan is depleted, you may feel depressed and tired. Low tryptophan (along with low levels of other essential amino acids) may be implicated in disease.

Serotonin is versatile. It has varying degrees of influence on a host of functions in your body and brain. Within your body it may modulate such conditions as **fatigue,** body temperature, and **pain.** Within your brain, for example, a low level of serotonin may be associated with certain thoughts, moods, emotions, and behaviors such as anxiety, fear, apathy, self-esteem, anger, violence, and aggression. On the positive side, it is suspected that a well-regulated level of serotonin helps with feelings of well-being, relaxation, and positive thinking. It may have influence on your appetite and facilitate restful, deep sleep (melatonin).

*Serotonin's pre-cursor and MVP is the amino acid tryptophan, which has a challenge reaching the blood-brain barrier (only about 1% makes it), is the least plentiful of all the amino acids, and yet is crucial for overall well-being (T. Malterre, personal communication, 2015).

Remember, you manufacture your own serotonin in two places: your brain and your secondary brain (your gut.) The majority of it is in your gut where it acts as both a neurotransmitter and a signaling mechanism. In your gut, serotonin regulates GI motility (how fast food moves through the intestinal tract) as well as **perception of visceral pain**. In the process, it also communicates with your primary brain. Knowing this, you can see why symptoms of IBS and FM might occur in the absence, or overabundance, of serotonin in your gut. If you have symptoms such as pain and diarrhea, you might have too much serotonin. With constipation*, you might not have enough serotonin, or be producing enough tryptophan, its precursor.

I believe CFS/SEID may be a disorder of the gut or brain. Perhaps my gut or CNS were disturbed due to stress, prescription drugs, antibiotics, or anesthesia. These scenarios may have disturbed the delicate balance of bacteria and/or perhaps inhibited amino acid or folate production via the shikimate pathway (Samsel & Seneff, 2013)? Perhaps white matter inflammation or poor vagal tone resulted. Perhaps it was a *neurotransmitter imbalance*, or oxidative stress and subsequent mitochondrial dysfunction. In any case, for me, the result was atypical fatigue. Were my crucial serotonin levels affected?

So what causes fluctuation in serotonin levels? There are reasons that trigger unusually high levels of serotonin such as medications, illegal drugs, and supplements, including possible interactions among those substances. Too much serotonin can cause inflammation as well. While *poor diet and chronic stress* can decrease serotonin levels, **Vitamin D** levels may **positively raise serotonin levels** (Medical Xpress, 2014) as well as influence gene expression and social behavior (Rutberg, 2015).

Several chronic conditions share a common link with chronic stress. IBS seems to be triggered by stress. Also, chances are likely that stress may be involved in the initiation of clinical depression, CFS, etc.

Here's the rub: The stress hormones, adrenaline and cortisol, and even insulin (take note pre-diabetics and people with metabolic syndrome) *actually cause your brain to release serotonin*. But if this release continues, then overtime, *your serotonin stores can be depleted*, which is not a good thing. Is such depletion the same as down-regulation? So we observe a vicious cycle. How doe we move out of this storyline? Self-care.

*Magnesium is the best support I know of for this condition. Try magnesium oxide and/or malate.

Is this why people with CFS, etc. have low melatonin levels, because they have *low serotonin stores due to severe stress*? Is this a reason we can't sleep? Or, perhaps it is first a condition of low tryptophan in the gut, which then converts to serotonin, and then ultimately melatonin. **Scientists suspect that difficulty getting restorative sleep could be due to inflammatory cytokines that reduce 5-HTP levels.** Cytokines also increase *norepinephrine* levels that are excitatory to the nervous system. Does this in turn reduce melatonin levels? What is the chain reaction that ensues?

I know 5-HTP is a game-changer for me. It helps me sleep deeply, and get more restorative sleep, like I used to enjoy when I was young, before I had chronic fatigue. This is just one of many reasons I use 5-HTP. Not only does it help **raise serotonin levels** significantly, it helps with sleep by **increasing melatonin levels dramatically** (by up to 200%). "5-HTP is [also] needed to heal the intestinal barrier … and tryptophan equals gut integrity" (T. Malterre, personal communication, 2015).

Self-Care to Heal from Chronic Stress

It is important to note that stress may cause disturbances in the **hypothalamic-pituitary-adrenal axis** (HPA axis.) As we have discussed, this axis has many functions such as assisting with digestion, mood, and sleep. **It plays a large role in contolling reactions to stress.** But constant stresss of any kind may promote dysfunction in the axis. Also, it seems that the axis may up-regulate at first, then down-regulate with fatigue. **It also up-regulates with clinical depression.** It may affect vagal tone. Disturbances due to stress can affect your hippocampus, **neurotransmitter levels like serotonin**, as well as affect you hormonally and metabolically.

What this means is that in people with CFS, for instance, the HPA axis may produce *less of the stress hormones* such as *norepinephrine and cortisol*. This is why spirulina helps me so much. It contains the essential amino acid phenylalanine and the amino acid tyrosine, which are precursors to *norepinephrine*, which naturally increases my energy and mood. Spirulina is also high in organic iron and B vitamins, which help to fortify the nervous system.

As we mentioned, *in reaction to activation of the stress response*, **serotonin is released.** This occurs via stimulation of the **vagus nerve** by deep breathing. Deep breathing tells the vagus nerve to *send a calming message to your nervous system. What are some ways to cultivate deep breathing?* Meditation, mindfulness, walking, yoga, Tai Chi, Qi Gong, massage, warm baths, exercise, sex, using biofeedback (HeartMath), being creative, enjoying nature, being with your loved ones and pets, engaging in prayer, going to counseling, using essential oils, lighting candles, and making social connections, etc.

I can't recommend yoga or HeartMath enough. You can literally calm yourself by being aware of what stimulates you, i.e. paying attention to biofeedback and consciously slowing your heart rate through deep breathing. Yoga stimulates your parasympathetic nervous system through pranayama (breath work) and/or vinyasa which connects breath with movement. You move but stay calm, which is a godsend for anyone with CFS, etc.

Again, this whole process of calming the nervous sytem is known as *The Relaxation Response*, a term coined by Herbert Benson (1975). His research showed that even short periods of meditation and deep breathing can alter the stress response in the body and may reduce pain levels. He found that your *MIND* is incredibly powerful in not only calming you, but ***also influencing expression of genes related to stress and inflammation.*** It is repetition in music, yoga, massage, or meditative chanting or breathing, for example, that calm the mind land body. See Chapter Four for more details.

Need extra help in addition to the foregoing suggestions? Try Seriphos (it stabilizes your HPA axis), Milky Oats, Rescue Remedy, L-Theanine, GABA, or passionflower, but always check with your health practitioner first.

Fatigue and Depression

Scientists are still not sure what causes depression, just as there is no agreement about the reasons for CFS symptoms manifesting in people. Perhaps these stumbling blocks exist because we need to look beyond science for full answers. But even within the world of systematic knowledge, there is a solid foundation of research that is starting to paint a clearer picture of the fundamentals of how clinical depression may unfold. Here are some basic facts and theories and insight into new theoretical assumptions and a new possible model of depression.

Depression affects almost 10 million American adults each year, which is about 5% of the population. Compare that percentage to that of people coping with CFS worldwide which is estimated to be 1-2%. While the numbers are higher for major (clinical) depression, there may be some common ground which I will explain in a bit.

Major depression goes beyond the blues. Anyone who experiences at least five of the following telltale symptoms (including loss of energy or fatigue) for two weeks or more on a consistent basis *may* be diagnosed with clinical depression:

Signs of Clinical Depression	*More Signs*
Depressed mood	Feeling worthless
Insomnia or excessive sleep	Frequent thoughts of suicide
Appetite or weight changes	Attempting suicide
Reduced interest or ability to	Agitated behavior
enjoy activities	Slowed behavior
Feeling guilty	*Loss of energy or fatigue*

Perhaps even more revealing is the *experience of depression*, which has been described as *the color draining out of everything, a flattened experience of the world, a foggy head, and a* "dull nothing" (Slater, 2013). Plus, of course, there is accompanying fatigue. I've also heard it described as a black hole.

This is my experience with depression of this nature. As I mentioned in Chapter One, when I took Naprosyn, sold over the counter as Aleve, I felt as if I were continuously falling down a black hole. I had no motivation to get out of bed. It was one of the worst times of my life, in addition to coping with chronic fatigue and domestic violence. I have definitely experienced depression from life's challenges. However, my stories don't define me, except I survived and I'm here. If you're alive, you're doing well. Keep going. You matter ...

Stress and Depression

While causes of depression are unknown, observations have been made about the relationship of stress to clinical depression: The HPA axis is known to be affected by several types of stress, including *oxidative, inflammatory, and psychological stress* which can result in dysregulation of the axis leading to either *hyper* or *hypo* activation of glucocorticoid (GC) receptors, damage to the brain, and inflammation. What may be especially relevant is how HPA dysregulation may occur more frequently in teenage girls coping with interpersonal stressors (Broderick & Blewitt, 2010). It also is noted to occur more often in children of depressed mothers. Researchers see a causal relationship between HPA axis dysfunction that increases over time, and the unfolding of depression in teens and adults (Guerry & Hastings, 2011). However, longitudinal and multidisciplinary studies are needed.

Other effects of stress include neurotoxic harm to the hippocampus, i.e., the possible brain damage mentioned previously. Also, prefrontal cortex immune variations may occur.

There may be compromise of the telomere/telomerase maintenance system.* It is important to mention the telomerase maintenance system because it has to do with cell replication and integrity, and maintaining chromosomal stability. It is recognized as a factor in early childhood stress and development later down the road of chronic conditions such as CFS and clinical depression (Kananen et al., 2010). For more on this topic, see *Early Stress and Chronic Illness* in this chapter.

Chronic stress can also impact the cardiovascular, neuroendocrine, immune, and metabolic systems. DHEA is diminished, along with antioxidants such as either Vitamin C or E, and anti-inflammatory cytokines. All of these factors may have bearing on a person's well-being and *possible development of depression.*

Other factors in the *relationship between depression and stress* may include depletion of the neurotransmitter levels of dopamine *(needed for pleasure)*, serotonin *(the feel good neurotransmitter)*, and norepinephrine. Of course, genetic predisposition and hormonal imbalances of the individual affect personal reaction to stress and *susceptibility to depression.*

Changes in cortisol levels - the main *glucocorticoid* - can result in changes in neurotransmitter levels of serotonin and dopamine which can, in turn, lead to *depressive symptoms.* Healthy neurotransmitter levels are critical to well-being.

The result of on-going stress can be cellular damage and physical illnesses. It has also been implicated in other chronic conditions where depression has not been diagnosed, but may have similar outcomes.

A New Theoretical Model of Depression

It could also be that in the future, the depression model may be better classified as a **whole body condition**, as opposed to a mental health disorder.

Included in this **proposed reclassification of** depression would be acknowledging that **specific interlinked biochemical processes** may play a role in the pathogenesis of stress-related depression, which itself may occur incidentally with other possible comorbid stress-related conditions such as Type II Diabetes, stroke, metabolic syndrome, cardiovascular disease, Alzheimer's, and accelerated aging.

*"A telomere is a repeating DNA sequence. ... telomerase, also called telomere terminal transferase, is an enzyme made of protein and RNA subunits that elongates chromosomes by adding TTAGGG sequences to the end of existing chromosomes. ... if telomerase is activated in a cell [vs. cellular aging or senescence], the cell will continue to grow and divide" (Aten, Kuo, & Questell, 2007).

Chronic stress has been implicated in the development of clinical depression (Zuckerman, 1999). Chronic stress can lead to high cortisol levels that may up-regulate the HPA axis. It is becoming clearer how much chronic stress plays in the unfolding of disease, or, rather, how we – or our bodies – react to chronic stress.

If we remember the field of psychoneuroimmunology, and the interplay of brain, body, and psyche, we may begin to see how every system in our body is interconnected, and how the breaking down of a system would affect our entire being.

Zuckerman states "stressful events play a key role in the development of mood disorders." In fact, Zuckerman says that "nearly every study relating negative life events to the onset of depressive episodes finds that there is an excess of such events occurring prior to the depressive episode as compared with their incidence in non-depressed control groups" (p.187). Stressful or traumatic events are implicated in the onset of CFS as well, and may lead to kindling. We will discuss this concept again more coming up here soon.

We've said that telomere cells are very important. Why? Because they are like the tip of a shoelace in that they keep our chromosome structures from unraveling (**like Zeb's stripes in the graphic**). Thus, telomeres help protect our genetic information. We also know that telomeres get shorter overtime for various reasons. In fact, leukocyte telomere shortening has been observed in *non-depressed individuals* due to oxidative stress which can damage enzyme telomerase in certain cells.* If a similar result is found in *stress-related depression*, then depression may be linked to the same biochemical pathways that lead to **whole-body diseases**.

Potential Treatments and Interventions for Depression within the New Model

Potential treatments and interventions mentioned in conjunction with the theoretical model of depression as a *whole-body condition* are varied. Some methods would include lifestyle interventions such as stress management, behavior change therapy, mind-body habits, exercise therapy, and environmental enhancement.

*"Cellular aging, or senescence, is the process by which a cell becomes old and dies … it is due to the shortening of chromosomal telomeres to the point that the chromosome reaches a critical length" (Aten, Kuo, & Questell, 2007). http://learn.genetics.utah.edu/content/chromosomes/telomeres/

Some biomedical treatments are being tested and include supplements for energy or to **boost antioxidant levels**. Other possible treatments include *anti-glucocorticoids, calcium blockers, glutamate antagonists, telomerase activation*, etc. A key point is that any **stress-related illness** may occur at a cell level specific to a given person, meaning that treatments must be tailored to the individual. This is what functional medicine does: it tailors treatments to the individual. It personalizes medicine.

A Connection between Depression and CFS?

It's taboo, in the CFS community, to say there might be a link between depression and CFS. However, there may be a connection between the two conditions in the realm of childhood and adolescent nervous system development. There seems to be a pattern linking childhood stress, trauma, abuse, and neglect to the etiology of clinical depression, CFS, and PTSD later in life.

Although a close connection between depression and CFS hasn't been previously seen in studies, we know it's common for doctors to tell patients who may have CFS that they're *just depressed*. However, as we discussed, clinical depression itself may be headed toward being reclassified as a whole-body condition. And, as I've mentioned, with both CFS and clinical depression, there seem to be similar patterns of **HPA axis reactivity** (up or down regulation) and **telomere shortening** during childhood and adolescence.

What about *auto-immunity*? As mentioned, there is research and expert opinion that CFS may be an auto-immune condition and some proof that clinical depression may also be linked to auto-immunity, which would make sense if it were also a whole-body condition. With both disorders, there have been some reports of circulating auto-antibodies in the bloodstream. Commonly, *immune dysregulation* is found in people who have *clinical depression and/or CFS*. Other possible links include **elevated inflammatory cytokines and C-reactive protein** (CRP).

Thanks go to *Joey, Cari, and Rachel* for the link to a *NY Times* article on treatment of depression. Please take time to read *Post-Prozac Nation: The Science and History of Treating Depression* (Mukherjee, 2012). Joey, Cari, and Rachel are founders of the website *www.AnyTreatment.com* dedicated to tracking, healing, and living well with chronic illness, and helping you find medical information you may need.

Looking back on it now, I had symptoms of a sensitive nervous system and an activated stress response system even as a child: I had severe stomachaches in social situations like camp and school. I always needed to catch up on sleep on the weekends, holidays, or vacation. And I was sensitive to chemical substances and chemical smells. Later in life, the stress of surgery and/or subsequent drug therapy may have put my body's capacity over the edge when it came to adaptively handling stress.

Was I born with a sensitive nervous system or stress response system (HPA axis) or did genetics and/or experience shape how my stress response system reacted when I was young, and how it reacts today?

This may be the most important section in this entire book. There is new research emerging which reveals a distinct pattern of how *early life stress* shapes and conditions the nervous system, i.e., how it perceives and responds to threats in the environment. Early trauma and other stressors in a young life, including the nature of care given to the child - especially experiences of deprivation - may greatly influence the potential to develop chronic illnesses down the road, when coupled with environmental factors.

Chronic illnesses of all kinds are implicated, including not only CFS, MCS, MS, PTSD, FM, and chronic depression, but also Type I Diabetes, Parkinson's, RA, Sjogren's, hypertension, heart disease, chronic pain conditions, and high cholesterol, just to name a few.

Doctors have been telling us to avoid *negative stress*, that it's bad for our health. Turns out, they are exactly right. The twist is that stress of any kind (including social, mental, emotional, physical, and environmental) when coupled with an already conditioned stress response - attenuated by early trauma, stressors, or sub-par caregiving - can prime the body, i.e. set it up, for developing a chronic condition.

 How does this happen? What can you do about it? There are plenty of steps you can take to help yourself, including practicing mindfulness, cultivating coping skills, and a mindset focused on adaptive flexibility.

ritarussell.wordpress.com

Turns out that *early trauma* and/or other *early stressors*, e.g., poverty, abusive household, illness, neglect, poor caregiving, violence, etc., may shape a developing nervous system in such a way that leaves a child feeling threatened and in a *state of survival*. The need to survive day to day often carries with it a feeling of being locked in *fight or flight* mode as opposed to being in a stage of growth and recovery, such as The Relaxation Response mode.

An early stressor, or early trauma, may *condition the HPA axis* to respond in fight or flight (or *freeze*, as *Peter Levine* points out - coming up next in this chapter.) Following the freeze, there may be a latency period when that early stress is reinforced by more stressors, coupled with a tendency to continue to see life as a threat or as something to survive.

Essentially, early stress in life may reduce the **neural plasticity** of the brain, including the stress response system (the HPA axis), and how it responds to stress later in life. Chronic stress - particularly early childhood and even adolescent chronic stress - may also damage or kill nerve cells, and even suppress or switch off genes that are responsible for the regulation of your stress response system.

If this is so, how can one turn on that gene expression again? By cultivating *The Relaxation Response* (coming up in Chapter Four). Also, since the brain is plastic (a strange word to use, in my opinion, but perhaps not in context) then the brain can make progress. See *Mindfulness and Post-Traumatic Recovery* coming up in this chapter.

Finally, it is possible that there can be a stressor that is big enough - say a virus, an illness like the flu or Epstein-Barr, a divorce, a car accident, or, as in my case, a ski accident with subsequent surgery - to push one's **already attenuated nervous system over the edge**. What might happen next? The person may be vulnerable to developing a full-blown *chronic condition*, depending on genetic predisposition.

In summary, early stress can prime the pump and possibly cause susceptible children to develop chronic illness down the road, if/when triggered by a later, major stressor, and depending on genetic makeup.

In this section, we are discussing early stress and trauma among the young, and I want to re-introduce the concept of **kindling:**

> Kindling was originally discovered in 1967 by Graham Goddard while studying the effects of electrical stimulation of the amygdaloid complex in the brain on learning in rats. Similar to the work of Eric Kandel, he found that long-term, low intensity and intermittent electric shocks to their brains caused rats have spontaneous, epileptic-like seizures – even when no stimulation was given.
>
> [Likewise], limbic kindling is a condition where either repeated neurological exposure to a sub-threshold stimulus (i.e. one that does not produce problems), or a short-term high intensity stimulus (e.g. brain trauma), eventually leads to a persistent hypersensitivity to that stimulus. (Gratrix, 2014)

PTSD is a disorder we commonly associate with adults, but one that can affect children and teens as well. Any individual, of any age, who suffers from PTSD may not only relive traumatic experiences over and over again, but **may be conditioned to similar stimuli**, such as a slammed door, which calls to mind the original trauma. Acute or intermittent stressors may then set off a chronic hyper-arousal of fight or flight response and send one off into the land of illness. Chronic inflammation and/or overstimulation can lead to the symptoms we recognize such as Th1 to Th2 dominance, lowered antioxidant levels, and poor mitochonrdrial function (Gratrix, 2014).

It is natural for us respond to and/or remember events that are emotionally charged. This can be a good thing, or in the case of PTSD and other mind-body conditions, not always so desirable. What can we do to help ourselves when stressors present themselves (as they always will)? With both memory and kindling, it is possible for us to *train our brains* to concentrate on creating positive pathways and memories. See PTSD coming up in this chapter for discussion of what might create PTSD and what you can do about it.

Concepts known as *attachment** and *self-regulation* may also play roles in how the nervous systems of genetically susceptible individuals may respond to their environments as children and how they may develop chronic illness when they are older. *Attachment* can be understood as the care and bonding that takes place between infant and caregiver for survival. It can also be understood as a deep emotional bond formed between sentient beings.

This early period of care and connection is critical to the infant in countless ways. Yet, we look at the human lifespan and we realize that attachment is so much more than just for infant survival. Attachment is how we find trust, support, emotional self-regulation, even health, growth, and the feelings of love. We all experience attachment with one another, at every stage of life, as we form relationships.

*Attachment is a theory developed by Ainsworth and Bowlby (Broderick & Blewitt, 2010).

Emotional *self-regulation* is eased and assisted by attachment. The ability to self-soothe our own emotions and reactions is assisted by the quality of our attachments. However, if the nervous system is out of balance, it can be challenging to self-soothe. "Because of the prolonged reabsorption phase following fight/flight, a high degree of sympathetic activation reduces the ability to self-soothe and self-regulate" (Porges, 2001). *Note: Activating your vagus nerve through yoga may help you self-regulate.*

Stephen Porges uses the term *sympathetic activation,* which refers to the heightened activity of the nervous system, specifically the sympathetic portion that controls heart rate, breathing speed, etc. The point is that it can be difficult to *self-regulate our emotions and well-being** with frayed nerves and a keyed-up body.

Thus, **traumatic stress** could be the very reason we don't naturally know how to take care of ourselves. Regardless of the difficulty, I wish to underline the importance of practicing self-care in healing any kind of chronic condition. We must practice what perhaps our bodies and nervous systems are not used to, in order to regain equilibrium. As you can imagine, it is vital to teach children about self-care, starting at an early age when the nervous system is particularly sensitive. Also, keep in mind that the nervous system starts developing before we are born, continues to be shaped during the first several years, and is "still maturing into our teen years" (Coppola, Singer, & Ombelets, 2014).

The nervous system is like a spider's web: It can be strong, flexible, and adaptive, especially when nurtured by supportive care-giving (unsupportive caregiving can be a major stressor all on its own). On the other hand, it also can be influenced by stressors that agitate the web (kindling). So, imagine a web is agitated by acute or intermittent stressors. Whether it's the nervous system of a child or an older person, a web that has been touched by stress or trauma is not broken. Let me be clear. *We are not broken.* Webs can be rewoven.

We can continually renew ourselves in most situations, I believe. Practicing self-care and having positive experiences with others can go a long way toward achieving renewal in body and mind. We know the brain is adaptable (plastic or flexible), meaning we can grow and change. As mentioned, this phenomeon is known as neural plasticity.

*Activating your vagus nerve through yoga may help you self-regulate and may affect your microbiome too.

The brain can and does adapt. In fact, *developing your right brain*, i.e., your creativity, along with cultivating The Relaxation Response may help your nervous system heal and find balance again. Why is the right side of the brain so important? For one thing, **creativity is closely associated with The Relaxation Response.** Harnessing The Relaxation Response can change everything. It can take your tightly-strung nervous system and literally allow it to rest and recover from imbalance caused by recurring stressors.

Anything that reduces your *allostatic stress load** is going to help you. Why? Because high allostatic load may hurt your chances of being able to handle future stressors. In addition, when you develop the Relaxation Response you may increase vagal tone, measured by heartrate variability, and find your way back to a vital, dynamic balance.

Further, creativity and touch can help us heal and feel whole again. See *PTSD and Memory* coming up in this chapter. Plus, learn how to become increasingly aware of and foster your mind-body connection, so important because we realize the intimate interaction between our mind, our body, and our symptoms and experiences.

Childhood Trauma and Risk for CFS

The University of British Columbia's Greg Miller, PhD, explored how early childhood experiences influence adult health. In an article by Beth Azar from the American Psychological Association, Miller is quoted as saying: "Early life adversity tunes the immune system to be vigilant for stress and a little **tone deaf to cortisol**, the hormone that helps manage inflammation, so the pro-inflammatory reaction can procede unrestrained" (Azar, 2011). To review what we've said about the role of cortisol, you'll remember that an activated HPA axis is generally one of the hallmarks of clinical depression. An *up-regulated* HPA axis results in excess release of cortisol, which may be a factor in the etiology of depression. At the other end of the HPA axis dysregulation spectrum, i.e., *down-regulated*, is hypocortisolism, which may be a precursor or indicator of CFS.

---

*Allostatic stress load is the physiological cost of chronic stress on the body, coined by McEwen (2000). http://allostaticoverload.com/load.html

In both clinical depression and CFS, research has pointed toward the possible major influence of *early childhood stressors*, i.e., abuse, trauma, neglect, etc., as contributors to the dysregulation of the stress-response system of the HPA axis. In addition, CFS has been linked with PTSD, which also has the biomarker of hypocortisolism.

Actually, it is also known that *childhood chronic or serious illness* may be the single most influential factor affecting telomere length as an adult (Price, Kao, Burgers, Carpenter, & Tyrka, 2013). Remember telomere length has a bearing on protecting our genetic information by keeping our chromosome structures from fraying. We also know telomeres get shorter overtime for various reasons. Shortened telomeres are believed to bear heavy negative influence on our health: http://learn.genetics.utah.edu/content/chromosomes/telomeres/

Let's talk about clinical depression for a moment again since we know early childhood stressors can play a role in its development. With depression, the HPA axis is affected and it up-regulates, which leads to higher levels of stress hormones. As we mentioned, the HPA axis can also get *stuck* in either up-regulation or down-regulation. Scientists are trying to figure out why the HPA axis does this, along with ways to help influence it to balance out again.

Do serotonin levels affect the upregulation of the HPA axis in depression? Or is depression more connected to how the HPA axis may up-regulated due to chronic stress, which, in turn, may inhibit new brain cell growth? The twist is, that serotonin may mediate new brain cell growth. Like CFS and FM, depression is still somewhat of a mysterious condition. It involves a system, and systems require synergistic healing. Mindfulness and MBSR (mindfulness-based stress reduction) have both been effective in helping people with depression. Just like with PTSD, sometimes medication is beneficial and necessary. There is always help and hope.

Please read *Toward a New Theory of CFS* in this chapter for more information. Also see Chapter Four on utilizing the *Relaxation Response* and other techniques to regain harmony in your HPA axis. Lower levels of serotonin can make it harder to respond to stressors such as an infection or even something like exercise. Again, ring any bells?

Did the stress of surgery affect the delicate balance in my brain or body or was it kindling from trauma that created my symptoms? Either way, the result for me was chronic fatigue. In others, imbalance may manifest as IBS, or FM, or depression depending on genetics and environmental influences. Is there a connection between chronic or acute stress and these conditions? *Science and medicine say yes, emphatically.*

And on the energetic level, what role does *joy* play in all of this? Serotonin is known as the *feel-good* neurotransmitter. In my experience, in general, the more you *feel good*, the healthier you are. Joy may put you into The Relaxation Response which is where healing can occur. See *Energetics vs. Genetics* in Chapter Five.

Communication is key to health. Your nervous system needs both stimulation and inhibition to stay in balance and to send and receive messages. When we become out of balance, our body's feedback loops and control mechanisms may be impeded, leading to poor health, i.e. imbalance.

What are your checks and balances? Probiotics? Deep nutrition? Stress Management? Self-Care? Yoga? Community? What does your body tell you? What do your rational brain and your intuitive brain (enteric) tell you to do next?

What is the solution? Start with awareness. Tune in and listen deeply to your body's messages, whatever they may be, or whatever the mixed signals may seem to say. Listen deeply to your body and honor it. It is on your side. See Chapter Five on *Riding the Wave of Health* for details.

To conclude this section, please make note that there is a clear pattern linking early childhood stress, trauma, abuse, and neglect to the central etiology of clinical depression, PTSD, and CFS later in life. We did not previously see a connection between depression and CFS, for instance, but the similar early patterns of HPA axis reactivity and telomere shortening in childhood and adolescence, in both disorders, may prove to be a rich area of further research.

More research is yet to be done, as well, on trauma and traumatic recovery. In the next section, we will explore the identity of trauma by looking at stress, kindling, dissociation, powerlessness, and fear.

As described in the previous section, *researchers* are seeing a connection between *childhood trauma and the possible subsequent development of CFS.*

The absolute expert on trauma is Peter A. Levine. If you haven't read his book, *Healing Trauma* (2008), I encourage you to do so. His companion book, *Waking the Tiger* (1997), is also excellent. However, I strongly encourage you to read *Healing Trauma* first, if you have been dealing with the aftereffects of trauma or PTSD and have experienced a negative impact on your health or life. In *Healing Trauma,* Dr. Levine outlines twelve steps for healing trauma. It's not psychotherapy. It's called *somatic experiencing therapy*, developed by Dr. Levine and it's similar to somatic coaching explained in Chapter Five. I have found yoga to work as well. It releases emotions/memories from your fascia.

I believe it is crucial to understand the nature of trauma and how it may contribute to or unravel the fabric of health and well-being:

"Trauma is about thwarted instincts. Instincts, by definition, are always in the present [moment]…With the full presence of mind and body, we can gain access to **the source of our own energy"** (Levine, 2008).

So what is trauma exactly? It's not necessarily what you might think it is. It is post-traumatic stress disorder (PTSD), but it encompasses much more. *I believe trauma is anything that takes you out of your body, and keeps you there indefinitely.* It's what causes you to *dissociate*, which is the opposite of being *mindful.* Dissociation is a protective mechanism of the central nervous system. When we feel overwrought by stimulation, we tend to fade or withdraw from the stimuli. We dissociate from our senses and life.

For me, as I've related, there were events and circumstances that brought trauma into my life: rape, a ski accident, surgery, abuse and violence in adulthood, etc.

The more I think about it, the more I suspect that surgery was a source of trauma for my body. I believe this was my tipping point that then set my body up to overrespond to other, even minor, stressors. This is a wild concept to me. I was unconscious during surgery. How could my brain have perceived surgery as a threat to my safety or well-being?

For some reason, *my primitive brain* (my amygdala) and perhaps my unconscious mind (my body) reacted strongly to being *put under* and to the aftermath of surgery, i.e., anesthesia wear-off, pain itself, ingesting prescription drugs for pain and ibuprofen for swelling. Then again, the explanation of the trauma might be as simple as just the process of going through surgery and recovery. If you add the notion of *kindling*, it makes sense that my nervous system reached a tipping point.

As for the event involving rape as a child, I only have vague memories of what happened to me with that group of kids. I have pieced together a lot of it, but much of it remains blocked from my conscious memory. I do remember … field, girlfriend, separation, two boys. It's interesting how something I cannot remember much about has had such an impact on my life. It's hard to fight something you can't see. But I can feel the effects in my body. *My body holds the memories* and tells me what it needs to let the trauma of the events be released.

Regarding the circumstances of my ski accident, is it possible that the accident was the result of a spiritual crisis? *Did I push myself so hard I had to fall down in order to wake up?* I most definitely was not present that day. My choices went directly against my instincts. Intuition told me to check my ski bindings, but I brushed it off. I always told people that it felt like I had been *pushed* when I fell. Of course, the logical explanation is that my ski got caught on a ridge of ice. I developed a fear of skiing and I operated from that place of *fear* for years. I also drank coffee that day. So the rational explanation is that my nervous system was on overload and that I was young, inexperienced, and I made a mistake. This is actually the reason I believe. I choose not to condemn myself for not being present that day. Yet, can it be that the spiritual and rational reasons are one and the same, ultimately? I fell down and then I woke up. This ski accident was my impetus, my big opportunity to wake up and begin to live more consciously.

Remember that the body perceives and processes all stress as the same and in the same way. Stress is stress to your body, whether the stress is physical, mental, emotional, spiritual, etc. However, what matters most is not *why* your body reacts to an event as stressful and traumatic. At the end of the day, it only matters *how you perceive stress in your conscious mind.* You are not at the mercy of trauma and stress. They are not more powerful than you. YOU are in control of how you feel.

If it is true that we're more powerful than trauma and stress, then why do we experience feelings of fear and powerlessness and why do we suffer as a result? Suffering is resistance to what is occurring. This notion is at the heart of Buddhist teachings, and I address suffering much more in Chapter Five. But, let's explore further here the two concepts of *powerlessness and fear*, and is there a connection between these states of being and the resulting symptom of *chronic fatigue*?

I believe there are many facets of chronic fatigue: physical, mental, spiritual, and emotional (especially grief). What I truly believe is happening is the primitive brain – for whatever reason – is stuck in the fight or flight mode. In short, it's stuck in FEAR. I do believe it is possible that the deepest level of the chronic fatigue condition *is related to fear and powerlessness*, as well as to their opposites: *courage and empowerment*. Of course, we must always consider the physical aspects: nutrient/enzyme deficiency, having a more *sensitive nervous system*, hypocortisolism, mitochondrial dysfunction, etc. And, as I've said, the physical, mental, emotional, and spiritual levels of chronic fatigue may indeed be intimately related. But, being in a state of fear – for whatever reason – has powerful results on the physical body.

In terms of trauma, many of us may find our relationship boundaries are weak, if fear and powerlessness dominate our emotional landscape. In fact, many of us who get sick easily have weaker boundaries, meaning we easily let into our worlds and energy fields all kinds of people including some with negative and/or toxic energy. We are all sponges for better or worse. Our energy fields expand or contract depending on with whom or what we interact. Think about it. When you allow people closely into your world who have unresolved issues such as an overly negative thinking, substance abuse, or unrelenting anger, you may be playing Russian roulette with your health. In fact, you may be a sitting duck for traumatic and stressful influences on your well-being - unless you protect yourself.

Of course, there are many factors that bear on how we react to stress and trauma, including PTSD, tending toward anxiety, rumination, etc. Plus, how greatly does being an introvert contribute to the way we perceive events? What about being a highly sensitive person? In any scenario, we are never at the mercy of trauma and stress. *Never.* As adults, we always have a choice to own our power and freedom.

According to Peter Levine (1997), there are three scenarios that can happen when faced with a stressful situation: fight, flight, or freeze. In the case of animals, they will sometimes freeze and play dead until their predator has passed. Whether or not they come out of the freeze is uncertain. If they do start to recover, the distinct pattern involves a very slow discharge of their *frozen* energy through shaking, trembling, and crying. Without completing the sequence of discharging patterns, the animal may die.

I've been *emotionally frozen* in certain situations and failed to act. Inaction almost always leads you down the wrong path, I believe. Looking more closely at this as I write it, I realize that being molested as a five year old probably had everything to do with being *frozen* and not taking action. What are you supposed to do when someone much bigger and stronger than you has physical control over you? You freeze and wait it out. Back then, I'm sure that was all I could do.

Inaction in a violent marriage, however, was a mistake and cost me much of my thirties. I should have filed for divorce or annulment after the first sign of violence. However, let me say that my description of my ex-husband's behavior and its subsequent effect on me isn't a reflection of how I feel about him. What I believe about him is what I believe about all humankind. *I believe we are not our behaviors.* Our behaviors are a reflection of what has happened to us, primarily. I don't hold him responsible for my illness. He was a victim of fear and violence in his past. I feel compassion for him and hope he finds healing and his way back to the light. For my part, I've forgiven him.

> *To forgive is to set a prisoner free and discover that the prisoner was you.*
> ~ Lewis Smedes

> *Forgiveness is the first step towards healing.*
> ~ Mark Twain

Remember the notion Peter Levine (1997) calls *undischarged traumatic stress?* When we have frozen memories of trauma, they stay trapped in our nervous system and can cause stress. Our goal is to release negative energy. Dr. Levine talks about the concept of uncoiling the stress response and moving out of the frozen state. FM can be seen as a tight coiled stress response or constant pain. On the other hand, CFS can be seen as a flattened-out stress response or constant fatigue.

I've felt both the coiled and the flattened stress responses because my nervous system, perhaps like yours, can alternate between the two extreme states. And I also know that in both states, stored stress begs to be discharged.

What our body needs or seeks is **dynamic** balance. In medicine, there is the notion that homeostasis is NOT what the body seeks. Fluctuations in health are normal. But the body craves stability, I believe. It craves a steady rhythm – much like a song or heartbeat - and a healthy, sustainable pattern of living.

The body does not rest in homeostasis, or stay stuck in one plane of balance, but rather enjoys a vital, dynamic, energetic balance. This doesn't mean you can't have positive stress, excitement, and challenge. In fact, your mind/body thrives on them. See *Stress, Coping, and Adaptive Flexibility Practices* coming up in this chapter.

Fatigue and pain are signals your body sends, telling you something is wrong. Sometimes our symptoms are also the result of our habits that no longer serve us. Our body is talking to us either way. If old habits are harming your health, retrain your body's landscape! Release those charged or trapped (frozen) emotions. Bring in, instead, *mindfulness*. Yoga and massage are great ways to release frozen energy as well.

Cultivate positive emotions and look at life through a positive lens. **Interpret life as a challenge not a threat**. If you fail to discharge the negative energy, your body may be like an engine running on overdrive all the time. With ME/CFS, it kind of feels like burning out your pilot light or losing your *chi*.

Then again, we never really lose our *chi*. The universe is made up of energy. The universe - one song - *is* energy. There is an infinite supply that simply changes form. It is just about tapping into the supply, or learning *how* to tap into the supply. This isn't woo-woo, it's physics.

In the case of people who have PTSD, their *primitive brains* may be on overdrive, fueled not only by direct memories of traumatic events, but the *kindling effect* of those events that keeps them dangling on the ledge of traumatic stress. In the case of CFS, that traumatic stress may lead to symptoms of chronic fatigue, etc.

When I experienced low energy, I often found myself apprehensive of other's intentions. This reaction stemmed from my past experiences with trauma/PTSD. When I felt this way, I challenged myself to think that I'm *not* different from others, even though I may feel that way in the moment. My body and spirit are endlessly resilient. I tell myself the world is a safe place. I can make it safe by *practicing* boundaries. I also remember I am connected to Source at all times, and I am safe.

How do you practice boundaries? Only let those into your heart - or territory - who earn your trust. Live from intention vs. absorbing other people's energies. Set boundaries ahead of time by telling people what does and doesn't work for you. And you can give warnings if someone crosses the line with you. If they cross the line once - or whatever your limits are - they are knocked out of your circle of trust.

PTSD – Post Traumatic Stress Disorder

Under the label *PTSD,* some 400,000 veterans have qualified for government benefits. The collective term, *Gulf War Syndrome,* embraces many conditions that might lead to PTSD. Considering what US military personnel endured - including being enveloped by dense plumes of smoke from burning Kuwaiti oil wells, absorbing the enormous stresses of war in a desert environment, and being exposed to extreme violence, etc. - it's no wonder many of those involved in the Gulf War got sick and are still fighting illness today.

We are discussing trauma and PTSD here. When the body is exposed to severe trauma, it may react like a rubber band that gets stretched too much. What happens to the rubber band? It shows fatigue and may break. In the body, severe trauma can cause a decrease in cortisol levels. Low cortisol levels are a classic sign of severe chronic fatigue.

As we've discussed previously, severe trauma can remain in the brain and body for a long time. For instance, **as a residue of physical abuse, I am easily sent into a reactive state, meaning my primitive brain startles easily** and often perceives threat, even when there is no threat. This is a normal reaction, one of self-preservation. It is also a sign of PTSD.

Yet, my body also tells me what it needs in order to accomplish the release of the memory. The keys to freedom are all inside of me. How so? I listen to my body's cues about what leads toward lower or higher energy. I try to expand instead of contract. I let my symptoms guide me to health. I practice yoga to release trauma. See Chapter Five for more details on transformation and letting go of fear.

Let's talk about the primitive brain. **The primitive brain is fueled by emotionally charged memory.** This is survival mode, and probably serves a very important purpose. The problem is when we don't have to be in survival mode, but the primitive brain may not understand this simply based on cues from our environment that it interprets as dangerous or threatening.

Trauma bypasses the prefrontal cortex (the modern brain), which is why trauma gets so easily conditioned and remembered. It's like **trauma has a short-cut access to the primitive brain,** or a back-road access. Again there is undoubtedly a reason for this - it can keep us safe in future dangerous events - yet it doesn't seem to serve us very well for everyday living or when we want to cultivate social interaction.

PTSD and Traumatic Stress

He broke my heart and then he broke my body. He knocked me out of bed. I felt nauseous. He slammed me against the wall and I lost my breath. He struck my jaw and the force flung me several feet across the room. I had a purple bruise on my left jaw, which I covered with makeup. I later found out he had cracked my back molar. He pinned me against the bed and smashed my glasses into my face. I had a black eye for days. My sister saw it and I told her I ran into a wall.

I write these words here because they happened. But I leave them here too. There is no room for these memories in my life.

You cannot underestimate the lasting impact of trauma. It can literally trap you in your body for years. It did that for me. When I was living with an unpredictable, abusive man, I felt *frozen* in my body, paralyzed by fear and exhaustion. My body and mind were both racing - literally, figuratively - telling me to get out! But I was indecisive, and frozen if you will. I was torn between what I still felt as love for him and my fear for my physical safety.

Instead of leaving, I fell ill. That was my subconscious solution to a seemingly unsolvable situation.

The **amygdala** region of the brain seems to **remember events that are emotionally charged.** So, one key to interrupting this pattern may be to remove the emotional attachment to old memories and/or current events that may trigger our stress points over and over again. How does this work?

First of all, let's consider the mechanism which may cause us to re-live old traumas. **Current events that may seem unrelated to the old trauma can remind an individual of the original traumatic event.**

When that happens, it may trigger an excessive release of stress hormones. **This release, in turn, can overly-stimulate the amygdala**, which then causes the release of even more stress hormones. At this stage, the body can go into **over-drive, and hyper-vigilance**. Recognizable symptoms may include a racing heart and/or galloping thoughts.

An example of this pattern might be the following: A military service person, severely wounded by a car-bomb in Iraq, returns to civilian life.

However, every time the veteran hears a loud noise - perhaps a car backfires or a door slams - the veteran automatically reacts with hyper-vigilance just as if it were the car-bomb all over again.

The veteran may lapse into an emotional flood dominated by a re-play of part or all of the original traumatic event. Or, the individual may suffer from sleep disturbances, including dramatic nightmares.

Remember, we have already established that PTSD, ME/CFS and FM patients seem to have suffered a high incidence of physical and emotional abuse, whether stemming from war time engagement, home or work life, student bullying, gang activity, economic deprivation, etc.
Trauma is stored in your body. It is stored in your fascia, a crystalline type structure that holds memory. How can we disrupt the pattern of stored trauma rising to the surface and haunting us over and over again? Yoga and massage release emotion stored in our fascia. By releasing emotion and memory in our bodies, and using mindfulness to connect with our breath when we sense danger or threat, we can begin to heal our brains and bodies.

Yoga helps me to literally release stored-up memories and
feelings through physical movement and mindful breathing.
What that means is I am able to return to the here and now.

According to Dr. Deborah Sweet, you want to **reintegrate your memories** in order to release trauma:

> You may not know that the right side of the brain has no sense of time and this is why we experience symptoms of trauma long after the incident is over. Trauma gets **stuck** in the right hemisphere. When we reintegrate memories in our lives, we release the trauma bringing ourselves back into present time where we have more control. (Sweet, 2015, paragraphs 4 & 5)

Research indicates trauma and stress shrink the delicate hippocampus. (McEwen, 1999). McEwen's research on stress and the hippocampus is very enlightening and gives us another reason why brain plasticity is so relevant: **stress can literally affect the structure of the brain**. But so can experiences, practices, and circumstances that are healing and restorative like yoga, connection with others, positive thinking, and most importantly, perception of life. But with that being said, **focusing on positive emotions** and the fact that our brains are plastic (resilient) means we can do a lot to work with the symptoms of PTSD.

According to Dr. Richard J. Davidson, and as reported in Erica Goode's article in *The New York Times*:

> Dr. Davidson and colleagues found that regions of the right prefrontal cortex are active during emotional responses involving anger, fear and sadness. The left prefrontal cortex appears to be more active in association with positive emotions, like feeling enthusiastic and upbeat ... It wasn't clear what factors accounted for the differences in brain activation and immune response, but environmental and genetic influences might play a role. Still ... the findings offered hints to how a person's mood might ultimately affect susceptibility to illness. The right prefrontal cortex, for example, communicates with certain types of immune cells, and stress appears to alter the functioning of a chemical messenger, dopamine, in the region. [Also], the right prefrontal cortex interacts with the HPA axis, a major player in the body's stress system, which in turn is linked to the immune system. (Goode, 2003, paragraphs 6, 13 & 14)

Cognitive Behavioral Therapy (CBT), Exposure Therapy, EMDR, Group Therapy and brief psychodynamic therapy are types of therapies known to be effective with PTSD. **The most success may be seen with CBT**, but try anything.

Dogs can also act as a buffer and boundary for people with PTSD.

Medication may assist the primitive brain and may help control major symptoms that curtail functioning. Of course, I always recommend the natural route like yoga and mindfulness, but you must do what works best for you. Do you whatever will give you your life back, even with a new normal.

In summary, we may be able to reintegrate memories to release trauma. We also may be able to cultivate the right brain to help heal our nervous systems. The right brain governs much of our self-regulation. When we can self-regulate our emotions we feel healthier, more balanced, and less reactive. To cultivate creative abilities, consider such activities as drawing, painting, dancing, or even listening to music. Engaging in creative activities helps re-integrate our brains and helps strengthen the connection between our primitive brains and our prefrontal cortex, or the modern brain.

The right brain also may be fortified by developing and expressing empathy for others, by engaging in full body experiences like yoga, dance or sex, and even by play and touch. I know I crave touch and never seem to get enough. I instinctively know touch heals my body. Touch (positive, of course) has been shown in attachment theory to soothe the nervous system. I also crave music and can feel it integrate my body. Please see Chapter Five for further tips.

Also, try to keep in mind this potential benefit to your health: by releasing stressful emotions you may notice that you naturally create more positive energy within yourself. For more discussion of this phenomenon, refer to the up-coming section *Hypothalamus: the Bridge between Mind and Body.*

One of the biggest ways to remove the emotional attachment created by traumatic stress is through **mindfulness**. Mindfulness also encourages brain plasticity. Mindfulness has been shown to be effective for several conditions including eating disorders and hyper-arousal in PTSD, among others. While it is still being studied, and has not been studied for PTSD associated with trauma, it may nonetheless be very effective.

Mindfulness and Post-Traumatic Recovery

While some people may fall prey to traumatic stress, others may use it as an opportunity to grow. This opportunity – or growth prospect - is known as post-traumatic recovery. Personally, I've fallen victim to traumatic stress, but I've also benefited from post-traumatic recovery. When I've **mindfully**, or intentionally, been present in circumstances, they have changed for the better. Remember this: **trauma lingers in dark corners, but presence shines a light on fear.**

Mindfulness is most often described as being about *presence, acceptance, curiosity, and non-judgment* of your circumstances. It's about being *open-minded* to your reality, just as it is. Presence = Power and Progress.

For me, I take the concept of *what it means to be mindful* even further: Mindfulness to me is about noticing any pattern I'm in and then observing that pattern from a non-judgmental place. So it's mostly about noticing my patterns but from a place of complete acceptance. This takes away any sense of fear or guilt. It removes the emotional charge and when the emotional charge is erased, oftentimes the pattern just naturally starts to change. You can change just by being present!

Just noticing patterns from an observational point of view is not only beneficial, but comforting to me. I don't tell myself I have to change my patterns, just notice and observe them. Presence = Change.

In addition, neuroscientists are finding that new pathways are the key not only to changing health habits, but in healing psychic wounds from trauma ... and even taming addiction. **Mindfulness is the key that unlocks the door to presence and power.**

Stress, Coping, and Adaptive Flexibility Practices

Adaptive flexibility can be understood as being able to drop a coping strategy that is not working and instead adopt strategies that are effective for one's own unique needs and circumstances.

Let's consider the roles of practices such as mindfulness, self-care, stress management, self-efficacy, mind-body fitness and biofeedback in mitigating the effects of chronic stress in those with clinical depression, CFS, PTSD, or any other type of chronic condition or life event.

We can start by turning once again to the practice of being mindful.

In my life, I've grown into the belief that mindfulness is about being grateful for my life exactly as it is. In fact, I give thanks for blessings, experiences, and challenges I've had. I've learned that the only way I prefer to thing about the past at all is in the **frame of gratitude**.

My goal is to practice awe and gratitude every day.

Gratitude is about waking up to the inherent wonder of your life. You'd be surprised what you can be grateful for … someone's eyes, laughter, gifts, or humor. And when practicing gratitude, you may find it heals your past and fills your life with color.

I have discovered that mindfulness, practiced in conjunction with gratitude, allows me **to make conscious space** for my life to not only **be** what it is, but to grow and flourish into what it desires to become …

Also, to me, there is no better feeling than **being open to the mystery of life**. Gratitude allows me to surrender to the mystery of my life and to explore where serendipity may take me. I feel as if I'm *connecting to the flow* and the grand adventure of my life as it unfolds in each graceful moment. Here is what mindfulness has done for me and what it may do for you as an *adaptive practice*:

~ Mindfulness leads you deep into the core of your existence as a sentient being on a tremendous journey into the mystery of love and being exquisitely alive ~

When I practice mindfulness, it is also my time - through gratitude - to communicate with and/or worship the universal divine as well as the divine within me. It feels good to acknowledge all of life and to honor my own life. **I consider it self-care.** Mindfulness keeps me present, and presence is how I feel connected to Source, mystery, and power.

Here are additional, specific adaptive flexibility practices which may help you to engage in living mindfully:

Shine your light. Think positive thoughts. That which we shine a light on is not only illuminated, it is also diminished in its power if it is dark energy.

Acknowledge your past in Gratitude. Any situation is an opportunity to learn and grow. That which we acknowledge loses its power over us, including the possibility of diminishing traumatic stress. Live in the Now.

Build new memories. If we keep building new, positive memories instead of lingering on old, traumatic ones, our brains, lives, and our nervous systems have a fighting chance of healing.

In the end, mindfulness may help you cope with what affects or has affected you. Perhaps we can't erase all old memories, but we can create new ones to ease the pain of the old, and *give precedence to the memory of health.*

In fact, mindfulness, in its original meaning, denotes a **lucid state of being**. "Mindfulness, as a state of being, originally referred to a lucid awareness of what is occurring in the phenomenological world or development of one's own memory" (Chiesa, 2013).

Further, *memory* or *remembrance* can be defined as an "understanding of what is occurring outside of conceptual or emotional classifications" (Chiesa, 2013). I interpret *emotional classifications* as referring to how one perceives life. When it comes down to it, how we perceive life is everything. Perhaps it's not so much genes or environment, as it is ultimately how we *interpret experiences and circumstances* that matters most.

Even more so, when we "let go" of our anxiety, we can relax into a creative way of being. "By yielding to the right, creative side of the brain we actually restore balance in the brain. This allows access to the mind-body connection to [aid in healing]" (Mackenzie, 2006).

Another coping and adaptive flexibility practice which might help you move into traumatic recovery is **stress management**, which is under the umbrella term of self-care. Once again we must take into account the idea of *perception*. Remember, we said that *how we perceive life* is critical to our health. So, how do you perceive stress? Is it possible that the cultivation of *eustress*, and by that I mean positive stress, can help you interpret stress as an opportunity to grow?

> Can our perception of stressors influence one of the main stress-response systems in the body, that is the HPA axis, or even influence the experience of traumatic stress as being experienced or even re-interpreted as traumatic recovery? (Broderick & Blewitt, 2010)

Here is *Herbert Benson's* take on stress, as described in *Outside Magazine's* article, *The 5 Step Self-Improvement Overhaul*:

> Stress inspires performance and efficiency," says Herbert Benson, professor at Harvard Medical School and founder of the Mind/Body Institute. "But," - and here's the catch - "only to a point." Benson studied that point for 36 years to understand the dynamics that underlie human stress, relaxation, and aptitude. What he found is that by pushing ourselves to the brink of a freakout, then retreating to a calming activity, we can induce a transformative relaxation response that propels us to the height of our capabilities. When stress sets in as we begin a challenging endeavor, hormonal releases lead to improved focus and creativity. Push too hard for too long, however, and you'll pass a critical juncture and go from feeling motivated and alert to anxious and incapable.

But stop just short of the crash and turn to a mellowing activity - exercise, artwork, whatever works for you - and you'll kick off a biochemical reaction that delivers a momentary buzz and new insights, followed by a period of lasting superior performance. "You want to get as close as possible to peak stress levels," says Benson, who details the strategy in The Breakout Principle (Scribner). "With enough trial and error, you'll learn where that place is." (Skolnick, 2007)

Self-efficacy is another coping mechanism and adaptive flexibility practice. A sense of **self-efficacy** refers to the degree of **confidence** a person has in his/her ability to get things done. In short, it is confidence in one's self and abilities. How we feel in both body and mind can have influence on our sense of self-efficacy. Thus, **the way we manage stress** can be a source of greater or less self-efficacy.

Individuals who focus on both psychosocial experiences as well as health behaviors "may see an increase in adaptive flexibility" (Bonanno, Papa, Lalande, Westphal, & Coifman, 2004) and a decrease in the effect of sensitization to chronic stress that can play a role in the development of disorders such as clinical depression, CFS, and PTSD. Also see the informative article in Harvard Medical Health Letter (Understanding the stress response, 2011). *Consider the following definitions:*

"Stress is defined as stimulation - as too much or too little" (Moore & Tschannen-Moran, 2010). Feeling "stressed" is feeling out of control. Perceive control and shift your reality and experience of what is "stressful" into what can propel you forward.

Eustress can be defined as a sense of calm and mastery. It could also be described as flow, where one's skills match one's challenges, i.e. stressors in this study (Csikszentmihalyi, 1990).

Self-efficacy (Bandura, 1997) *can be defined in the following ways:*
"Believing one has the capacity to be successful in future endeavors based on modeling or vicarious experiences, physiologic or affective states, verbal persuasion, or having the confidence to know one will be successful based on previous, mastery experiences" (Moore & Tschannen-Moran, 2010).

The HPA axis is known to be affected by stress (including oxidative, inflammatory, and psychological) which can result in dysregulation of the axis - either hyper or hypo activation of glucocorticoid (GC) receptors - also known as hypercortisolemia.

Does our perception of stress affect telomerase activity in the neuro-immune system or stress-response system? Does our degree of self-efficacy alter HPA axis reactivity or the telomerase maintenance system? What roles do self-efficacy, positive eustress, health behaviors, and psycho-social factors play in traumatic recovery?

Voluntary participation in activities such as biofeedback, cultivation of positive emotions, engaging in physical exercise, seeking social support, and other forms of stress management may improve self-regulation of emotions and self-efficacy. Increasing eustress and self-efficacy, in turn, may affect the equilibrium of the HPA axis and result in telomerase maintenance and stabilization or reversal of symptoms in conditions such as PTSD, clinical depression, and CFS.

Finally, although much theory does suggest it is helpful to allow oneself to process a traumatic event, there is also empirical evidence that it may be healthier to focus on optimism, to engage in distraction from the traumatic event, and to just look forward to the future.

There is hope. *There is always hope.* Those who hurt you bear karma, which is not your business. You are not the abuse, the violence, or the angry words of others. Detach from suffering.

Your heart is cocooned in metamorphosis. Your body is wrapped in angels' wings. Your soul flies on the wings of transformation. Fly home.

Mind, Body, Spirit and Your Health

Your mind, body, and spirit might operate, in synch and in balance:
awareness (mind), wholeness (body), and peace (spirit)
Balance is not life balance. Life is unpredictable. When you live on the edge of your potential, you are not always in balance. However, you can be in balance with routines that keep you focused such as meditation, spiritual practice, or mind-body fitness such as yoga.

Balance is the feeling you get when your body, mind, and spirit are synched up in unison. It's when you realize you are living at your highest potential and are genuinely psyched to be alive. It's the sense of peace that floods your spirit when you see early spring shoots coming from the ground and reaching toward the sun.

The balance and web of mind, body, and spirit is hugely important. In fact, realizing this connection can be a major **game changer** for you in mastering your health. Why? Because **well-being is mind, body, and spirit**. All three must be activated and in balance so that health can flow. Also, you can affect well-being by touching just one area of the web: mind, body, or spirit.

Let's focus on just **mind and body**. Mind and body may, in fact, be the same entity. Most neuroscientists would disagree. They say we have a brain, which they study, but not a *mind*. Yet there are many people, including myself, who have experienced the mind as separate from the brain. Even the famous neuroscientist, *Candace Pert,* who wrote *Molecules of Emotion* (1999) believed in a **mind-body field**. She theorized that our bodies are our subconscious minds (Pert, 2004). What did Pert mean? I believe she meant that the thoughts we think subconsciously - are actually the body itself. Your "sub-conscious mind" is what your body "thinks." This process is intuitive, automatic, and primal. Please see Chapter Five for further discussion.

While that alone is a heady topic - your body is your subconscious mind - our focus here is on the interface between mind and body, which includes your brain, in my opinion. What is that interface? What balances energy?

Focus on the Hypothalamus: A Bridge between Mind and Body?

The hypothalamus contains **oligodendrocytes** (which form myelin), **microglia** (immune cells), and can activate inflammatory signals in response to stimuli (Thaler, Choi, Schwartz, & Wise, 2010). What role does chronic inflammation play (stimulated by irritants or chronic stressors) in conditioning the hypothalamus to potentially activate the brain's immune system, and even lead to chronic brain immune activation? Is this similar to the concept of kindling? In addition, since the hypothalamus is also the emotional center of the brain, what role does it play between mind and body? What role does it play in energy balance and homeostasis?

> Rigorously evaluating the progression of the inflammatory signaling cascade within specific hypothalamic cell types is a key next step towards resolving the paradox surrounding the effect of inflammatory signaling on energy homeostasis. (Thaler, Choi, Schwartz, & Wise, 2010)

The hypothalamus is part of several axes and there are multiple axes in the body. Three of them are the hypothalamus-pituitary-adrenal axis, the hypothalamus-pituitary-thyroid axis, and the hypothalamus-pituitary-gut axis.

(Image: Marc Baron, Clker.com)

Its role may be crucial in signaling the brain's immune system to **chronically activate** in response to chronic inflammation, fueled by stimuli and stressors.

The hypothalamus "transforms emotional response into physical response" (Mackenzie, 2006). It's the emotional headquarters in your brain. Is it the gateway to your physical body? What is the mind-body exactly anyway? Is it one and the same or are the two just linked? See Chapter Five for details.

As a possible bridge, or gatekeeper, between emotion and physical response, the hypothalamus plays out this role through *neuropeptides* that communicate perceptions, or emotions, between your brain and your body, including your gut, organs, and immune system. Remember that neuropeptides, made famous by Candace Pert, are chemical messenger hormones.

> Molecules known as neuropeptides link our thoughts and emotions to every part of our bodies…our thoughts and emotions can even switch genes on and off [and] can cause new areas of growth in our brains, which eventually leads to changes in our bodies. The entire body is actually hardwired to feel every emotion. (Hamilton , 2008)

Here's a further clue to contemplate based on our current conversation:

~ *Your hypothalamus controls your energy levels* ~

This clue may be hugely important for those battling chronic fatigue.

The hypothalamus also manages your appetite, digestion, body temperature, body fluid balance, blood sugar, adrenals, lungs, heart, in fact the entire circulatory system, and reproductive functions. Your hypothalamus is the main link between your nervous system and your endocrine system (read: *psychoneuroimmunology* or PNI.) It is an "essential mediator of the sickness response" (Thaler, Choi, Schwartz, & Wise, 2010), which may lead to a **negative energy balance** (more coming up on this subject in this chapter).

Your hypothalamus communicates with your pituitary gland and works hard to coordinate circadian rhythms, **homeostasis**, hormones, etc. It is profoundly connected with other parts of your brain, including your limbic system (read: the emotional and primitive brain which includes the amygdala), sensory regions, autonomic zones, and cerebral cortex, to name some areas of the central nervous system.

The hypothalamus is responsive to light and scents. I have been light-sensitive for years, and my sense of smell has also been heightened. Additionally, the hypothalamus is alert to the presence of *cytokines*, which is important because cytokines can damage the hypothalamus. It also has sensing neurons that may detect leptin, insulin, ghrelin, glucose, and micro-organisms.

Finally, the hypothalamus is a **major player** in the **stress response system** and **controls long-term reaction to stress**. In fact, it is the main control center for the stress response of your neurotransmitters, glands, hormones, etc., and actually acts to counterbalance stressful events by releasing serotonin, an inhibitory neurotransmitter. The amygdala is the body's internal alarm system, and the hypothalamus communicates with the amygdala. When we're out of balance in any way, the hypothalamus can become stuck on *up or down-regulation regulation*. If the hypothalamus is gatekeeper between body and mind, how does the hypothalamus interpret signals from stressors and communicate with the rest of the body? How may inflammatory signaling from the hypothalamus contribute to symptoms?

> Inflammatory signaling in the hypothalamus as an essential mediator of the sickness response … rigorously evaluating the progression of the inflammatory signaling cascade within specific hypothalamic cell types is a key next step towards resolving the paradox surrounding the effect of inflammatory signaling on energy homeostasis. (Thaler, Choi, Schwartz, & Wise, 2010)

As mentioned, "inflammatory signaling in the hypothalamus [is] an essential mediator of the sickness response –the anorexia, cachexia, fever, inactivity, lethargy, anhedonia and adipsia that are triggered by systemic inflammatory stimuli and promote negative energy balance" (Thaler, Choi, Schwartz, & Wise, 2010). Is this "sickness response" (which we will be discussing further) just another word for CFS? Research says no (Morris, Anderson, Galecki, Berk, & Maes, 2013), but there may be more of a link than current research suggests. In kindling, the amygdala may remain *stuck on red alert*. Yet, what role does the hypothalamus play in this process and the subsequent symptoms of fatigue, brain fog, etc.? What is the interplay between emotions, chronic stressors and irritants, and the subsequent chronic inflammation that the hypothalamus may signal to the brain's immune system to stay chronically activated? Is there any similarity to limbic kindling, which also includes a hypersensitivity to stimuli? Which comes first? Chronic inflammation or hypersensitivity? In any case, how does one ***recondition the immune and/or stress response system*** that is chronically activated? If hypersensitivity, it could be due to the innate SPS trait.*

> Always keep in mind that there is a beautiful inter-play unfolding in your bodymind and within your spirit at this very moment. May you continue to experience an exquisite set of feedback loops that create a lush landscape and full symphony of health within you.

> The hypothalamus obeys commands of the amydala and insular … chronic activation of the amygdala can lead to high cytokine levels, mitochondrial dysfunction, latent virus re-activation, excess of nitric oxide, oxidative stress, more allergies and sensitivities, including hypersensitivity of the nervous and immune systems. [The point is to get back into] balance so the body can get into the self-healing process. (Gupta, 2015)

*See page 204 for much more information on the SPS innate trait and Highly Sensitive Persons (HSP's)

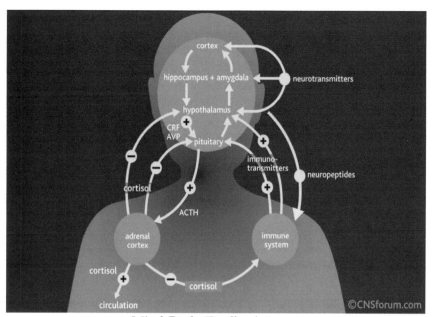

Mind-Body Feedback Loops

Mind-Body Feedback Loops image used by courtesy of CNSforum.com

Your Nervous System and Stress Response System

As you may notice, a lot or all of the conditions we have been talking about have one thing in common: your nervous system. *The nervous system is the first thing to develop in your mother's womb.* A healthy nervous system that develops when you are young is, I believe, a big part of what keeps you well.

Your nervous system also influences all other systems in your body, as well as all of your organs, glands, and tissues. When you realize the *power* of a balanced nervous system, you begin to see how imbalances can lead to Parkinson's, Alzheimer's, CFS, MS, etc.

Perhaps you are familiar with the various nervous systems:

Central Nervous System (CNS)

 Brighthub.com

Peripheral Nervous System (PNS)
sensory division of PNS
motor division of PNS

Somatic Nervous System (SNS)

Autonomic Nervous System (ANS)
sympathetic division of ANS
parasympathetic division of ANS

Enteric Nervous System (ENS) -
neurotransmitters in the gastrointestinal
system

Here is a detailed look at how the intricate architecture of nerves is laid out in the body:

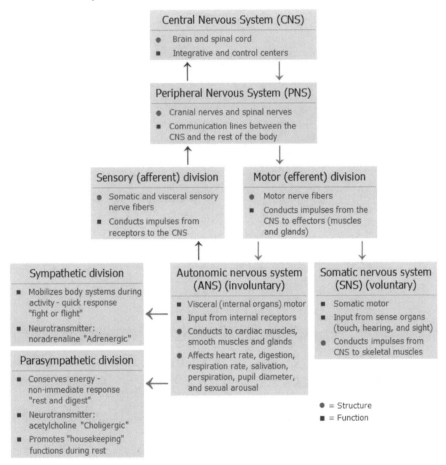

Nervous System Flow chart used by courtesy of My-MS.org

A nervous system's information is communicated through feedback loops to organs, glands, tissues and cells by the hormonal system. Thus, we are made aware, once again, of the intimate connection between the hypothalamus, pituitary, and adrenals, not to mention the immune system, central nervous system, and psyche!

The **sympathetic and parasympathetic** are divisions of the *autonomic nervous system* (automatic - beyond conscious control.) The sympathetic division is activated during stress, even positive stress, known as **eustress.** It then increases heart rate and blood pressure and can even halt peristaltic action in your digestive tract. Sound familiar?

When the parasympathetic division is activated, you move into rest, your appetite may return, and your heart rate and blood pressure tend to go down. Also, the immune system may have a better chance of reaching homeostasis, which can be due to a reduction of and regulation of inflammation by your vagus nerve.

Your SNS and PNS have opposite functions, yet work in synergy together. This is the point of recovery: to achieve balance again, and synergy between two opposing forces. This is one of the main goals, I believe: to recondition your nervous system, slowly over time, so it reaches dynamic balance.

To help activate the parasympathetic division, try **slow, deep breathing** (try even to hold your breath a few seconds on the inhale and exhale). You will activate your vagus nerve, which starts in your brain and travels all the way down to your organs. It releases a neurotransmitter known as acetylcholine, which tells your body to relax. Stimulating your vagus nerve through slow, deep breathing calms your hypothalamus along with your entire stress response system. You can then move from fight or flight, or the sympathetic response, to rest, relax, and digest, or into the parasympathetic state.

Other ways to enjoy the parasympathetic state are: yoga, and any type of meditation such as sitting, gazing at a candle, or walking. Other helpful parasympathetic activities are enjoying music, making love, or anything that is repetitive and puts and keeps you deeply in the present moment. One of the most popular is looking at baby animals on the web (especially cats!). Any of these actions, or others like them, may change your physiology and deliver you **transformative moments**. What a gift. As I have mentioned, the parasympathetic state is also known as The Relaxation Response.

What may be the most important point in all of this, however, is the function of the **vagus nerve** in calming your stress response system. The vagus nerve is one of the main components of the parasympathetic state. It travels from your brainstem all the way down to your stomach, and into other organs such as your heart, lungs, GI tract, and pancreas.

If you look closely at that last sentence, you see how chronic stress may affect all these organs and systems in your body. The vagus nerve also communicates with your immune system, and plays a role in decreasing inflammation by encouraging the HPA axis to release anti-inflammatory cortisol. There are many reasons to **activate and heal your vagus nerve** and **restore vagal tone.**

I believe it is one of the primary keys to feeling better.

As I mentioned earlier in this chapter, when your autonomic nervous system (ANS) is dysregulated, or out of balance, it may lead to the formation of chronic conditions.

This phenomenon can occur because of interplay between **biology and biography**. Think of **biology** as your genetics, and **biography** as your environment, including how you perceive stressors in your environment.

Recall the field of **epigenetics**, which includes factors **above or beyond genetics**. It has been shown by research that our thoughts, which are translated into emotion and then translated again into physical response, can and do influence our biology, i.e. our genetics.

How can this be if the stress response system is part of an automatic response system, i.e. seemingly beyond our control?

Some bodily processes *are* beyond our control. However, our thoughts are in our control. And since everything is interrelated - mind and body - we have more control over how we perceive stress, and even in deciding to allow it into our lives, or not, than we may realize.

To me, the nervous system seems like a violin: some of us are the high notes and some of us are the low notes. Perhaps high and low notes could be compared to the chakra system (see Chapter Five).

Here's the thing: We all - *and everything* - balance each other out.

Perhaps those of us who vibrate at the high notes (HSP's, etc.) are already strung very tightly, and vibrating at an already very high level (note: I don't mean we are "high strung" nor better than anyone else).

Perhaps extra pressures of stress, stimulants, trauma, viruses, sugar, etc. may cause us to reach critical mass, i.e., get stuck in the stress response. This may, in turn, manifest as pain and/or fatigue.

In turn, the pain/fatigue may block the free flow of energy throughout the meridian system. See Chapters Four and Five for details on meridians and your energetic body.

The Sickness Response:
CFS, Autism, Depression, and Fibromyalgia

"Sufficient evidence is now available to accept the concept that the brain recognizes cytokines as molecular signals of sickness" (Dantzer, 2009).

The **sickness response** is a non-specific immune response to stress that is activated via the **brain-immune loop** designed to fight infection. So, your brain and your immune system are connected, and signal one another through a bi-directional feedback loop. To be clear, we already have reported that hormones affect neural activity and vice-versa, as has been proposed by traditional PNI - psychoneuroimmunology. Now we can add that the **immune system seems to affect neural activity** and vice-versa, meaning there is a bi-directional loop involved.

Everything is interconnected and behaves as such, both on the micro levels, in your body, and on the macro levels, in the universe.

Symptoms of the sickness response include many of the same found in M.E./CFS such as: fever, less appetite, increased release of cortisol, pro-inflammatory cytokines, altered liver response, neuroendocrine changes, added anxiety, sleeping more, and, yes, lower energy levels.

Medical professionals have usually considered the sickness response as being par for the course, meaning it was nothing major to worry about. Today we are critically examining the phenomenon of the sickness response and what may be really going on.

The sickness response is activated by **signals from your hypothalamus**. As we've been discussing, explorations into the role the hypothalamus plays in ME/CFS, PTSD, and even RA and FM may be extremely relevant to mitigating these conditions.

Additionally this process involving the sickness response seems to be connected to depression, and even other forms of chronic illness, according to Dantzer (2009):

> Depression has some very similar characteristics to The Sickness Response, and may be at least in part influenced by pro-inflammatory cytokines, triggered by immunotherapy or psychosocial stressors, or inflammatory disorders ... depression itself can be accompanied by altered immunity, including activation of the innate immune system, further increasing the proinflammatory cytokine load. (Dantzer, 2006)

Not only is there a connection between depressed mood and the sickness response, but there also seems to be a link with the **stress response:**

> Depressed mood produces all the same behavior changes as both the sickness and stress responses-changes that conserve energy and keep people out of harm's way. ... Evidence for connecting depression with the sickness/stress circuitry comes from studies in animals and humans. For example, studies of patients receiving interleukin-1 to fight cancer found that they developed severe depression and, vice versa, people with depression have elevated cytokine levels. (Azar, 2001)

We also know that the sickness response activates your stress response system. According to Steven Maier, stress can literally be another form of infection (as cited in Azar, 2001). In short, stress can make you sick.

Doctors have been warning us about stress for years, although the flip side is that we are often ignored when we don't feel well and it can't be traced to anything *concrete*. We may now have evidence as to why. Is it as simple as ME/CFS really being the sickness response? As mentioned, not according to research, but could the stimuli or irritants that lead to chronic inflammation (that triggers the sickness response), lead to white matter damage and the symptoms found in neuroinflammatory disorders? In my experience, the simplest answer is often the answer. We will discuss this more in the last section in this chapter. First, Blaylock discusses microglia (the brain's immune cells), an activated immune system, and autism:

> You see, the brain has a special immune system that operates through a unique type of cell called a microglia ... These tiny cells are scattered throughout the brain, lying dormant waiting to be activated. In fact, they are activated by many stimuli and are quite easy to activate. For our discussion, activation of the body's immune system by vaccination is a most important stimuli for activation of brain microglia.

> Numerous studies have shown that when the body's immune system is activated, the brain's immune cells are likewise activated ... The brain's immune system cells, once activated, begin to move about the nervous system, secreting numerous immune chemicals (called cytokines and chemokines) and pouring out an enormous amount of free radicals in an effort to kill invading organisms.

> Unlike the body's immune system, the microglia also secrete two other chemicals that are very destructive of brain cells and their connecting processes. These chemicals, glutamate and quinolinic acid, are called excitotoxins. They also dramatically increase free radical generation in the brain ... The problem with our present vaccine policy is that so many vaccines are being given so close together and over such a long period that the **brain's immune system is constantly activated**.

Check out this article on how inflammatory disease may cause fatigue:
https://www.sciencedaily.com/releases/2009/02/090217173034.htm

This has been shown experimentally in numerous studies. This means that the brain will be exposed to large amounts of the excitotoxins as well as the immune cytokines over the same period.

Studies on all of these disorders, even in autism, have shown high levels of immune cytokines and excitotoxins in the nervous system. These destructive chemicals, as well as the free radicals they generate, are diffused throughout the nervous system doing damage, a process called bystander injury ... Vaccination won't let the microglia shut down. In the developing brain, this can lead to language problems, behavioral dysfunction, and even dementia. In the adult, it can lead to the Gulf War Syndrome or one of the more common neurodegenerative diseases, such as Parkinson's disease, Alzheimer's dementia, or Lou Gehrig's disease (ALS). (Edwards, 2015)

Here's the really fascinating and trippy part about the sickness response:

According to Robert Dantzer (2004), "sickness behaviour is mediated by proinflammatory cytokines that are temporarily expressed in the brain during infection. These centrally produced cytokines are the same as those expressed by innate immune cells and they act on brain receptors that are identical to those characterized on immune cells."

However, cytokines don't cross the blood-brain barrier, a fact we mentioned earlier in the section on inflammation. So how do the signals from your immune system get through to the brain? **Via your vagus nerve, and via neurotransmitters called paraganglia** (Edwards, 2006).

Even more fascinating is this, "according to Maier: If I cut your vagus, your brain doesn't know you're sick" (as cited in Azar, 2001). Is it becoming clear? Your vagus nerve plays a critical role in health, along with your hypothalamus. Can yoga alter the course of inflammatory signaling in addition to improving vagal tone (which would be measured by heart rate variability - HRV)?

We still have much to learn about the possible connection between pro-inflammatory cytokine signaling, The Sickness Response, and their potential roles in neuroinflammatory conditions:

> Very little is known about the contribution of immune-cell trafficking in the brain to the activation of pro-inflammatory cytokine signaling and its behavioural consequences, even though this is likely to be important in CNS diseases. For example, depression is a highly prevalent co-morbid condition in multiple sclerosis ... At the basic science level, it must be recognized that research into cytokine-induced sickness behaviour is still in its infancy. (Dantzer, O'Connor, Freund, Johnson, & Kelley, 2008)

Many people who have experienced some type of recovery from ME/CFS swear by yoga. But what if you have *fibromyalgia* and a great deal of associated **pain**? Can you benefit from certain yoga movements? It will depend on trial and error. Try poses to see if you can tolerate them. You may be able engage in some yoga, and most certainly in the meditative aspect of yoga. Tai Chi or Qi-Gong may be a better fit with many of the same benefits, i.e. improved neural signaling, and increased vagal tone. What may be most important to understand about pain is the **role of pro-inflammatory cytokines**:

> In chronic pain conditions, such as fibromyalgia, the assumption that is classically made is that neurons cause the problem. That is, the uncontrolled pain must be due to malfunctioning neurons in the pain pathway. I will offer a radically different view. That is, that non-neuronal cell types called glia may be the root of the problem. Spinal cord glia (astrocytes and microglia) are immune-like cells which release an array of neuroexcitatory substances when these cells are triggered to activate. Key among these spinally-released substances are the proinflammatory cytokines: Interleukin-1 (IL1), interleukin-6 (IL6) and tumor necrosis factor (TNF). Evidence accruing across multiple laboratories over the past decade provide compelling support that activated glia, and their proinflammatory cytokine products, are key players in the creation and maintenance of diverse pathological pain states. This profile suggests novel approaches to pain control where spinal cord glia and their proinflammatory cytokines are the therapeutic target, rather than neurons. (Watkins, 2004)

Watkins also discovered that pathological painstates may be created by **viruses, nerve damage**, and other processes that, again, tap into the glial pathway and release proinflammatory cytokines (Edwards, 2006). The goal is to disrupt the action of pro-inflammatory cytokines or to interrupt their signaling. Cytokine-suppressing drug therapy, lifestyle therapy that cultivates positive habits and emotions, and mind-body fitness may be some such ways.

Adrenal Fatigue…Or?

There is still a grand divide between alternative and mainstream medicine on most fronts of how to practice medicine and what constitutes healing. Thankfully we now have integrative medicine that bridges this gap to a certain extent. But alternative and mainstream medicine more often than not do not see eye to eye, although the practice of CAM (complementary and alternative medicine) shows progress in modern medicine. But, there is still plenty of controversy. For example, there is a debate between mainstream and alternative medicine over whether or not *adrenal fatigue* is a real condition.

Much of the conventional medical community claims there is no such thing as adrenal fatigue. They say that either you have an irreversible, auto-immune, endocrine or hormonal disorder - called adrenal insufficiency - or that your adrenals are just fine. There is no in-between. They do not believe that your adrenals can become fatigued due to undue stress, etc.

Although I tend to relate to alternative and integrative thought, I believe mainstream medicine is right about adrenal insufficiency, to a degree, at least.

Alternative practitioners say there's a range of symptoms in the gray area between adrenal insufficiency and perfectly functioning adrenals: chronic fatigue, exhaustion, low blood pressure, appetite loss, weight changes, dizziness, depression, salt cravings, abnormal sleep and menses cycles, headaches, confusion, irritability, brain fog, cravings for stimulants, and hypoglycemia to name some of the symptoms.

Alternative practitioners **label this fatigue** as *adrenal fatigue syndrome (AFS)*. But, AFS is said to be only an **internet disease** by the public-education affiliate of The Endocrine Society. I am not a fan of putting down internet research. Yet, often, we find only partial facts that paint only part of the picture. Complete facts give us answers we can act on.

Others claim it is not the adrenals alone that become affected, but rather the entire HPA axis. This is the theory I subscribe to, after much research of the literature and first-hand experience. The end result, in any case, is that the body insufficiently produces the conditions needed for energy, and produces a ton of symptoms as well.

There are three types of adrenal insufficiency. The primary kind is a disorder of the adrenals themselves. So when about 90% of the adrenal cortex is damaged and **cannot produce enough cortisol** and probably not enough aldosterone, then the condition is considered primary adrenal insufficiency, which is also called **Addison's disease.**

Secondary adrenal insufficiency is due to inadequate secretion of the *adrenocorticotropic* hormone (ACTH) by the pituitary. In response to receiving ACTH, the adrenals make the cortisol hormone. Cortisol levels and ACTH levels are closely related. If the pituitary does not secrete enough ACTH, it affects cortisol production in the adrenals.

Then, there is **tertiary adrenal insufficiency** also known as
hypocortisolism. Here is Dr. Lena Edwards on this subject:

> Research has shown that the most common cause of low cortisol states is
> hyperreactivity of the HPA axis to the negative feedback induced by
> hypercortisolism. Essentially, cortisol rises, the central nervous system
> responds and acts to lower cortisol, but the control is never removed once
> the brake has been applied. A patient can have symptomatic low cortisol
> without having Addison's disease! (Edwards, 2011)

The condition involving low cortisol is what some alternative practitioners
believe is because of "adrenal fatigue." Low cortisol states may lead to deep
fatigue, but the condition is *governed by the hypothalamus, not the
adrenals.* Recall that the hypothalamus controls energy levels.

Their belief may still serve a role since many modern medicine practitioners
believe there are only Addison's Disease or Cushing's Syndrome and *no grey
zone* in between when it comes to adrenal insufficiency. Please see the book
Adrenalogic, for much more information on hypocortisolism.

About twenty eight million Americans deal with **hypothyroidism, another
major cause of fatigue.** Many people also have what is called **sub-clinical
hypothyroidism,** also not acknowledged by the conventional medical
community, as it is *often not detected.*

Clearly we need to be *open-minded and respectful* of people who are not
feeling well, whether or not their condition is recognized by modern
medicine.

The HPA axis is known to be affected by stress (including oxidative,
inflammatory, and psychological) which can result in dysregulation of the axis
- either hyper or hypo activation of glucocorticoid (GC) receptors - also
known as hypercortisolemia. Does this mean that the stress response system
reaches a new set point after having gone through severe or chronic stress?

We have explored many theories of chronic fatigue and ME/CFS/SEID.
The following section includes some of the main theories and highlights that
stand out to me. While research is still unfolding, immune markers have
been found (coming up) and we are getting closer to understanding, I believe.

Toward a New Theory of ME/CFS

Before we dive into talking about a new theory of ME/CFS, there are two recent events in the ME/CFS community worth mentioning.

The first event involves the renaming of ME/CFS. After careful deliberation, the Institute of Medicine (IOM) has given a new name to ME/CFS: it is now called *Systemic Exertion Intolerance Disease (SEID.)* While I'm not fond of the name or the limited criteria surrounding it, there are some crucial benefits, which are the following:

Due to this name change, it is anticipated patients will receive better diagnoses, treatments, and acceptance. Research effort will increase.

> Beyond encouraging physicians to take the condition seriously, diagnose patients and treat their symptoms, the panel also intends for the document to spur more research funding. As more information becomes available, both the diagnostic criteria and the name are expected to evolve. The goal is to identify markers in the patient's blood or body tissues that can be used both to diagnose the illness and as targets for treatment. Indeed, the report calls for a re-evaluation of both the definition and the name in "no more than five years." (Tucker, 2015)

As you can imagine, this name change should positively affect health policy and clinical trials. Plus, as noted above, the name and criteria may be temporary as we learn more about the condition. All in all, the changes are very good news.

The second major event that happened recently is extremely relevant on several fronts. You may remember that Dr. W. Ian Lipkin, of Columbia University, was part of the multi-center group that ruled out two viruses as possible causes of ME/CFS (Lipkin, Alter et al., 2012). In 2015, Lipkin and a distinguished research team identified distinct immune markers that point to ME/CFS - or SEID - as a biological disease and not a psychological one.

> Researchers at the Center for Infection and Immunity at Columbia University's Mailman School of Public Health identified distinct immune changes in patients diagnosed with CFS, known as myalgic encephalomyelitis (ME/CFS) or SEID. The findings could help improve diagnosis and identify treatment options for the disabling disorder, in which symptoms range from extreme fatigue and difficulty concentrating to headaches and muscle pain. These immune signatures represent the first robust physical evidence that ME/CFS is a biological illness as opposed to a psychological disorder, and the first evidence that the disease has distinct stages. (Lipkin & Hornig, 2015; Lipkin, Hornig et al., 2015)

I have two points to make about the foregoing research. First, a psychological disorder is no less important than a biological one since the brain and body are intimately connected. In fact, isn't the brain part of our biology? I hope so. I'm tired (perhaps pun intended) of people judging others who have mental disorders.

With that being said, although we don't have biomarkers yet, I believe we are closer to finding some, perhaps like hypocortisolism and the immune signatures that Lipkin and his team discovered. I've always felt from my own experience that this was a biological condition. As I've stated, the fatigue was *not all in my head.*

But let's bring it back to the positive as we explore more about what a new theory of ME/CFS may look like. We've made real progress as of late. Part of that progress is remembering the roles **brain plasticity** and the **application of mindfulness** may play in recovery from ME/CFS, or for anyone facing any chronic condition or any life circumstance.

In fact, we have many skills and tools at our disposal. Mindfulness (Hölzel, Lazar, Gard, Shuman-Olivier, Vago, & Ott, 2011), positive psychology, and neuroplasticity (Shaffer, 2012) show such promise on so many fronts including health and well-being, memory, learning, relationships, self-acceptance, and much more. **This is the era of neuroscience and we're edging toward the era of mind-body medicine.** Further, the study of the microbiome is a whole new frontier of medicine.

We're making strides in alternative, integrative, and mainstream medicine. I'm hopeful for our healthcare system, although it's currently far too complicated. Mostly, we need to take responsibility for our own well-being. This is one gift of facing a chronic condition: it gives you the opportunity to become conscious of your life and well-being. **How can we move toward a new theory of ME/CFS? First, we need to be open-minded to both theories as well at to the experiences of patients.** Here is a theory of CFS by Dr. Richard Van Konynenburg (2003), followed by my own thoughts:

> It looks as though CFS onset occurs when a person with a certain genetic makeup is subjected to a long-term combination of various types of stress. The result is that the HPA axis and the sympathetic nervous system respond to stress by becoming up-regulated for a long time, raising the secretion of glucocorticoids, adrenalin and noradrenalin, and these cause a Th1-to-Th2 immune response shift.
>
> (Something Dr. Sternberg didn't discuss, but which I think comes into play, is that there is a depletion of glutathione, partly as a result of oxidation of some of the adrenalin and noradrenalin to form o-quinones,

which are detoxed in Phase-II using glutathione. Glutathione depletion also promotes the Th1-to-Th2 shift.)

As a result of the shift to Th2, the body does not have effective defense against viral or intracellular bacterial infections. Several ... viruses (such as Epstein-Barr) are present in the cells of the body of most people in the latent state. They become activated and produce infections. The immune system attempts to respond, but is not able to do so effectively because of its suppression by the HPA axis and sympathetic nervous system. In its attempt, it further drains the body's supply of cysteine to make glutathione, robbing the skeletal muscles of their supply, as Bounous and Molson hypothesized. The muscles thus go low in glutathione [and low in ATP?], and the oxidizing free radicals there (including peroxynitrite) rise in concentration, blocking their metabolism and producing fatigue. Later in the pathogenesis, the HPA axis becomes blunted or down regulated. I think this occurs because of a direct attack on the hypothalamus. I don't know whether this is due to toxins, pathogens or oxidizing free radicals, or some combination, but elevations in all of these are known to result from glutathione depletion, and the hypothalamus is not protected by the blood-brain barrier. Even though the HPA axis becomes down-regulated, there is still not an effective Th1 response to attack the viral infections, because of glutathione depletion at this point. However, the down-regulated HPA axis now opens the PWC up to inflammation, and this explains things such as the high prevalence of Hashimoto's thyroiditis and elevated antinuclear antibody. The PWC thus ends up with the worst of both worlds, with no effective protection from the viruses and the intracellular bacteria, or from inflammation.

I think this makes a believable front end to the story of how CFS gets going in at least the ... rapid onset cohort. It remains to identify genetic polymorphisms that predispose some to CFS when subjected to ... long-term stress. I suspect the relevant polymorphisms will be found in... the operation of the HPA axis or the immune system or both [or how about in the liver?] It makes sense they would be located in systems involved in the early part of the pathogenesis of CFS in order to be accessed, and thus to be relevant to increasing the probability of going to onset of CFS. (Van Konynenburg, 2003)

I understand Dr. Van Konynenburg to be saying that HPA axis downregulation comes first, and then inflammation. I wonder if chronic inflammation/chronic activation of the brain's immune system comes first? Also, what about the role of the microbiome and how an alteration of it may disrupt immune and brain function/health?

What about the impact of detoxification on our genetic expression? As we consider theories of ME/CFS/SEID, I believe we must consider irritants, stressors, and environmental toxins, and how they may create chronic inflammation that lead to pathology. Here is Dr. Mark Hyman on the importance of glutathione and how impairment of glutathione production may lead to chronic illness:

Normally glutathione is recycled in the body - except when the toxic load becomes too great. And that explains why we are in such trouble...

In my practice, I test genes involved in glutathione metabolism. These are genes involved in producing enzymes that allow the body to create and recycle glutathione. These genes have many names, such as GSTM1, GSTP1 and more. They are impaired in some people for a variety of reasons. We humans evolved in a time before 80,000 [now 100,000] toxic industrial chemicals found in our environment today were introduced, before electromagnetic radiation was everywhere and before we polluted our skies, lakes, rivers, oceans and teeth with mercury and lead.

That is why people survived with the basic version of the genetic detoxification software encoded in our DNA, which is mediocre at ridding the body of toxins. At the time humans evolved we didn't need more. Who knew we would be poisoning ourselves and eating a processed, nutrient-depleted diet thousands of years later?

Because most of us didn't require additional detoxification software, almost of half of the population now has a limited capacity to get rid of toxins. These people are missing GSTM1 function -- one of the most important genes needed in the process of creating and recycling glutathione in the body. Nearly all my very sick patients are missing this function. The one-third of our population that suffers from chronic disease is missing this essential gene. (Hyman, 2011)

And, here is my theory about what may cause ME/CFS/SEID:
Acute or chronic stimuli/irritants may lead to nutrient depletion and chronic inflammation/activation of the brain's immune system. This may lead to oxidative stress and glutathione depletion, overstimulation of the HPA axis that results in up then down-regulation of the axis, a flattened-out cortisol response, white matter loss affecting neuronal signaling, and resulting fatigue.

When there is loss of myelin sheath, it can lead to a short circuit of electrical impulses. Neurotransmitters transmit signals between neurons, and the way they communicate is electrically. A large percentage of people who have MS also have chronic fatigue. Is there a connection here? Is it due to auto-immunity or lack of diversity in the microbiome? Is it due to a genetic vulnerability to chronic stress, perhaps exacerbated by weak links in their neurotransmitter systems? Is it due to neuronal loss? Is it a certain form or stage of the Epstein-Barr virus wreaking havoc on the central nervous system (CNS)?* Or, perhaps, it is just to due HSP's* being out of balance? *I am certainly not dismissing anyone's experience by saything this either.* Whether it's a virus, chronic stress/stimuli or irritants leading to chronic inflammation of the brain's immune system and loss of white matter - or something else - I believe fortifying the microbial interaction system with fruits, vegetables, herbs and possibly targeted pre and probiotics, removing irritants, and focusing/cultivating positive energy can affect immunity, gene expression and brain plasticity. This is what has worked best for me.

*Please see "Resources" and "Highlights" for more on HSPS's as well as The Epstein-Barr Virus.

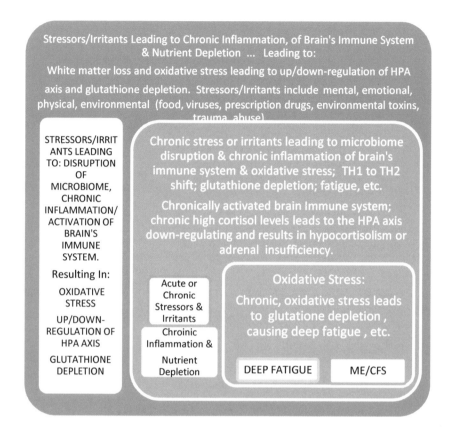

Stressors/Irritants Leading to Chronic Inflammation, of Brain's Immune System & Nutrient Depletion ... Leading to:

White matter loss and oxidative stress leading to up/down-regulation of HPA axis and glutathione depletion. Stressors/Irritants include mental, emotional, physical, environmental (food, viruses, prescription drugs, environmental toxins, trauma, abuse)

STRESSORS/IRRITANTS LEADING TO: DISRUPTION OF MICROBIOME, CHRONIC INFLAMMATION/ACTIVATION OF BRAIN'S IMMUNE SYSTEM.

Resulting In:

OXIDATIVE STRESS

UP/DOWN-REGULATION OF HPA AXIS

GLUTATHIONE DEPLETION

Chronic stress or irritants leading to microbiome disruption & chronic inflammation of brain's immune system & oxidative stress; TH1 to TH2 shift; glutathione depletion; fatigue, etc.

Chronically activated brain Immune system; chronic high cortisol levels leads to the HPA axis down-regulating and results in hypocortisolism or adrenal insufficiency.

Acute or Chronic Stressors & Irritants

Chroinic Inflammation & Nutrient Depletion

Oxidative Stress:

Chronic, oxidative stress leads to glutatione depletion, causing deep fatigue, etc.

DEEP FATIGUE   ME/CFS

So, why did I get sick after surgery? Was there a **breakdown** in certain systems and/or communication (signaling) mechanisms - between my *mind, brain, and body*? Or, was my body trying to just **signal to me** that it was out of balance? Whatever occurred, it's up to me to bring awareness to my symptoms. I try to listen deeply to what my body says at any given point so I make the best choices for my health and well-being. No matter my circumstances, I have chosen well-being.

Overwhelmed? Believe, me, I can relate. But, just remember, you have so much more control over your well-being than you think. Remember, this too: the dark night shall pass - it always does - and the road ahead is full of so much light ...

Madrid at Dawn: Zezao.com

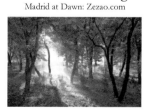

Chapter Four - How I Got Better:
Sacred Energy, Sacred Life, The Lights of Health

You already have the precious mixture that will make you well. Use it. ~ Rumi

What is the precious mixture Rumi is talking about? Rumi is referring to *vital, embodied energy*, also known as *chi* or *prana*.

If you feel you have *low* energy, and you want to get your *chi* back, here are some suggestions: do your best to *release* your emotional energy and *cultivate* your physical energy. Also establish clear boundaries, practice conscious self-care by taking care of yourself first, and manage and reinterpret your *stress* on all levels: physically, mentally, emotionally, socially, culturally, spiritually, and environmentally.

This chapter is about how I got better. It may be a different path for you. Either way, let's start with the basics ... your foundation of health.

Nutrition and Digestive Health

Natural forces within us are the true healers of disease. ~ Hippocrates

Hippocrates is the *Father of Western Medicine*. He believed the body needed balance in order to be well, including balance between mind, body, and environment. What is balance? You find balance when you have a great foundation.

Vitamins and minerals are the sparkplugs of your body's energy and metabolism, and the foundation of physical well-being, along with the all-important amino acids that create a healthy neurotransmitter system.

I believe much of the *chronic tiredness** we feel is due to depletion of crucial vitamins and nutrition, as a result of acute or chronic stress, inflammation, oxidative stress, etc. Such depletion, in turn, robs us of real, sustainable energy.
*Not to dismiss other possible causes like white matter loss, impaired neuronal signaling, etc.

Nothing tastes as good as being healthy feels. Yet the enjoyment of great, healthy food is also so good for you. Even more so, a big part of well-being is ideally enjoying the synergy of a heavenly meal, prepared by an inspired chef.

Nutrition is not glamorous, or a designer pill. However, it was nutrition and lifestyle ultimately - along with focus and faith - that helped me greatly to recover along my journey. Eating right and practicing yoga, as I learned to re-interpret stress, were all major parts in the process of healing for me. In fact, if I had to pick two things that support me to this day, it would be *mindset and digestive health*. They are the combined force of *bodymind* that consistently sets me free.

I have to eat well. Call it fate, luck, genetics, call it what you will. I call it a blessing in disguise. The fact is, if I eat well and avoid, on most days, ingesting anything artificial or artificially processed, then I do pretty well. If I start making poor food choices, I can get sick, or at least feel off which is not enjoyable.

Feeling well is an unmistakable feeling.

It feels like early spring green shoots reaching for the warm sun.

If I eat (and think) well, I feel well, which is really just experiencing the *pure vitality* of feeling vibrant in my mind, body, and spirit.

I value vitality these days. It is one of my main core values. Therefore, even in addition to eating well for the health benefits, the most important reason to me is that I feel better, I feel lighter, I feel more alive, present, and full of radiant vitality. *This is the feeling I covet.*

I value being inspired. Inspiration is what keeps my motor running. What keeps you going? When I do my part to stay healthy and alive, *I am on fire*, and I feel I can do and be anything.

Eating real nutrition is key to living my values: to being vital and feeling inspired.

I encourage you to consider eating well, for the benefit of your health and quality of life. Try to make real, live, organic, unprocessed food your staples. This small change can be the **tipping point** for coveted well-being.*
*Thanks to the amazing Caitlyn Boyle for this valuable tip: http://www.healthytippingpoint.com/

Eat Real Food to Reach The Tipping Point	
Food to Maximize	*Substances to Minimize*
organic foods, unrefined foods, raw foods, cultured foods, fermented foods, superfoods, expeller-processed oils, sprouted grains, legumes, seeds, if agreeable	refined or processed foods, *sugar*, low on stimulants, little to no preservatives, artificial or fake ingredients, irritants to you

Am I suggesting this is the only way to eat? No. What you eat is based on what you need and is up to your physical needs and instincts.

Eating for pleasure is important as well. Check out Marc David and *The Institute for Food Psychology* to find out more about the role of pleasure in metabolic health. You can listen to my interview with Marc David at *The Wellness Coach* on BlogTalkRadio:

http://www.blogtalkradio.com/thewellnesscoach/2014/04/10/speaking-with-marc-david-founder-of-the-institute-for-the-psychology-of-eating

Indeed, perhaps the most important part is to *relax* while you're eating. Yes, it is critical *what* you eat, but your *state of mind* during the meal is also vital. Have you heard about people who seem to be able to eat whatever they want and they are just so healthy? Perhaps they were super relaxed about what they were eating, so they absorbed more of the nutrients. Cultivating *The Relaxation Response* really does make a big difference in how we enjoy and absorb our food, as does eating mindfully and the intention to live well.

Remember: *Your body works on exquisite feedback loops of energy.*

Yet, anyone who is ill may not absorb nutrients as well. Perhaps it is because the digestive system, especially the small intestine, may have become compromised during the progression of your fatigue. And it is the small intestine which may be implicated in auto-immunity. See *Auto-Immunity* in Chapter Three.

However, it is known in medical circles that stress compromises digestion. Many of you, who have ME/CFS, notice this. Remember the hypothalamus controls appetite. If you're stressed by events, your appetite may be shut down. **Stress also robs your body of vital nutrients that contribute to energy like B vitamins, Vitamin C, magnesium, electrolytes, etc**. The good news is the digestive system and immune system can get better. It may sound simple, but it may be profoundly powerful to do your part to relax and stay calm so the digestive system can properly digest and absorb nutrition.

More on Digestive Health

Digestive health is critical. It is the seat of your power, the root system of your health, just like the root system of a plant or tree.

How can we maintain our digestive health? I've never been a big fan of giving things up, unless it's substances that clearly irritate my system. Instead, try to think in terms of amounts or substitution. I think it's important to find foods which may be better for you, to pinch-hit for a food which may not be supporting your health, even though you love it! You may find you like the alternate even more, with a few taste bud adjustments. There are many foods *that taste just as good as they are good for you.* Both aspects of food are equally important, that is they must taste good *and* support your health.

Perhaps over time, you will find you can come back to many of your favorite foods when your digestion is stronger, and *when you have truly relaxed and sunk deeply into relishing the present moment.* Meanwhile, do your best to *relax* and *trust* life. **Amounts matter too.** I have found that deep nutrition with just a ***small*** amount of healthy stimulation (acai, B Vitamins, chia, K. Ginseng) keep my nervous system running more smoothly. This is not my idea, although I have been doing it for years. It is based on the brilliant idea of Dr. Jon Kaiser and I have found it really works! The combo is: nutrients' cellular energy and stimulants as the spark plug that "lights them up" (Kaiser, 2014). You can read about Dr. Kaiser's exact theory* here: http://jonkaiser.com/

Did you know your digestive process can be up to 40% more effective when you enjoy your food? That means if food tastes good to you *and* if you are feeling free of stress (i.e. relaxed ☺) your digestion will run more smoothly plus you will gain the most nutrition from your food. We instinctly know this experience is true. It is also part of the wisdom taught in Food Psychology, along with lessons taught based on a growing movement to look at food from the holistic point of view. Please see *Resources* at the end of the book for information on Food Psychology and how it may benefit you.

Let's talk more about *taste*. Some of the best food I've ever tasted is organic. On the other hand, some food *tastes good* as a result of the unnatural, excitatory nature of how it has been force-grown, processed, and produced. Make no mistake about it: processed food has been carefully crafted to *taste good* to your palate and your brain. Yet many of these types of foods, like *refined table sugar, MSG, and aspartame,* are called *excitotoxins*, and although they may taste good initially, especially when combined with other foods, *they can and do inflict havoc on your body.* Why? Because excitotoxins excite and overstimulate your brain unnaturally, and often artificially … consuming excitotoxins is a slippery slope. Be prepared to face the consequences.

*He recommends mitochondrial nutrients with various stimulant medications (Kaiser, 2014).

Food is a chemical. Once you upset your brain and body chemistry, you are at the mercy of where your body is until or unless it can regain balance again, primarily through breath, sleep, or exercise. Once you ingest something, it literally has biochemical power over your body for hours, if not days. Why take the risk? Of course, none of us live in a vacuum, and we all wish to enjoy life. I get it. But, healing requires making empowered choices. I have found that when I make conscious, empowered choices, well-being follows.

Regarding food choices, you will be forced to tolerate the experience of whatever chemical reaction ensues. That is what happens to your stress response system with excitotoxins like **refined sugar** or **MSG**. Also, by way of comparison, we may experience similar, excitatory responses when we live in a state of acute or chronic stress, etc.

But back to excitotoxins. Excitotoxins also can mess with your delicate neurotransmitter system, throw your HPA axis off-kilter, **may damage your white matter - through glutamate excitoxicity -** (Matute & Ransom, 2012), and overtax your liver, resulting in chronic low blood sugar.

You may enter a biochemical realm where your body is constantly asking you to self-medicate with more of what you consumed: sugar, caffeine, or any substance that irritates your body. Refined carbs can have the same impact on you as well (pastries, bread, etc.).

First of all, it's not your fault, and, no, you're not an addict. The last thing you need is another label slapped on you. It's a biochemical imbalance in your body. And, believe me, I know what it's like to feel the after-effects of choice I have made, like eating chocolate* for "energy."

Secondly, it's up to you to consider not ingesting irritating or refined foods, and explore substitutions like carob for chocolate or quinoa for grains. Consider avoiding white flour, high fructose corn syrup (HFCS), trans-fats, hydrogenated fats, artificial flavors, colors and sweeteners, MSG, and stimulants like refined sugar, and maybe caffeine or other irritants, depending on your chemical makeup. The good news is that there are many foods you can eat that create feelings of *well-being* but without serious side effects.

Refined foods steal away your power.

Refined foods can deplete your nutritional reserves - the **sparkplugs** of your energy. They can leave you exhausted. **Exhaustion is powerlessness,** on all levels of being. If you're not in your own power, you cannot experience true well-being. I explore this concept much more in Chapter Five.

*I use only milk or white chocolate, focus on liver health, and cardamom oil to help process caffeine ☺

There may be a fine line between *health and sickness*. But there is an enormous difference between *vitality and disease*. Many have never experienced true vitality. I wonder if it's a largely unknown state of being due, in part, to numbing our bodies with food grown with pesticides and injected with hormones. Do we eat essentially *dead food* and thus miss out on the true vitality of life?

How can you experience what it means to feel alive if what you consume may promote disease?

For many, eating is recreation. However, when you're facing daunting health challenges, food is much more than recreation. In fact, it may become your primary source of medicine. ***Food is your pharmacy, it your ally.*** What worked for me? *I listened to my body.* It told me what to do and what to eat in order to get better. *I let my body's needs lead me back to health.* Here are lessons my body taught me along the way:

Lessons Learned from My Body Which May Help You
Pay attention to every single thing you put into your body. Does it make you feel better, worse or neutral? Does it give you *real* energy or steal energy away?
Focus on *what makes your body thrive right now.* What makes you feel the best so you can do the most?
Know the difference between *cravings* - which are triggered by malnutrition (like craving chocolate because you are deficient in magnesium you should ideally be getting from leafy greens) - and what your body is asking you for to thrive.
There is a diet custom-made for you and only your body can tell you what it is. Genetic testing can tell you what you polymorphisms are, but your body knows what it needs.
Listen closely to your body.

Let's talk more about cravings. If your body is low in magnesium, you may crave chocolate. Dark chocolate has a higher level of magnesium than most any other food except seaweed. In reality, you are craving magnesium (Sircus, 2009). Yet, if you consume large amounts of chocolate to fulfill your craving, you may be robbing your body of other essential nutrients. I am saying this for my own sake. ☺

Speaking about cravings, let's talk about sugar again. ☺ Sugar competes with a very important energy nutrient: Vitamin C. They have similar chemical structures and therefore compete with one another for entry into our cells. Linus Pauling determined that white blood cells need high doses of Vitamin C. When we consume large amounts of sugar, we may be curtailing how much Vitamin C can reach our cells.

Also, **sugar robs energy - *including electrolytes* - from us**, more than almost anything else. Not only is it considered an excitotoxin that directly impacts the brain, but it is also an **anti-nutrient**. It robs us of vital minerals and B vitamins. Sugar is also *sneaky*. It raises neurotransmitters *artificially high* at first - making us feel great - but then ends up depleting them, leading to an energy deficit that leaves us fatigued, anxious, even impatient. Does this sound familiar?

Refined sugar is not the only type of sugar to monitor in your diet. I also recommend you reconsider *agave*, even though it tastes amazing and is popular as a substitute for other sweeteners. I do make an exception, once in a blue moon, for desserts like the fabulous ones my sister makes! However, agave is high in *fructose*, which is considered a toxin, or poison, to the body.

Free-form fructose is another sweetener to monitor, especially *high-fructose corn syrup*. There is solid research revealing how destructive free-form fructose* can be in the body. Please watch Sugar: The Bitter Truth by Dr. Robert H. Lustig, a link to which is given in the *Resources* section at the end of this book. He is a great resource on obesity and refined foods.

Many of us use sugar or other substances as a means of coping with life. Everyone has their armor, how they make it through the tough times: sugar, wine, chocolate, etc. Instead of **consuming** something that you don't really need in your body, consider **exploring other ways to cope.** Try yoga, Qi-Gong, sleep, love, movies, games, nature walks, creative activities, or *helping others who are suffering.* Let tactics like massage, baths, pedicures, essential oils, or even *Rescue Remedy, L-Theanine, or Lavender* be your release or shields if you are extra sensitive.

There are many healthy ways to cope that can help you to **thrive and not just survive.** Again, this is known as self-care and even traumatic growth for those who have faced abuse or trauma. You can thrive!

*Please see *High Fructose Corn Syrup* in the *Resources* section for information on NAFL (pg. 431).

But let's not focus on what you can't have or don't want to eat while you're healing. Let's focus on what you can or wish to eat so you heal and thrive.

To me, healthy food tastes much better than processed, non-organic food. You will notice that your taste buds may change over time. What doesn't necessarily taste good to you at first may taste amazing to you once your body chemistry evens out.

So, don't write off a food just because it doesn't appeal to you right away. It could be that it's not right for you. But it could also be because your body is out of balance. Trust your instincts and your impulses to try new foods and food combinations. Of course, your food should taste good. It should taste great! But it should be pretty darn good for you as well, indulgences aside.

For instance, *wheat grass shots* taste sweet to me. But, to you, they may taste bitter at first. This could be because your pH balance is off, perhaps due to body chemistry. We are supposed to be about 75% alkaline, and only 25% acid. Many of us are out of balance this way. The more alkaline foods you eat, the more your taste buds will change, and natural foods will taste better to you.

The first time I tried *spirulina*, I took it at night and the B vitamins kept me up. It didn't taste very good to me either. But over time, I have come to appreciate the taste and the natural, sustained energy it gives me is a godsend. Spirulina is naturally high in B vitamins that are so crucial for feeding, maintaining, and building your nervous system. It is also a natural, potent anti-inflammatory. It is one of my "go-to" supplements. I take it primarily in tablet or capsule form these days. But I still take it in powdered form as well. Vanilla also really masks the taste of green superfoods in general. You could also try carob-mint or cacao-mint flavored Spirulina by Pure Planet.

B vitamins in their real, organic forms make a difference. I recommend spirulina that comes from Hawaii, as it also has a higher beta-carotene content (it has to protect itself from the intense sun down there) and it is also fed by deep ocean water to up it mineral content, etc. Plus it is more "fresh" than spirulina from the mainland like California, in my opinion.
My body can tell the difference immediately. Hawaiian spirulina is also high in organic iron and GLA. Spirulina, also stimulates the production of norepinephrine* in the brain which leads to more **real energy** in the body.

*Vitamin C also increases norepinephrine (May, Qu, & Meredith, 2012), and it also fortifies your adrenals. I take natural vitamin C complex for true energy support when I'm "tired." It works well for a day or night-time lift in energy levels for me. I also use 5-HTP for nighttime energy support, as it raises serotonin levels, which can be depleted by stress. It also produces melatonin, the hormone for sleep. Manage high cortisol, as it can lower your melatonin levels.

Why I Love Hawaiian Spirulina

High in B vitamins including *potentially human active B12**, crucial for feeding, maintaining, and building the nervous system
High in Iron & Protein
Great natural source of sustainable energy

Potent anti-inflammatory and abundant source of gamma-linoleic acid (GLA) which may help reduce inflammation

Spirulina helps produce the chemical *norepinephrine* that is *a cousin to adrenaline;* it gives you tons of real, natural sustained energy
without causing the body to crash and burn later

Works as a natural anti-depressant; produces *phenalyanine and tyrosine;* the latter is also an appetite controller

May detox the liver due to high levels of magnesium.
It is also vital to have enough magnesium in the system to convert the Vitamin D we get from UVB sunlight into a usable form.

Rich in glutathione; may assist the liver in detoxing

Hawaiian spirulina is high in organic iron and may have unusually high beta-carotene content since it must protect itself from intense Hawaiian sun.
It is fed by deep ocean waters, which may increase its mineral content overall.
It may be *fresher* than mainland spirulina. My body knows the difference.

Finally, strange as it sounds, one of the things I love about spirulina is its deep, rich color.
Its color has a positive affect on me.
It has what I call blue-green energy, just like the energy of our planet.

As you explore and experiment, keep in mind that your body is unique to you. In fact, everyone's body is unique because it has a specific signature code. This means that different foods work for different people. Spirulina works for me, but it may not work as well for you. You want to figure out what foods *make your body sing,* a beautiful idea expressed by *Ani Phyo,* well-known author, organic chef, and advocate for healthy eating. One of her latest books, *Ani's Raw Food Essentials: Recipes and Techniques for Mastering the Art of Live Food* (Phyo, 2012*)* may help you.

*The B12 may or may not be human active form. Also, earlier research on the benefits of phycocyanin (found only in spirulina and cyanobacteria) includes: preventing liver & kidney damage, neuroprotection, & its benefits as a potent water-soluble antioxidant. The latest research shows that: "phycocyanin may have anti-inflammatory activity through the suppression of nitric oxide, prostaglandin E-2, tumor necrosis factor alpha and the Cox-2 enzyme. This anti-inflammatory mechanism 'may contribute, at least in part, to its anti-hyperalgesic activity.' Hyperalgesia is an increased sensitivity to pain" (Cyanotech, 2009).

Nutritional genomics states that we all have variations or polymorphisms in genes passed down through generations which are potentially triggered by our modern diets, or chemicals in the environment. Different races can have different genetic susceptibilities as well.

Graphic Courtesy of National Human Genome Research Institute

For example: many prescription drugs are metabolized by cytochrome P450 in your liver. Many people have varying polymorphisms of this very important family of enzymes, which metabolize up to 80% of drugs prescribed today (Chhabra, Reed, Anderson, & Shiao, 1999; Zhou, Liu, & Chowbay, 2009).

However, as dominant as our genetics are, there is another powerful player called *environment.* According to Dr. Jose Ordovas, biochemist at Tufts, "the gene is the gun, but the environment is the finger on the trigger. [Gene mutations] have been with us for thousands, or in some cases hundreds of thousands of years, passing from one generation to the next, because until now, our diet didn't trigger any negative effects" (as cited by Kahn, 2005).

As powerful as genetics are, Dr. Ordovas - biochemist at Tufts University - suggests that what we eat creates our own **internal environment** that either nurtures our health, or that may pull the trigger to set in motion our genetic vulnerabilities.

Further, Bruce Lipton (2008) reminds us in *The Biology of Belief,* that the **environment of our own mind** is more commanding than even our very influential genes. This is also known as epigenetics, again which means above and beyond genetics. Deepak Chopra says it beautifully: we can't change our genes, but we can change the way our genes express (Yeanoplos, 2014).

Look, I get it. It can be so hard to change eating habits.

It's really not about giving up most foods as it is about maximizing what your body loves, and minimizing what is irritating. Learn to prep and source food, like I did. I read books, watched cooking shows, acquired a Vitamix, a mini-prep cusinart, a spiralizer, etc. I love raw food like juiced greens, but many foods need heat to access nutritional properties and to enhance enjoyment. *It's about balance, fueled by instinct and passion.* My journey, like yours, is an *on-going process* to find what makes my body thrive and function at its *new normal* and highest capacity. More days than not, my body is now in *harmony.* ♪ It is in vital, dynamic balance by conscious choices I make each and every day, every hour, and even every minute.

The Upward Spiral of Health

I believe it is most definitely possible to feel well again. You may come across a *new normal*, but your new normal might even be a vitality that you've never known before. In fact, it is what happened for me. I was *well* before I got sick, but I wasn't *vital*. There is no substitute for vitality ... embodied *chi/prana* that flows throughout your whole being.

It took time to figure out my *upward spiral*. I did make improvement. I went from being exhausted and sick in bed to not feeling super well, but living life. However, it was obvious that my inflammation remained at chronic, low levels for years.** I was still "stressed out." *I was still stuck living in a place of fear and not living from a place of love, inspiration, and wholeness. In addition, I wasn't getting the deep nutrition I needed, despite eating well, i.e. refined food, top-soil depletion:* "What If The World's Soil Runs Out?" (2012).

What ultimately worked, over time, was real, deep, consistent nutrition and living a life that emphasizes positivity, inspiration, vitality, and dynamic balance. Every day is a bit different, fueled by a desire to thrive, be happy, and live at my highest level and potential. I try to keep "fatigue" out of my realm of thought. I try not to "fight fatigue." I eat well, *I do yoga, I do my best, I try not to stress*, I surround myself with positive energy, thoughts, and people.

Also, what do you tell yourself about energy? I tell myself energy is love, breath, it is electromagnetic, and it is renewable and sustainable.

I've eaten quite well since I was about 20. After I developed chronic fatigue the first time, I educated myself and I ate even better, avoiding processed, denatured food and irritants. My body finally reached homeostasis again. Most importantly, my cortisol levels had dropped and my glutathione levels had risen - and I looked and felt well. *I also realize now I am an HSP (pg. 204).*

With my second episode of illness, I revamped my diet even further, yet I still could not recover. As I've described, the allostatic stress load from multiple sources was just too high from never-ending: violence, sleepless nights, divorce, illness, loneliness, and laser treatments, even too much refined sugar. My stress levels - or reaction to my circumstances - were high, and I believe my electrolyte levels plummeted. I had to ultimately supplement to rebuild.

I had to change the way I looked at and lived my life. It was moving from fear to love and living in creative energy. *It was from eating real food.* It was also *a few key supplements* like *food-based minerals* (see pg. 291), Hawaiian spirulina, and real Vitamin C* that also *helped reset my body and nurture me back to whole once again.*
*Electrolytes (minerals w/an electric charge) conduct electricity in your body: they are electrical energy.
**I actually believe that hypocortisolism is a protective measure by the body to protect one from high cortisol levels. Cortisol can be extremely damaging to the system, and produce many of our symptoms.

There are many supplements that have been god-sends for me. I will be mentioning specific ones throughout this chapter and the book. Specific brands have worked for me so I mention them because **brands and retailers matter**. They matter because there are no uniform regulations on what we consume, so we need quality, transparency, and traceability in what we buy.

Yet: *I never talk about supplements anymore without also discussing food.*

As I've mentioned, it was a combination of things that helped me heal. *One of the biggest game-changers was incorporating raw and food-based supplements. I had severely depleted nutritional reserves, depleted by stress. I couldn't gain the upper hand, no matter how well I ate.* Yet eating real food matters. This is what works for me: live, organic, non-gmo foods, raw foods, greens, superfoods, less processed foods (this requires a conscious effort), as well as time, restorative exercise like yoga and Qigong, community, connection, and *a healthy, positive mindset.*

I was determined to feel better. What did it for me was grounding my body in deep nutrition, keeping my detoxification pathways open and my digestion running more smoothly (with leafy greens, supplements), and anchoring into love, faith, wholeness, inspiration, and connection.

I also had to figure out the best ways to restore good bacteria in my gut, by reducing my stress levels, including how I perceived stress. **High cortisol* levels may affect your gut bacteria and candida levels.** Sometimes we overlook the most **obvious sources of fatigue:** *chronic stress, low electrolytes, low Vitamin C levels,* etc. I will discuss this more coming up toward the end of this chapter. Friendly bacteria as a part of food, instead of isolated in a supplement, works really well for me, although some supplements also work. Some people also follow *The Body Ecology Diet.*

But keep in mind that it was *reinterpreting my stress levels* as well as *live food* and raw/food-based supplements that helped me gain the upper hand. Our reserves can become depleted by acute/chronic stress, which may lead to a compromised immune system, candida, chronic fatigue, and chronic illness.

There are many foods and supplements I use on a regular basis like Megafood food-based vitamins. I also use *CellFood,* and it *raises my energy levels,* consistently. Apparently, it increases oxygen in the body. To me, **oxygen is a nutrient.** Adding Cellfood to my diet is like drinking coffee, but without the side effects. It has added, natural minerals that may help to rebuild and stabilize the body. In the 1940s, *Everett Storey,* invented a proprietary, bioavailable oxygen formula and called it CellFood. Storey's scientific efforts to split water, so that the two gases were released into the body, were acknowledged by *Albert Einstein,* who was a colleague of Storey's. *High cortisol levels can be the result of many types of stressors including anger, irritants, synthetic chemicals, etc.

In addition, *VitaMineral Green* changed my life the first time I took it. I felt my body begin to *reset* itself. It was euphoric, similar to how I felt when I started using *Hawaiian spirulina*. It does take several weeks to months to receive the full benefit of any new nutritional strategy or supplementation, but the initial effects can be a real blessing. High quality superfoods and supplements can offer this benefit, I believe.

*They can **supercharge your cells** and raise your vibration of well-being.*

It can take years to develop nutritional deficiencies. Likewise, it takes time to repair deficiencies, and restore good health. In homeopathic circles, they talk about the healing cycle this way: if you've dealt with a condition for ten years, it may require ten months to make repairs, *in reverse order*. Reverse order means your *body deals with the most recent insult first* and works back to earlier injuries or impurities. I believe the body heals in linear and non-linear ways. Relax and open up to the mystery.

Let's talk some more about adaptogens, which help us *adapt* to stress and help us bring balance to our system. One such adaptogen is holy basil, also known as tulsi, which is one of the most powerful adaptogens, in my opinion, along with gota kola and Siberian ginseng. Siberian ginseng is another potentially great adaptogen. It seems to work for many symptoms of fatigue, as well as different kinds of fatigue, and may support energy levels in general.

I've heard maca works well, especially for men. It used to be too *yang* for me, although my body likes it now. If one is already chronically stressed, it may be best to avoid taking in excessive *yang* energy.

Remember, you want to apply the opposite energy to your system in order to restore balance.

I also love the adaptogen magnolia, one of two ingredients found in the trademarked supplement known as Relora. Magnolia is said to reduce cortisol levels. I take Relora often at night to help keep my body in balance, especially if I can tell my cortisol levels are a bit high.

I used American ginseng as an adaptogen during my first illness. I still love it, but it may have *phytoestrogenic* qualities and/or effects on my liver, which may cause inflammation. However, with Siberian ginseng, holy basil and gota kola, there are no side effects for me, at least.

Another important supplement may be *astaxanthin*. It has powerful antioxidant properties that **can cross the blood brain barrier.** This is especially crucial as the hypothalamus has been affected by, you guessed it, oxidative stress and possibly poor methylation as well. What helps repair or prevent oxidative stress? **Antioxidants. Most antioxidants don't cross the blood-brain barrier.** Astaxanthin has been reported to help with endurance and stamina. This does not surprise me at all when talking about poor mitochondrial function or other symptoms, which may be affected by oxidative stress as it relates to those with ME/CFS and other chronic conditions.

One of the biggest gains I made was when I discovered **Orgain nutritional shakes**. Orgain has no artificial sweeteners, preservatives, or colorings. All Orgain shakes are non-GMO, gluten-free and soy-free. They are chock full of organic fruits and veggies, as well as organic brown rice and organic fiber. They also have organic whey protein, which raises glutathione. Orgain was developed by *Dr. Andrew Abraham*, a trained physician, who had cancer. In 2008, after diagnosis, he underwent extensive treatment and was placed on a liquid diet. He needed a *nutritious protein shake* but couldn't find one. So he pursued pains-taking research and then formulated the first Orgain shake himself in his own kitchen, based on organic nutrition that is fortified with vital, tried and true vitamins and minerals. I love this shake!

I also love Starbucks Evolution Smoothies (these are non-organic, but work for me) for protein and electrolyte replacement, and CalNaturale Svelte Banana Crème protein shakes. Starbucks smoothies are a great alternative for busy people, looking to stay well on the move. Also, look for **My Perfect Protein Shake** on my website (see *Welcome* for the link). Again, I mention brands because integrity matters. Tranparency matters. Ingredients matter. I'm sharing what helped me heal, on a physical level. Of course, nothing works in isolation. I also had to cultivate other aspects of living as well: positive mindset, total nutrition, and whole bodymind self-care all went hand in hand. I have developed a sustainable way of living that works for me.

The sum total of what I'm sharing in this book is my own practice of *living a healthy lifestyle and lifestyle medicine, which has positively impacted my health and wellbeing.* As you develop your own **lifestyle medicine plan,** focus on what makes your body, mind, and soul thrive!

These are the keys to well-being: What is your *winning combination* with food? What unlocks your health and vitality? What makes your body *come alive*? Each of us has an energetic signature that is cultivated through food, love, relationships, etc. *Food and relationships* are both such intimate parts of our lives, and they can often make us or break us.

What builds your body and soul up toward the heavens, yet also roots you firmly in the ground? What *healthy cravings* do you quietly have that you ignore? If you have a subtle craving for strawberries, or squash, or a hug or a talk, don't ignore it. Act on it!

> *I embrace and follow my body's deepest desire for wellness and connection ...*
> *here-in lies the path of well-being*

Whew! Here you go. Embrace your health, the life you deserve. You can do it! It is so worth it. Real food tastes and *feels* way better, and the payoff is you get to actually function again and have a life, if this is your only **energy-deficit issue**. Even if it's not the *only source of your energy drain (there are other issues like chronic inflammation)*, you will be doing your body a huge favor by loving it, respecting it, and *trusting its cues.*

Trust is where health lies. Trust your body, trust in life, and trust in the higher good/God/whatever you want to call it. **Trust lies only in the present moment though.** When you say, *I Trust Life*, you sink into the present moment, and all is well, or will be well, both figuratively and literally. You become the hero or heroine of your own life when you drop into the present moment and **fight for your health and happiness.** Peter A. Levine (1997), author of *Waking the Tiger: Healing Trauma*, calls these types of efforts, **heroic energies.**

Your courage is your energy right now, along with your hope, and your faith in yourself and in a perfectly unfolding universe.

You might be wondering: **how do I do all of this, integrate all of these changes for real, for good?**

The short answer is **self-love.** See Chapter Five for details.

Let's talk about *trauma* for a moment because, as a concept, it has impact on this part of our discussion. Are you traumatizing your body over and over again, i.e., engaging in self-abuse, by feeding it negative energy, whether from hanging out with the wrong people, focusing on negative or limiting beliefs, or ingesting junk food, as in refined foods? If you answered, *yes*, to any of these thoughts, then consider this: When you let go of trauma, you sink into the present moment and free up and access your *real energy*.

And it is in the present moment where trauma - past, present, or future trauma - has no hold on you. Trauma is a major contributor to illness, pain, disease, and *fatigue*. Many people who have chronic fatigue have experienced trauma as well, for whatever reasons. Call it a double whammy, I guess. This is not true for everyone, of course. It has been noticed in research, however, as we discussed in Chapter Three.

There's a stigma against sick people that few acknowledge. It easy to understand why: no one wants to be reminded of his or her own frailties, weaknesses, and vulnerabilities. The stigma includes the misconception that people who are ill are also weak and powerless.

We all talk about desiring power. Some might say: **If I had power, this is what I would do; this is how I would change the world.**

The truth is, you have all the power you need, right now. You use your power wisely to **make choices every day about the products you buy,** and how you manage to feed and take care of yourself and your family, whoever they may be. **We were all born powerful.**

Healing (loving and accepting) yourself is powerful. Well-being is a positive choice. Joy and Happiness are always available to us at any moment...a heartbeat away.

Yes, the world is full of unfriendly chemicals and toxins. This is unfortunate. But you can't avoid life, or stop living, in fear of them. Do your best to avoid what you can in the way of harmful ingredients, additives, packaging materials, etc. *Be smart, read, educate and protect yourself ... demand transparency and traceability in products.* Two of the **best defenses are to create a positive mindset and to create a strong body that can resist and fight off chemicals, viruses, and bacteria *in the first place.*** True well-being is within your reach. The most important thing is that *you believe it.*

Don't ever take your eye off the jump. But if you do, forgive yourself and get right back on the horse. It doesn't matter if other people judge you. Judgment from others doesn't change your reality. What matters are that you stop judging yourself and stay focused on the positive. Staying positive is half the battle. Find your positive growth edge!

Actually, living in the positive realm of life is everything. It's literally a matter of survival. ***Positive energy is lifeforce.*** Ironically enough, there is an unbridled optimism that can come with facing illness, when you realize that life is indeed a gift and every second of breath is precious.

The Quick Fix vs. Sustainable Health

We've been conditioned to get what we want - *now* - in our culture! ***Instant gratification*** is the name of the game, especially in our hyper-tech culture. The problem with this view of life is that it's unsustainable. The body is a system that changes slowly over time like the subtle change of the seasons, minus acute changes or stressors.

Well, let me qualify that stance. Your state of mind* can change instantly. You can ***decide*** to have a healthy mindset and that can happen instantly. Now, I'm not talking about, say, needing help with clinical depression or schizophrenia, for instance. I'm talking about your daily outlook and your attitude toward others in your life, your conditioned responses to life in general, and your general frame of mind. Do you respond, generally, from a place of love or fear?

Health is both a *state of being* (mind) and a *way of being* (body.) Both the ***state of being healthy and the way of being healthy are a process and a lifestyle.*** They both encompass how you live. And, for the most part, they take time to develop. It takes **practice to live well.**

We always look for that magic pill. Deep nutrition is the closest thing to it. Except it's not magic, it's just real nutrition. For me, it's real food plus raw/food-based supplements. Sustainable health is: deep nutrition, managing stress, and avoiding irritants. Quality sleep and practicing self-care and cultivating a positive mindset are key too.

*You can decide to be positive instantly. Sustaining positivity takes practice which builds neuroplasticity.

We must learn to slow down, and show respect for one another and for ourselves. Well-being, just like spirituality, is a journey, not a destination … and not a random text, high, or IM. Consider slowing down to enjoy the ride of life and savor each precious draw of breath.

Five Keys to Sustainable Well-Being

Here is an article I wrote for *MindBodyGreen.com* and which appeared on May 7, 2012.

*There's a little known secret that the **natural high of good health** trumps all other kinds of highs, artificial or otherwise. The temptations of the easy high are everywhere. The problem is when you numb the hard stuff, and you end up numbing the good stuff too, like joy and progress. What's the alternative? The mellow rush that comes from taking consistent good care of yourself. Well-being is easier to achieve and maintain than you might think, and it can be your best ally in buffering the slays of this modern world.*

Good health may be your best armor in this world, but why does it seem easy for some people to maintain vibrant health, and more challenging for others? The key is in trusting life and letting down your guard, ironically, getting into the flow with healthy behaviors, and keeping at them until they begin to feel effortless. Just like a plane that eventually reaches cruising altitude, you too can reach the natural high of good health with practice. Here are five ways to naturally cultivate sustainable well-being in your life:

1. Get Positive about Expressing Yourself

Emotions are meant to be felt and expressed, not bottled up or suppressed. As scary as it can seem, expressing what you really feel, and being who you really are, affects the quality of your health dramatically. Suppressing emotions through addiction, soft or hard, just delays the inevitable, and literally stresses your body out in the process, which can break your body down. Consider the idea of creating or being positively addicted to something like music or sports that has the capacity to transform you, as opposed to annihilate you. Instead of dreading what you feel, try examining it, savoring it, or even honoring it. What you release, releases you, and raises the bar of your health threshold that much higher. It is very tempting to ignore our deep pain, but that only delays us feeling great. Pain is temporary. Vitality can be yours for life.

2. Reach Out… And Hang Out With Someone

Yep, you guessed it. Connection is crucial to health. In fact, it just may be the most important thing you do. John Travis says "Connection is the currency of wellness." Why? Because we're social creatures. It comes down to hardwiring. Why does connection work? Think about it: how does anything work in life?

Because it has something else to feed off of. How does a light burn energy? Because it is plugged in. We are all interconnected, whether we like it or not. We thrive when we connect not only with our own life, but the lives of others, and the world at large. What if you're a lone wolf? No worries. Just make sure you call or email someone once in blue moon. Most likely you'll be glad you did, and so will they. Who knows, you just might enjoy yourself too, another key to sustainable well-being.

3. Get in the Flow and Get Moving

We were designed to move. But movement should feel good, not be a chore. In fact, it raises more of the feel-good neurotransmitters such as serotonin and dopamine. Your own brain is your best pharmacy. It even has THC receptors (accessed naturally by the neurotransmitter anandamide - ananda meaning "bliss" in Sanskrit – or by allowing your kinesthetic awareness to take precedence along with deep, slow breathing). Consider what you truly enjoy, and then do as much of it as you can over the course of your day to keep your metabolism running on high, which is the whole point. Not only does what you focus on take focus, it takes shape according to the amount of time you engage with it. It's a law of physics: "...a body in motion tends to stay in motion." And the more you move, the more your body will ask you for what it needs nutrition-wise to sustain itself naturally. It's win-win.

4. Eat What Sustains You

Trying to figure out what to eat has become like trying to solve a Rubik's Cube. Instead, try following your body and your natural instincts. What food is your body asking you for, especially if you've been active? Try to only eat what makes your body **thrive**. What raises your energy levels when you eat and keeps them steady? What drops your energy immediately? What we eat is deeply personal, but it can also affect us deeply. A few things to keep in mind: maximize fresh food, eat both for pleasure and nutrition, and consume live, cultured foods that support your life-force and the living system that is your body.

5. Get Outside and Get Back Into Nature

According to Richard Louv, author of **The Nature Principle**, nature makes us more intelligent and creative. But more urgent is that we need nature. We need the electromagnetic energy of the earth and sun, and the rush of the ocean and shelter of trees to balance out the mesmerizing, technological pull of the screen. We need the wide, beautiful distraction of nature to alleviate the mental fatigue of circuitrized modern life. We crave "...the living dream that we share with the soaring hawk" (**The Spell of the Sensuous** - David Abram), the cadence of whale song, and unbroken stretches of beach scattered with shells and enigmatic life. Being outside calms and soothes the stress response and recharges you naturally. Looking for a sustainable, healthy high? Look no further than the unpaved path outside of your door.

Below is a chart, courtesy of *AmazingGrass.com,* illustrating how similar our own hemoglobin (read: blood) is to chlorophyll. Chlorophyll has been called *sun energy* among other beautiful terms. We need sun exposure (directly, I believe, although in moderation) for synthesis of Vitamin D, which acts like a hormone in the body and is absorbed for up to 24 hours through the skin after exposure to sun. Consuming chlorophyll is probably our best bet to further reap the benefits of this amazing star of light and life. Note the similar molecular structures of hemoglobin and chlorophyll in the chart below.

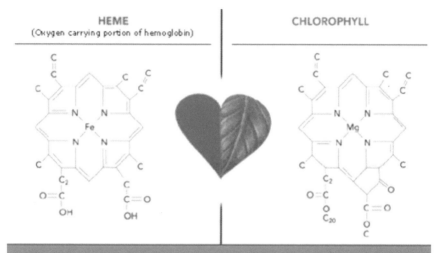

Note how hemoglobin and chlorophyll share an almost identical molecular structure. This explains why chlorophyll is so readily assimilated into our blood stream and our bodies are able to utilize its powerful properties. With the addition of chlorophyll into our diet, we are consuming the very essence of life's energy. Essentially the "blood" of plants is absorbed into human blood, which transports nutrients to every cell of the body.

Many gracious thanks to http://amazinggrass.com/

What's one of the best ways to get chlorophyll? Green superfoods. Like other green superfoods such as spirulina and barley grass, *wheat grass* is extremely high in chlorophyll and is the perfect food to use as an example of *nutritional synergy.* Wheat grass is synergistic because it is more than the sum of its parts: it is nutrition gold. It's high in *folic acid* and may assist the methylation process. It's high in *B Vitamins* so it's great for sustaining energy and soothing the nervous system. It's high in *iron, Vitamin A, and enzymes.* It has *all* of the essential *amino acids.*

http://thechalkboardmag.com/50-reasons-to-drink-wheatgrass-everyday

Wheat grass is also high in *fiber* - more than an equal eight gram serving of oat bran. It is also considered a source of *leafy greens*. Greens are considered one of the most important food sources. The popular kale is also another source of greens. Also, because wheat grass is highly alkaline, it effectively balances pH in the body. It's high in *antioxidants* to strengthen the immune system and protect against oxidative stress. It's high in *Vitamin C* and may support your adrenals and may reduce effects of food sensitivities and allergies. This latter is my hypothesis, based on the fact that wheat grass strengthens your immune system of which over 70% is in your digestive tract. It also seems to help me be less sensitive to certain foods, which is a really nice potential benefit.

Can you see how wheat grass is a *whole food*? It follows that the benefits of wheat grass result from the *synergistic nature of whole foods*. Remember this: real, complete, synergistic whole foods are more than the sum of their parts. Well-being comes from a place of wholeness.

Linguistically, the word *health* means *whole* and *holy*. I use the word *holistic* when I talk about authentic health and well-being. To me, *holistic health* means these things:

Holistic health is the union of body, mind, and spirit.
Holistic health is the relationship you have with your body, mind, and spirit.
Holistic health is the relationship you have with others.
Holistic health is the relationship you may have with a divine source of energy.

Can I ask you some questions?

What is your relationship with your body? Are you friends with your body? Do you give it what it needs to thrive?

And your mind? Are you at war or at peace in your mind?

How about relationships with others in your life? Are they healthy relationships? Do they deliver joy and completeness both ways, i.e. between you and others? Personally, I feel a tie with all things - both living and inanimate. I practice awareness of this connection and do my best to honor it.

What about your relationship with a creative source, where life may have originated? For me, I've had experiences with what has been called God. Maybe this doesn't work for you. But can you feel some kind of connection to your spiritual self anyway, say through your creativity or your imagination? What is your concept of how life originated or operates? Can you feel a connection with that?

Synergy, then, is how health occurs, when the total is greater than the sum of its parts. A great example of synergy is the experience of listening to a symphony orchestra vs. hearing each individual instrument played on its own. In the hands of master musician, the sound produced on each separate instrument is *beautiful*, whereas, listening to symphonic music is *rapturous* and gives a sense of *coherence*.

Wholeness promotes synergy. Holiness is related to union and, to me, coherence. To me, coherence is feeling connected to the creative source of life. It is the feeling I experience in the state of real, authentic, holistic health that cannot be shaken by slights, by abuse, or by trauma. When you experience coherence you have the choice to tap into an infinite source from where we came, and trust that it is a place of infinite light and healing energy, because its very nature is creative.

When you *relax* into health, and trust the process of life from a holistic point of view, this is where and when health has a chance to emerge.

This tree/work of art is alive.

It is whole. It is holistic. It is holy.

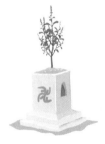

Tips, Supplements* and Recipes

First, consider investing in a Vitamix and a Cuisinart Mini-Prep. These are two powerful kitchen tools for making healthy, yummy food!

For my recipes, please go to the end of this section. They are listed under *Recipes I Love*. There you will find recipes for drinks, shakes, smoothies, snacks, and meals. Plus, I'm looking for *your* favorite recipes! Check out and send recipes to me at *PortlandWellnessCoach.com*.

But first, so you can pack up your *tool box of well-being*, here are *tool box tips* and *everyday tips* that may help your health:

*The Natural Foods Industry saved my life. I am not prescribing to you. Any products I mention are because they helped me. Find what works for you and demand quality, transparency, and traceability!

Toolbox:

Sweeteners

Little to No Refined Sugar ~ Hard, but you can do it! Try Truvia, stevia, or xylitol! There are so many alternatives now, making it a no-brainer and super easy to switch to healthier sweeteners. Your well-being is so worth it!!

Truvia ~ My go-to, favorite sweetener! I use it on cereal, fruit, in smoothies, cold herbal tea, etc. It works for my body!

Nu Naturals Pure Liquid Vanilla Stevia ~ This tastes amazing in tea, coffee, yogurt, pancakes, etc. I am sensitive to alcohol, but I tolerate trace amounts now, and it evaporates if you put it in piping hot water, or use to it to bake with, etc.

Toolbox:

Greens & Plants

Plant Nutrition ~ Green, clean, serene energy is my favorite kind of energy. Chlorophyll and blood are almost identical in cellular structure. You are made up of light energy.

Greens ~ Dark, leafy greens are full of magnesium and they make you feel so naturally good, and give you clean, green, calm energy! Did you know Wheat Grass is a leafy green? Wow!

Veggies ~ The more the better! They're alkaline and full of protein and minerals. Be creative. It's all about the synergy of how food works together to taste amazing and fuel your chi! Greens and veggies help me feel grounded with tons of energy!

Inside Your Home ~ Plants can remove up to 90% of VOCs. Try spider plants or ferns of any kind.

Bananas ~ I love bananas! They help with sore muscles if you have built up lactic acid from being active or have an overactive HPA axis, etc. They contain tryptophan, which converts to serotonin, the calming neurotransmitter. They're great for natural sustained energy yet calm you down at the same time. They're filling too. Bananas rock!

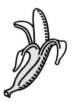

*Little to No Refined Foods ~ Try not to use refined sugar and flours.
I can tolerate **evaporated cane juice** now, but rarely refined sugar.
Refined sugar is stripped of nutrients, bleached, has the same density as
many drugs like heroin, and may have GMO's in it.*

*Raw Foods ~ **They are** naturally high in glutathione and enzymes,
and can be really yummy and give you loads of energy!*

*Plant-based foods ~ You guessed it. Give your immune system the
upperhand, and build a strong, unshakeable foundation of health!! :)*

Herbs ~ Herbs are food! Enjoy them often for your well-being!

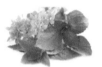

The beauty and power of herbs can change your life! Some Tips:

Herbs include: basil, borage, celery, chives, cilantro, dill, garlic, ginger, lemongrass, oregano, parsley, peppermint, rosemary, sage, savory, spearmint, stevia, sweet marjoram, tarragon, thyme, turmeric, etc. Consider exploring the origins of each herb and discover the exciting, exotic history that accompanies its journey through time and trade. Along the way, you may discover the health promoting qualities these amazing herbs possesses and how you can put those powers to work in your life. Discover the raw origins of life, health, and well-being!

Here's one example: Turmeric may be known to you as a yellow spice used widely in Indian cuisine. It's a tropical plant so you can cultivate it outdoors if you live in a warm climate. The plant grows a tuber, or rhizome, much like ginger does. It can take some 10 months for a new crop of roots to develop, and they are the part of the plant you will harvest. Turmeric may help address inflammation, just as chamomile and olive may do so as well. They are called immuno-modulators and they potentially can modulate an overactive immune system. Turmeric is also an antioxidant, and may have anti-cancer properties. To your health!

Andree Suddoo

*Follow The Danielle Lin show to keep up to date on health, products, and the natural foods industry.

Toolbox:

Herbs,

Essential Oils, and

Healthy Fats

Vanilla Bean ~ Fragrant vanilla beans grow on an herbaceous vine. Medicinally may ease stress and may have a calming effect on the body.

Lavender Oil by Silexan, or Calm Aid by Nature's Way ~ Essential oil formulas that may reduce physical and/or mental anxiety without making you sleepy. Check with your doctor first!

Good Fats ~ Essential Fatty Acids (EFAs) such as Organic Flax Oil, Evening Primrose Oil, and Borage Oil taste so good and are beneficial for you, your cells, weight, and immunity!

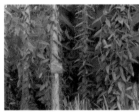 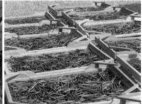

Vanilla Vines   Vanilla Beans Drying

Toolbox:

Probiotics Live Food, & Cellfood

Acidophilus Milk ~ High in protein which is crucial to heal your immune system. It has a nice, sweet flavor, and has Vitamin D added.

Noosa ~ One of my favorite yogurts (I love Wallaby & Chobani too) and chock full of live, friendly bacteria. So good, and so good for you.

Kefir and Liquid Yogurt ~ Try Organic Valley's liquid yogurt, Helios Kefir, and Nature's Way Primadophilus Optima Max Bifido. Probiotics support digestion and immune function.

Kombucha ~ As I understand it, Kombucha is converted caffeine and sugar. It still has an essence of black tea. I am sensitive to caffeine, but I seem to do well with this. I prefer Dave's Kombucha Tea. It comes in many flavors and has electrolytes too from added juice or superfoods.

CellFood ~ Bioavailable oxygen and trace minerals. I put it in milk, yogurt, herbal tea, Orgain, protein shakes, etc.

Toolbox: **Superfoods**	*Spirulina and Green Superfoods* ~ Nutrex or HealthForce Nutritionals offer the best spirulina, in my opinion. Other green superfoods include wheat grass, chlorella, E3Live, barley grass, blue-green algae, avocadoes, alfalfa, etc.
	Wheat Grass ~ I prefer Amazing Grass; Pines; wheat grass shots. *Vitamineral Green* ~ If you need a jumpstart for your health, this may be it.
	Chia Seeds - These seeds give me great energy without any stimulation. Great source of protein and fiber as well! Versatile in recipes too!

Toolbox: **Protein & Energy Aids**	*Amazing Meal* ~ Greens, superfoods, and great for energy!
	Orgain Protein Drink ~ An organic, non GMO, nutritional shake with 16 grams of protein and superfoods.
	NADH ~ May help supply energy. May aid some folks with Parkinson's. May help functionality of enzymes in the body. Stands for Nicotinamide Adenine Dinucleotide. Found in fish, poultry, and yeast-containing foods. Can take as supplement.
	Whole Eggs ~ Not only for protein, but for the production of adrenal hormones and stabilization of adrenals and thyroid.
	Tera's Whey Protein with Vanilla Bourbon ~ One of my favorite, bio-available protein powders. Clean, usable protein, mixes well, tastes good. May help with glutathione production for poor methylators. Now available in a grass-fed version as well.
	Sprouted Grains, Nuts, and Seeds ~ For protein, sustained energy, and fiber. Consider allergies, sensitivities and symptoms: MSHope.com

Toolbox: **Vitamins:** **Raw,** **Food-** **Based,** **Bio-** **Available,** **or** **naturally** **from** **Sunlight**	*Vitamin C ~ **Use real/bio-available** forms such as camu-camu, acerola berry, etc. This makes all the difference to me in terms of energy and absorption. I love Megafood & Planetary Herbals for real Vitamin C sources from which I see results!* *Vitamin D ~ Get outside and soak up some sunshine and fresh air for your body and soul. Important for Vitamin D and all around well-being. While you're out there, enjoy some moderate restorative exercise such as walking, tai chi, qi-gong, yoga, etc.* *Source of Life Vitamins ~ This food-based multivitamin has a microdose of Korean Ginseng, as well as spirulina, borage oil, etc. A great, general multi-vitamin that comes in powdered form as well.* *Vitamin Code Vitamins ~ Garden of Life; MegaFood Brand* *Real Food Organic Vitamins ~ Country Life; This raw-based multivitamin has just a touch of acai in its formula.* *Three great rmulti-vitamin brands. They all give me great energy!*

Toolbox: **Extra** **Nutrition** **&** **Digestive** **Health**	*Miso Ginger Broth ~ Trader Joe's: wonderful support for the digestive tract and may improve appetite. Wonderful product!* *Nutritional Yeast ~ High in glutathione and B vitamins, especially B12. I prefer the kind that is not fortified with **extra** B vitamins. It's harder for me to process for some reason. Whole Foods makes their own brand.* *Tazo Wild Sweet Orange Tea ~ Steep one bag in cold water for 6 minutes. I add CellFood, Truvia, one or two drops of liquid Stevia, and sometimes sliced lime or lemon. Fresh, live, soothing flavor and energy.* *L-Glutamine ~ May help repair/rebuild intestinal lining.*

Toolbox:	*Asthaxanthin ~ Crosses the blood-brain barrier (most antioxidants don't) to possibly combat oxidative stress. Also boosts energy levels naturally, perhaps because it is such a powerful antioxidant and may protect the cells of the mitochondria in your muscles from oxidation.*
Anti-Oxidant Stars	
Find your Upper, Anti-Oxidant Edge!	*Berries ~ The darker, the better. Wild blueberries are loaded with major antioxidants. Abundant in Maine and Eastern Canada! Wash and add to cereal, yogurt, or sprinkle with Truvia or some kind of natraul, allternative sweetner, and eat by themselves. Yummy!*
	Artichokes ~ Cut off stem and pop one in an inch of boiling water, and cook/steam until leaves are tender. It's done when you can pull out the inner petal! Eat the sweet, meaty part only, and discard the remainder of leaf. Pull the remainder of leaves from the base of the choke. Knife out the fuzzy part of the heart. You can eat all the rest, including the stem! So good and supports liver health & detoxification!

Toolbox:	*Organic Coconut Milk ~ For electrolytes, MCTs. I prefer the regular, organic kind that has not had any fat taken out of it. Great for Thai dishes! Try as a half and half substitute!*
Non-GMO, Organic Cereals	
& Other Yummy Foods!	*Organic Hemp Hearts ~ Yummy, healthy, and versatile! I put them in cold or hot cereal. Full of fiber! Organic makes a difference!*
	Nature's Path Gluten-Free Cereals and Granola Cereals ~ Guaranteed organic and GMO-free which makes a huge difference to my system in terms of non-gmo corn especially. Nutritious and delicious. I love these cereals. Yum! Still family-owned too!
	GlutenFreeda Packaged Oatmeal ~ Amazing flavors. The maple sugar may break down the oatmeal a little; making it easier to digest.

Toolbox:	*Amy's Frozen Foods* ~ *Anything made by Amy's is outstanding, not to mention healthy, and tastes really wonderful. They're also one of the few natural foods companies still*
Easy	*independently owned, often meaning higher standards and quality.*
Foods	
and	
Snacks	*Sahale Nuts* ~ *My favorite and they make them in many so amazing combos! Great for health nuts & food connoisseurs!*
	Greens Plus Bars ~ *Protein and superfoods, and alkaline, high-quality nutrition on-the-go.*

Toolbox:	*Valerian* ~ *Soothes nerves. and a source of GABA. It is also an adaptogen, which means it may support well-being while you sleep.*
Soothing	*Calms & Sedalia* ~ *Effective homeopathic stress relief.*
Tools for	
Nerves	*GABA* ~ *One of the main ingredients in valerian for calming your brain and body. You can buy it this way, as well, in isolated, pharmaceutical grade.*
	Sprouted Brown Rice ~ *High in B vitamins and GABA to calm the nervous system.*
	L-Theanine ~ *great for anxiety, yet doesn't make you drowsy. I prefer the kind actually made from green tea by Simple Truth.*

Green tea contains L-Theanine, which may calm your nerves. This may be suitable if you are not sensitive to caffeine. Rich in anti-oxidants too!

Toolbox:	*Perfect Calm by New Chapter ~ Perfect blend of herbs, nutrients, and adaptogens for managing stress levels and for balanced energy.*
Stress and Sleep	*Stress Assist ~ Has B vitamins and adaptogens; calms you down and energizes you all at the same time. Fabulous formula.*
	NutraSleep ~ Fantastic formula for either relaxing or deep, restorative sleep. I take it with 5-Htp for sleep. This is yet another helpful formula by Source Naturals
	Mood Up Stress Down ~ Raises energy while relieving stress levels. One of my favorites with added Vitamin D3.
	Theanine Serene w/ Relora~ A fantastic, synergistic blend of GABA, L-Theanine, and adaptogens like Holy Basil, and Relora (a standardized form of Magnolia.) You can take it at nighttime as it is great for sleeping. I take it by itself or with 5-HTP.
	Magenesium Malate ~ Great for energy, nerves, and elimination :) Solaray's Sleep Blend ™ SP-17™ I love this formula! for sleep!

Chia seeds are packed with omega-3 fatty acids, which are crucial for brain health. The seeds come from this flowering plant in the mint family. See below.

Toolbox:	*Gingko-Bacoba Quick Thinking ~ by Rainbow Light*
	Wonderful synergistic formula to assist with energy and brain power.
Brain Power	*SAM-e ~ Assists with dopamine production, a valuable neurotransmitter in the brain. Improved dopamine levels aid our cognitive function. May also help if you don't methylate properly.*
	Walnuts ~ Walnuts are rich in Omega 3 fatty acids that help our brains. Notice the walnut looks like a brain too! Hmm!

Toolbox:

Homeopathy and Flower Essences

King Bio Homeopathics ~ Water-based formulas. Wondeful if you are sensitive to lactose or alcohol-based homeopathy.

Natrabio ~ Adrenal and thyroid support formulas.

Homeopathic Chamomille ~ Great for headaches, anxiety, and teething for kids. Try Camilia by Boiron.

Homeopathic Arnica ~ Really helps with pain and fatigue.

Rescue Remedy ~ For stress, fatigue, pain, or the fear of pain. Superb for anxiety and trauma. Great for pets and plants, too. Rescue Remedy plus L-Theanine, PharmaGABA (at nighttime) and lavender oil all work wonders to calm down my HPA axis.

Flower Essences ~ Excellent for deep-level emotional healing.

Toolbox:

Detox

pH Quintessence ~ Supports the balance of your pH levels and may be helpful for Phase II liver detoxification. Proprietary formula includes alfalfa leaves and stems. May help your body achieve a more alkaline state.

Fresh Lemon Juice ~ I prefer to use fresh lemon juice (first and foremost) or some type or green superfood to help with Phase II liver detoxification. Lemon juice works very well and is gentle on the system. It is far more gentle than milk thistle formulas, yet very effective.

Toolbox:

Color

Color Therapy *~ Lavender, yellow, green, whatever gives you energy and makes you feel good! This tactic works in general. Do what makes you feel good to experience well-being!*

Mint *~ This literally wakes your brain and energy right up! Try mint in lip balm, in tea, or as an essential oil or supplement!*

Honoring and expressing my true emotions *~ Did I slip this in here? Yes, I did! Life is rich with colorful experience. Soak up, open up, and drink it all in!* ☺

Arnica, D-Ribose, Electrolytes ~ Tactics to support that "bottomed out" feeing for me are whole fruit/green superfood smoothies, and taking supplements like licorice or Vega's Electrolyte Hydrator. Replenishing nutrition and fortifying against stressors really works for me. Sometimes, I also take Siberian Ginseng or other adaptogens. Homeopathic arnica and Seriphos work great for me as well, for **when my body feels overextended**.

Kick-It-Biotic by WishGarden ~ My go-to herbal formula if I'm under the weather. I love so many of their formulas for stress, immunity, etc.!

Essential Oils ~ Essential oils are like tiny **jewels of energy**. They can lift physical, mental, emotional, and spiritual energy right up to the heavens! Vanilla, cocoa, and sandalwood are some of my favorites as perfumes. I like Simplers Botanicals, Valentina's and Pacifica's Island Vanilla roll-on/spray.

I love Aveda's natural perfumes (amazing, natural scents and Aveda is based on Ayurvedic medicine) and also blends that have cocoa/citrus. S-Limonene - found in citrus - has been shown to improve moods and may affect neurotransmitters (Daniel, 2013; Zhou, W., Yoshioka, & Yokogoshi, 2009).

I put therapeutic blends on my wrists, and they uplift my mood and energy levels. Cocoa and citrus oils like wild orange give me energy earlier in the day, via transdermal application (vs. being absorbed by the liver), while other blends calm me down later in the afternoon/evenings with chamomile, etc. Ask me what I use! Use caution taking GRAS therapeutic grade oils internally. Consult with a qualified, certified aromatherapist.

Possible Properties of Wild Orange Essential Oil

Antibacterial	Carminative
Antidepressant	Choleretic
Antifungal	Digestive
Anti-inflammatory	Hypotensive
Antioxidant	*Sedative (calms you down)*
Antiseptic	*Stimulant (may support energy)*

You can also diffuse essential oils throughout your environment (car, home, office) with a diffuser. This is my favorite way to use them, beyond transdermally, which is absorbed straight into the skin. Use *caution* if taking internally (therapeutic grade only, only certain kinds, not evaluated by FDA).

Scents can be powerfully energizing. Try linalool (lavender), citronellol, limonene (citrus), and geraniol.
Research on essential oils: http://www.ncbi.nlm.nih.gov/pubmed?term=essential%20oils
*One blend I love has a synergistic blend including rose, sandalwood, and cocoa - which lifts my energy earlier in the day. It also has *ylang ylang*, which has been shown to lower cortisol levels (Daniel, 2013). Powerful effects of D-Limonene: http://goo.gl/LbbslS

Essential oils are known to have antidepressant effects (Komiya, Takeuchi & Harada, 2006) as well as antiviral and antibacterial properties (Wu, Patel et al., 2010).

Green Grapes ~ Grapes are one of my favorite fruits. They consistently raise my energy levels. Grapes have many micronutrients including B1 (for energy) and B6, Vitamin C, manganese, potassium, and Vitamin K. They're chock full of phytonutrients, resveratrol - great for longevity - and are low glycemic. They're also natural diuretics, and draw toxins from the body in a mellow way. And **_grapes are berries,_** which are good for your immune system, nervous system, and they lower inflammation. They fight oxidative stress and raise your blood glutathione levels. Grapes are one of my go-to snacks! But remember, always buy _organic_ grapes! I love raisins too for energy!

5-HTP ~ This is my _medicine_ at nighttime. I use it for more energy (as it creates serotonin, which stress depletes, and to help me sleep more deeply. It lights up the signal between the hypothalamus and adrenals. It also creates up to 200% more natural melatonin in the body. Those with high stress levels and/or fatigue often have high cortisol levels at night, and therefore lower melatonin levels. Melatonin signals your body to sleep. Other techniques to foster sleep include slow breathing, which activates the vagus nerve.

Other tactics ~ _My body is extra sensitive to the effects of stress, so I was low in vital minerals and electrolytes. What solved this for me were Megafood's Calcium, Magnesium, and Potassium and Solaray's Sleep Blend SP-17._ I was then able to sleep deeply and my energy levels recovered during the day. _My body needed extra nutrition I just couldn't get otherwise (our top-soil is depleted and stress also depletes crucial nutrients which we need to heal and be well). Deep nutrition can make such a powerful difference. I couldn't gain the upper edge until I supplemented. You could also try Alteril or plant melatonin like Herbatonin. Other tactics for sleep include tryptophan,* PharmaGABA and standardized valerian. Valerian works like natural valium - to calm both body and brain. I use a citrus essential oil blend on my feet to relax. Also, consider hormonal balance. Talk to your practitioner about hormones, as they require specific dosing. I use Vitex/Black Cohosh to balance progesterone levels,_ and watch estrogenic foods. I take each night as it comes, and do my best to keep my stress levels down during the daytime. _Everything is interconnected: daytime choices and activity affect sleep patterns and cortisol levels. You can sleep well!_
*I am also sensitive to tryptophan, so I use Black Cohosh instead, which may increase Trp levels.

Low Stimulants Tip ~ I used to do just fine with chocolate before I got sick. But after my first round of chronic fatigue, I avoided sugar and chocolate. When I started eating it again, my toleration was okay, although not what it was before my ski accident. But remember that stimulants can be interpreted by your body as stressful. And you know that on-going stress is a form of trauma. You want to let your body and your HPA axis heal and rest as much as possible from acute stress. *What I've found is that it's* delivery and amount *for me.* Very small amounts of healthy stimulation seem to work for me.* *Too much stimulation affects my HPA axis & my liver doesn't detox estrogen well.

Be aware that caffeine is estrogenic, as well as some herbs, etc. Seek cortisol and hormone balance. It can be a fine line, and balance is different for everyone. I use Estrotone by Gaia to stay in balance hormonally, along with watching my cortisol levels carefully, through diet, yoga, and mindful living. I love Aveda's *Comforting Tea* and Tazo's *Wild Sweet Orange Tea* (I also travel with the packets, as they are small, and give me consistent energy via mint, citrus, & licorice). I love vanilla rooibos tea, too. My **go-to low/healthy stimulants** are *Orgain (acai), Nature's Plus Vitamins, SweetLeaf Chocolate SweetDrops*, Green Plus Chocolate Bars, chocolate lip balm, cocoa absolute in high-quality essential oil blends (ask me what I use) and *raw vitamins with acai.*

I often also take Spirulina tablets/capsules for B vitamins and iron. Trader Joe's has small tablets for traveling. Another new favorite is Fo Ti. This gives me consistently good energy. **This is my winning formula:** deep nutrtition (food and raw/food-based quality herbs and supplements), practicing self-care and stress management, and avoiding irritiants to my mind and body. This is how I have found my upper edge of well-being to get and stay well!

Tips about Other Supplements and Foods I Love:

Busy Brain Release by Rainbow Light/Imagine Soups/Solaray JetZone/Seriphos/Amy's (still family-owned), MegaFood

Kevita/*Lara Bars/MyChelle/New Chapter/The Honest Co. MSM/Liverite/Tart Cherry for natural melatonin/Nature's Way

Raw, Organic Proteins: SunWarrior, Amazing Grass, Garden of Life Spike Vegit Magic /Trader Joe's Super Seed & Ancient Grain Blend

Omega 3's Nordic Naturals ~ Omega 3's are a studied and proven supplement. They keep inflammation in check and aid the health of every cell in your body. *You must have cell integrity to be well.*

Cold pressed juices and drinks - Suja, Forager, and Evolution

*I eat healthy grains in moderation and food bars only occasionally, as they can be high in sugars, etc.

Adaptogens ~ Adaptogens work because of hundreds of unique *phytochemicals* found in them. Theoretically, adaptogens can help your body *adapt* to non-specific stress over time. Here are the ones *most recommended for chronic fatigue,* with some descriptive notes to follow:

Grounding Adaptogens

- [ ] Licorice
- [ ] Ashwaganda
- [ ] Siberian Ginseng

Uplifiting Adaptogens

- [ ] Gota Kola
- [ ] Rhodiala
- [ ] Fo Ti

Grounding Adaptogens

- [ ] Maca
- [ ] Holy Basil (uplifiting also)
- [ ] Korean, Chinese, & American Ginseng (cooler)

Relaxing Adaptogens

- [ ] Magnolia
- [ ] Damiana
- [ ] Valerian

Ashwaganda ~ Great if you're not sensitive to nightshades. Some other nightshades include tomatoes, potatoes, eggplant, sweet and hot peppers, paprika, cayenne, pimento, and even ibuprofen and tobacco. Look for any member of the *Solanaceae* family, and remember that food sensitivities can cause and/or increase your symptoms of fatigue, arthritis, and *affect your immune system.*

Damiana ~ Known to have adaptogenic properties which may relieve anxiety, nervousness.

Fo Ti ~ One of my favorites for a burst of energy! Great for hormone balancing!

Ginseng, American ~ Helpful if you don't have liver detox issues, where you may or may not be able to break down the estrogen-like properties. However, it can work well for energy on exhausted days.

Ginseng, Korean and Chinese ~ These are generally too yang for me, although *small doses work well*. But many people seek them out.

Ginseng, Siberian ~ Great overall tonic for both brain and body. It supports energy levels anywhere in the body. It is said to especially support and fortify the adrenal glands.

Gota Kola ~ One of my go-tos for physical or mental energy along with Fo-Ti. Works well if you are "tired but wired." Good for vein support too.

Holy Basil (also known as Tulsi) ~ One of the most effective adaptogens. Has menthol properties to wake up your brain. Seems to support deep, physical energy. Holy Basil (Tulsi), Gota Kola, and Siberian Ginseng are three of the most consistently recommended adaptogens for chronic fatigue, hypocortisolism, CFS, etc.

Licorice ~ Works well to raise cortisol levels; helps inflammation when due to low cortisol; also works well if one feels the *bottom dropping out*. May be contraindicated for those with high blood pressure or other cardiovascular issues. May help liver disorders. Helps with feeling "bottomed out."

Maca ~ Too yang for me, but works well for many people and perhaps especially for men. So if you have a more yang constitution, maca may be a great choice to support energy levels.

Relora ~ A combination of Phellodendron amurense and Magnolia, two Chinese botanicals used as adaptogens. You can find this in Theanine Serene w/Relora by Source Naturals.

Rhodiala ~ May support mood in addition to energy levels.

Some Recipes I Love

<u>Snacks</u>

Fruit & Protein Snacks

~ Sliced, organic apple
Two tablespoons of Adam's Natural Crunchy
Peanut Butter & sprinkle with Truvia

~ Organic Strawberries & Truvia to taste
~ 6-12 Organic, Hawaiian Spirulina Tablets
~ Eden Foods Tamari Almonds - *Spirulina is high in protein and gives you great energy! Almonds are so healing!*

*Protein Shakes

Good Morning Sunshine
1 Odwalla Mango Tango (mango is low glycemic) or 2 cups lowfat, organic milk or Kefir
1 Organic Orange, sliced (the whole orange, including rind)
3-4 cups water
6-8 scoops Vanilla Protein Powder (I use Tera's Whey Bourbon Vanilla – they also make a grass-fed kind)
2-3 tablespoons Organic Flax Oil
Vanilla Stevia and Truvia to taste - I use Whole Food's Vanilla Stevia packets

Make sure to cut up the orange well. Put all ingredients into your Vitamix. Blend on variable, 8-10 high, then move to full speed on 10 for a few minutes. *Yum!*

Superfood Banana-Strawberry Smoothie
2 cups Vanilla Kefir
2 cups 1% Organic Milk
2 organic bananas
1 cup organic strawberries - washed
2 Tbsps. Vitamineral Green
2 Tbsps. Hawaiian Spirulina*
½ cup water
½ bottle of a Mango Tango
6 drops of Cellfood
Vanilla Stevia to taste
Truvia to taste

Blend in Vitamix on variable/10 for 2 minutes. I put the whole strawberry in, even green tops for tons of energy and added nutritional support!

*I've found *vanilla* really balances out the taste of green superfoods like spirulina. :)

Pancakes

I use Pamela's Baking & Pancake mix (gluten-free), add in 2 eggs, lecithin, bananas, flax seeds, & stevia!
I use organic flax oil and stevia as syrup! I like Zema's too!

*Look for *My Perfect Protein Shake* on my website: PortlandWellnessCoach.com on the "Welcome" link! Send me your recipes too via my website!

Organic, Non-GMO Cereal and Raw Bagels

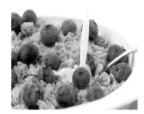

I love cereals like Nature's Path gluten-free granolas. I pair cereal with kefir, Truvia, Tera's Vanilla Whey (for extra protein) and raisins for a burst of natural, sustained energy!

I also adore gluten-free raw bagels by Easy Living Foods! I put Trader Joe's light butter on them, Truvia, and sometimes fruit-only preserves. Cage-free eggs are great partners for bagels, my absolute new favorite combo!

Drinks

Aveda's Comforting Tea – I was thrilled to discover this amazing, healing tea by Aveda (the name is derived from the word Ayurveda). It is healing and soothing, and it tastes mild. Great support for well-being!

Roobios Tea - One teabag organic Roobios, steeped for 6-8 minutes, add creamer and stevia to taste - I use 4-6 drops of liquid stevia and one packet of Truvia.

TAZO Wild Sweet Orange Tea - Steep one bag in cold water for 6 minutes. I add CellFood, Truvia, 1-2 drops of liquid vanilla NuStevia, and lemons, etc.

Spa Water - Fill a pitcher ¾ of the way with fresh water. Cut off the stems of 6-8 organic strawberries, and slice up half of an organic cucumber and place it in the water. Cover and let steep in the fridge for at least an hour. You can add lemon slices, etc.!

Meals

Raw Spaghetti Pasta Meal

Prepare raw yellow squash by cutting into long, thin spaghetti shapes, using a spiralizer.
Dressing: Pre-chop a few organic, raw cashews and place in Cuisinart. Add 2 tbsp. apple cider vinegar and ¼ cup extra virgin olive oil. Blend all dressing ingredients. Season with Braggs Amino Acids as needed.

Eat light, fresh, live, whole food (aim for 90% of food choices) to raise your vitality and well-being naturally and effectively!

Pesto Avocado Meal

1 handful of fresh, organic basil leaves and stems
1 cup extra virgin olive oil
1/3 cup apple cider vinegar
1 cup raw cashews, walnuts, almonds (more alkalizing) or pine nuts
1 tbsp. parmesan cheese (optional) or add some sea salt
Blend all of the above 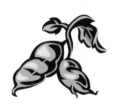 ingredients in a Cuisinart
Cut up one ripe, organic avocado. Spread pesto over
avocado and enjoy!

Sprouted Tofu and Avocado Meal

1 block of medium firm sprouted tofu, chopped. I use Wildwood.
1-2 chopped organic avocadoes
Season mixed tofu and avocadoes with Braggs amino acids and juice
squeezed from 1-2 organic lemons. *Option to add in organic, free-range eggs.*

A Sweet Way to Get More Energy

I have always had a craving for sweet foods. While I avoid refined sugar, I believe there is a reason I crave sweet foods: it raises my serotonin levels. Sweet foods stimulate ATP (which is not only a source of energy, but is also an intercellular signal) in your taste buds, which stimulates the release of serotonin (Choudhari & Roper, 2010; Kinnamon & Finger, 2013). I love sweet potatoes, cashews, fruit with stevia, and mixing stevia and hemp milk as a natural way to improve my energy levels. This works especially well for me late in the day! Stimulants produce serotonin too, but you are more likely to experience a crash afterwards. I prefer to use mint and healthy sweet foods as much as possible to give me a boost of energy naturally and effectively and minimize stimulants as much as possible.

Wheat Grass Shots* & Apple Cider Vinegar

Fresh wheat grass is powerful on so many levels, but it helps my energy tremendously and keeps my liver running smoothly. For the road, I use Amazing Grass packets, but I try to get fresh shots at Jamba Juice. You can grow your own wheat grass too! I love Bragg's apple cider vinegar as a drink for tons of energy and immune support. I put a shot in a glass of water and sweeten with 1-2 packets of stevia (Truvia for me – find what works for you!).

* Consider fresh citrus juices to assist in Phase I detoxification but watch your blood sugar. I don't juice citrus every day, but fresh citrus & wheat grass can support liver well-being.

What I Do on Days I Wake Up Tired

If I wake up tired for whatever reason, and my body's energy doesn't *even out naturally* after an hour or so – which it usually does these days - I use tactics like raw/food-based vitamins, superfoods, DMAE, Fo Ti, Gota Kola, Wheat Grass shots/Orgain/or healthy versions of chocolate. I also love NOW peppermint gels with ginger and fennel. Mint seems to reduce brain inflammation* for me, which improves my energy levels. *I target gut and brain inflammation, and liver health first, as these may be primary sources of fatigue issues. With deep nutritional support, I stay energized. For me, deep nutrition was the answer.*

Every day I do the best I can *to feel the best I can* in a healthy, sustainable way. I support my body vs. over-stimulating it. But, if I get overstimulated, I take **magnesium malate and L-Theanine** to keep my nervous system in balance and fortified, and Theanine-Serene, 5HTP, and black cohosh (I like Target's Up & Up) at night. Most importantly, I don't worry about what I had to do to thrive and survive that day. I also love JetZone, which has homeopathic arnica and Kali Phos. in it. It helps restore my energy levels and reduces lactic acid in me. It's a winning combo and a homerun for my body. What are your homeruns? Some of my homeruns are Orgain, Cellfood, Megafood, protein shakes, stevia, yoga, greens, green superfoods, chia seeds, milky oats, inspiration, connection, Qi-Gong, mindful living, music, nature, and LOVE.

The Symptom of Zero Point Energy - Your Turn-Around Point

I have been many times in a place where I had absolutely *zero energy*. Now, I can see this place is a blessing in disguise. Why? Because I believe the body is naturally trying to **conserve energy in order to heal and reboot**. *You are tired for a reason.*

Here's the good news: zero point energy can actually be your turn-around point. What comes after zero energy? The return of energy, potentially. At least, this is what happens for me, consistently. As you experience this place of zero energy, **pay close attention to what your body needs and desires.** *This is the best tip I can give you for chronic fatigue:* support your body's energy needs by balancing downtime with purposeful, passionate living. **Find balance between support and stimulation.** See if your energy/nervous system bounces back like a rubber band. When you hit rock bottom - the only way to go is back up again. Your healing symptoms may be excruciating, but they have awoken you and pulled you back into your body. As you become more aware and present to your pain and/or exhaustion…as terrible as you may feel…you are feeling, and that is the silver lining. The night is always darkest before the sunrise, which is always coming. For most problems, I believe, the solution is somewhere in the problem. If CFS is an imbalance (of chronic inflammation, etc.) then the solution is balance again. Relax and let your body reboot. Find that sweet spot between calm energy and positive stress. Rest, but also seek support and positive energy: food, company, purpose.

*Chronic inflammation & low energy may be due to a chronically activated immune system, including the brain's immune system. We have immune signatures & blood markers thus far (Lipkin & Hornig, 2015).

The other side of no energy is energy. This is not a simplistic solution. It is the nature of energy. It naturally ebbs and flows. I believe the feeling is just much more pronounced if you have chronic fatigue (again, we don't know why – perhaps due to an imbalance in the HPA axis, or gut flora, which affects brain function or chemistry). I am not belittling what you are experiencing either. Remember, I have experienced this too. I am talking about physics and energetics. It's about surrender vs. resistance. It's about releasing contracted energy (fear-based) and expanding into positive energy.

When you feel low energy at any given point in time, ride it out, and try to *find a place between rest and positive eustress* – relaxed, positive energy and supportive energy (from purpose, support, nutrition, anything that lifts you) and let your body reboot and gain positive ground. If you pay close attention to the subtle messages of your body, you may sense an instinctive call/voice asking you to listen, relax, and get back into the flow of life and well-being.

Homeostasis vs. Stability

We can lose and gain ground in life, in health, and it is normal, it is just the nature of life, which is change. Nothing is static, health is not static …

Well-being, however, and the choice to be well in mind, can offer a source of stability in this ever-changing world. We can choose joy over fear …

Fluctuations in health are normal, homeostasis is not, like constant fatigue.

But the body craves stability, I believe, rhythm, a healthy pattern of living that is predictable. Your body and mind crave rhythm, balance, and stability.

So what do you do when presented with the **seemingly static problem of chronic exhaustion?**

Of course, we have explored potential theories and causes of chronic fatigue. This chapter has been exploring possible support via nutrition, and, coming up, self-care, stress management, and cultivating a positive mindset.

For you, dear reader, here in the moment, reading this section in the book, here is a possible suggestion for your immediate sense and experience of chronic fatigue. I believe that for most problems, the solution is somewhere in the problem. The key is to **slow down enough and tune in to pick up on the frequency of the solution to your current challenge**. *What would give your body stability right here in this moment?* Whatever it is, do that …

Even in the darkest of times, my soul and body craved stability and the impetus for healing. **The will to feel good is strong.** *Never give up hope.*

Journal Entry

My fatigue began as a result of surgery. My symptoms pretty much stayed as they were until I got into natural living. Even then, my body was sensitive, and I got tired easily. On some level, my bodymind may have sensed I was in danger, or it interpreted the events of injury, surgery, drugs, and rehab as stressful.

Perhaps my body interpreted surgery as trauma or I was just over-stimulated from being an HSP. I began to heal after surgery, because of my diet and lifestyle, but then I was triggered again by severe emotional and physical distress. Only this time, I wasn't under the knife.

The question is, why did it take me so much longer to recover the second time? I believe it was due to the trauma my mind held about my marriage, both the violence in it, and the breaking of sacred vows, of my trust in love. This is where the mind comes into play. I had to figure out how to heal, trust, and love again.

In other words, *I had to release fear in order to heal.* I had to move away from interpreting life as stressful, despite my primitive or unconscious mind. Either that, or, *I was just being a naturally normal, highly sensitive person (HSP).*

Either way, my goal was to walk a path that would interrupt the homeostatis of fatigue and other imbalances, while allowing my bodymind to regain balance and *the truest stability of living fully and deeply in the ever-present moment ...*

I had to learn to reinterpret stressors as opportunities to grow and even flourish. Even as an HSP, I had to learn to re-interpret stress ...

I had to enter a new paradigm. I had to take a deep breath, trust, and *let go into FLOW.* There is either fear or flow. We choose the path...

I had to release fear and inhabit love, energy, inspiration, and *every electric moment of life.* I transformed my fear into passionate energy.

I had to find *new stability in my positive growth edge,* where there is no stable ground but the energy and transformation of LOVE

What is Stress Exactly?

Overwhelming stress can break down the body's protective mechanisms.
~ Hans Seyle

Distress is anxiety-producing, eustress is energy-producing. ~ unknown

Stress is an innocuous word with massive implications. It's talked about much, but understood little. Maybe we need a new word for it to signify the severe impact it can have on upsetting the balance of the body. Here are some things we do know:

- *Stress is the body's non-specific reaction physically, mentally, or emotionally to* **change** *in the environment. (This definition is adapted from* Stress without Distress *by Hans Seyle, 1974).*
- *Change* is everywhere.
- *Change* is the only guarantee in life.
- *Change* is the number one condition of life.
- In order to manage *stress*, you must learn how to welcome and navigate *change*.

Dr. Hans Seyle (b. 1907-d. 1982) was a pioneer in the study of change and stress. In 1936, he began developing his theories and he defined three stages of human reaction to change and stress: the *alarm stage*, the *adaptation stage*, and the *exhaustion/depression stage*:

> The Third Stage: HPA Axis Depression: With repeated exposure to a stressor, thus prolonged cortisol elevation, the hypothalamus and pituitary lose sensitivity – thus the system never turns off, ultimately exhausting the HPA axis. Left unbalanced, it can have a diverse and irreversible impact on the body. (Schuler, 2016)

Since the time of Dr. Seyle and his *General Adaptation Syndrome (GAS)* theory, further research and data has accrued on the subject of stress. In my opinion, the ultimate goal for *all of us* is to interpret the majority of situations in a positive light in order to cultivate *eustress* - or good stress - as opposed to interpreting events as *stressful*, which may ultimately lead to imbalances in the body, mind, and well-being.

What are some sources of stress?

- Divorce
- New job
- Job Security
- Personal Finances
- Loss of a loved one
- Difficult co-workers
- Acute or chronic illness
- Caretaking/Raising a family
- Troubles with a relationship
- Moving to a new town/home
- New responsibilities/clients at work

Here are some symptoms of stress:

- Fear
- Worry
- Anger
- Anxiety
- Fatigue
- Heart burn
- Depression
- Eating poorly
- Skin problems
- Upset stomach
- Shallow breathing
- Weight fluctuations
- Chronic inflammation
- Being overly reactive to others
- Inability to concentrate for long stretches
- Loss of sleep, low quality sleep, nightmares

The following are some conditions associated with chronic stress:

Asthma	Multiple Sclerosis
Allergies	Lupus/Fibromyalgia
Hypertension	Type II Diabetes
Heart Disease	ME/CFS/SEID

- Chronic stress upsets internal health mechanisms such as your immune system, endocrine system, digestive system, etc. which may set you up for acute, chronic, and/or degenerative illnesses. It may affect your health by **affecting your immune system** (including autoimmunity and Th1-Th2 shift). *How?*
- Stress may impact the immune system (which the field of psychoneuroimmunology tells us is influenced by the nervous and endocrine systems) leading to **white blood cells downregulating their cortisol receptors.** According to Miller, Cohen, and Ritchey (2002) this "reduces the cells' capacity to respond to anti-inflammatory signals and allows cytokine-mediated inflammatory processes to flourish" (as cited in Segerstrom & Miller, 2004).
- In turn, this may lead to subsequent non-specific inflammation implicated in conditions like MS, RA, and heart disease. In fact, there may also be "increased antibody production to [a] latent virus, particularly Epstein-Barr" which is consistent with a Th1-Th2 shift (Segerstrom & Miller, 2004).

There are multiple factors involved in what makes stress so damaging. When we get *stressed out*, our *fight or flight response* is activated. Our adrenals pump adrenaline, giving instant energy to deal with the *emergency* at hand. This is fine in the short term, especially if we are being chased by a tiger, real or imagined. But a prolonged stress response is a recipe for disaster. If you feel stressed on your daily commute, or get anxious each time you talk to your partner, then your adrenals are working overtime. What should be a rare event becomes chronic. And chronic stress means elevated adrenaline levels, which results in raised cortisol, which may lead to fatigue if cortisol levels ultimately fall too *low*. This is when you reach for sugar, coffee, chocolate, or all three stimulants. So here is the sequence in diagram:

Elevated Adrenaline→Raised Cortisol→Cortisol Crash→Fatigue→Stimulants

Stimulants do not contain energy.
Instead they make the body use the energy it has at a faster rate. ~ unknown

Overstimulation only makes the problem worse. Because stimulants force the body to use energy faster, *and* because they force the adrenals to produce even more adrenaline, too much creates an *energy debt* in the body. Having too much (or too little) cortisol in your system is *not* a good feeling. Cortisol is necessary, and it keeps inflammation in check. But too much cortisol can affect your immune system. Too little cortisol can result in low energy and inflammation as well.

Overstimulation can keep your body in a state of fight or flight, which means you can't heal as well. In other words, too much stimulation may tend to keep you in a state of chronic stress. Chronic stress is basically trauma, and, frankly, who wants that for their body or mind? Yet, a little stimulation is good. *Again, it's about finding that sweet spot between stress and eustress, relaxed energy and positive eustress.*

Sometimes trauma stems from relationships or other wounds and the emotions attached to them. Some sources of stress are unresolved emotions like fear/anger. Our bodies and minds are intertwined via neuropeptides and neurotransmitters. If we are harboring feelings like hate, anger, or sadness, we may be doing damage to our bodies by not processing our emotions. I use yoga to process emotions, as they are stored in the fascia of our bodies. Fascia is a crystalline structure that holds memory. By practicing yoga and QiGong, I am able to keep my body cleared of the build-up of emotion as it passes through me.
http://www.drnorthrup.com/tag/fascia/

Techniques like EFT (Emotional Freedom Technique) or *EMDR* therapy *(Eye Movement Desensitization and Reprocessing)* may be helpful. During EMDR therapy, the patient may be able to process and resolve lingering trauma. Many people swear by EFT too. Other techniques that might help release emotions include **massage** - which *also keeps fascia healthy like yoga and processes emotion* – acupuncture, stretching, art, music, walking or dog/animal therapy. Our bodies were designed to keep energy and emotions flowing. Find what works for you and try to engage in those activities regularly to stay well and stay in SYNCH.

Stress is a given in life and work. (I understand many of you may not be currently working or able to work. *Never feel shame* – I have been there – and check out my *Empowerpreneur* program on my website.) As we've noted, *a little bit of stress is good* as it can keep you on-target to meet deadlines and perform well. And when you're in the flow, you perceive stress as *good stress* – what keeps you alive/thriving. *Hans Seyle,* the endocrinologist who coined the word *stress,* also coined the word *eustress,* meaning *good stress.* The word *eustress* has two parts: *eu* means *good* in Greek, and the second part - *stress* - is obvious. As we quoted at the beginning of this section, eustress is energy-producing. *Eustress* on the job, at school, or at home is a life-affirming, positive factor.

But excessive worrying about your work performance or conflict with co-workers or family is mostly a lose/lose situation. The bad news is that you can't control other people's actions, or what they think of you. The good news? You *can* control your own actions and take measures to reduce stress. Try these ideas: breathe slowly, take regular breaks, go for short walks, get some fresh air, and keep your blood sugar levels stable. Not only might your creativity and productivity increase, but you could find yourself getting along with people better. Other people's actions? Let them roll off your back if you can. Relationships both personally and professionally are worthwhile and essential. Remember to breathe, smile, relax, and roll with it ...

Whatever is causing you stress, nine times out ten it will find a way to work itself out, whether or not you are worrying about it. In fact, it tends to work out better if you aren't worrying. *Relax into well-being and the FLOW of life. Move out of fear-based living and into the ZONE ...*

Don't stress, progress! Stress can be your growth edge!

The Art of Self-Care and the Practice of Well-Being: Self-Care and Holistic Stress Management

Holistic stress management is about conscious living.

It is vital to find ways to stay calm and focused no matter how crazy life gets. That means we need to practice and prioritize our self-care and stress management skills. In view of that need, I've developed a six point system that you may find to be of use in your daily life:

S.T.R.E.S.S. MANGAGEMENT ™

- ➤ **Support**   Connect with living beings: family, friends, pets
- ➤ **Trust**   Let go of what you can't control; have faith in yourself
- ➤ **Relax**   Practice yoga, deep breathing; seek nature often
- ➤ **Exercise** Reduce insulin and adrenaline; be as active as you can
- ➤ **Sleep**   Build a strong foundation with restorative rest
- ➤ **Sound Diet** Control blood sugar levels with healthy eating

---

To get you started, let's do a brief overview of the six points of this S.T.R.E.S.S. Management plan.

Support: What does support look like? It looks like the people around you: family, friends, professional people, teachers, etc. It is a healthy habit/practice to connect with others. Connection is everything.

Connection is the currency of wellness. ~John Travis

We are not meant to go through this life alone. We need each other, whether we like it or not, or care to admit it. If you need someone to talk to, don't be afraid to ask for time to talk. If you need help, ask for it. Pets give great support as well. If you live alone, consider a pet.

Trust: Trust is crucial to health. If you don't trust in a higher power, find someone or something you can believe in. First and foremost, believe in yourself. Having faith that everything is going to be okay is crucial in managing stress levels. Faith isn't just something you have, it's something you exercise. *Faith is a spiritual muscle.* You can't control everything that happens around you. Trust that other people can take care of some things as well. Delegate power, when you can. And trust that everything is okay, even just as it is.

Relax: Slow down. Take deep breaths. Nothing is so important beyond life itself. Healing happens in a state of deep relaxation. Try getting into rhythm with nature. Nature is the best stress reliever ever, I think! Nature heals and moves at her own pace, and yet gets everything done. You have more time than you think. Relax.

Either melt or disappear into stress or flower into eustress*
*Eustress: stress that is deemed healthful or giving one the feeling of fulfillment.

Exercise: If you have trouble exercising regularly, you might enjoy having a dog. Dogs need to be walked once or twice a day, every day, rain or shine. Dogs are also amazing therapy for trauma and PTSD.

Sleep: When you retire to your bedroom sanctuary, being able to let go and trust that you are going to have a restful night is a big part of sleeping well. You want to sleep deeply so that you recharge your body/rebuild your system. If you have sleep problems - for whatever reason - find a way to solve them. Sleep is crucial to your overall health and in managing stress. There is much more on the importance of movement and restful sleep coming up in this chapter.

Sound Diet: Eating fresh fruits and especially eating greens and vegetables are the cornerstone* of a sound diet. Try exploring the many variable, sensuous tastes food has that can satisfy your appetite and need for variety. However, if eating well is a habit you haven't mastered yet, be creative! Keep nourishing snacks available. Learn to

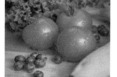

cook, create, and prepare food. **Invite people over for gatherings that focus on food and connection**. *There is always a reason to get together and celebrate life and each and every unique day.* Food is fuel, yes, but when it is prepared with love and intention - and with the intent to unite people and share stories and experience - it becomes alchemical.

*I spent time at an eco-resort in Costa Rica, at a place called The Iquana Lodge. They served us simply the best food I have ever had: my symptoms virtually went away, and I felt so much more vitality in general. They served us primarily local, fresh, plant-based food and I believe it raised not only my antioxidant levels, but improved the diversity of my microbiome. The power of real food, and particularly plant food (herbs, salads, vegetables, and whole fruit) cannot be emphasized enough. Your body was meant to be whole. Feed it real food and give your body a fighting chance to regain equilibrium, and fortify/repopulate your immune system.

The Relaxation Response

Everything you do can be done better from a place of relaxation. ~Stephen C. Paul

If you're looking for an exact opposite of the stress response, you'll find it in what is called *The Relaxation Response*. As we've discussed, it's a term coined by *Herbert Benson* in 1975. His groundbreaking research showed that even short periods of meditation, with repeated slow/deep breathing, can alter the stress response.

Benson found that any type of meditative, repetitive activity may activate the parasympathetic nervous system, which allows the release of hormones and neurotransmitters such as oxytocin, endorphins, and dopamine that enable our bodies to heal.

> [There are] two steps usually required to elicit the relaxation response. They are: (1) the repetition of a word, sound, prayer, phrase or muscular activity and (2) when other, everyday thoughts intrude, there is a passive return to the repetition. (Benson, 1975; Hoffman et al., 1982)

Healing happens in a state of deep relaxation. In fact, Benson's research showed that the *mind is powerful* in not only being able to calm us down, but to *influence expression of genes related to stress and inflammation*. You can read about a collaborative investigation conducted by members of the Benson-Henry Institute for Mind/Body Medicine at Massachusetts General Hospital (MGH) and the Genomics Center at Beth Israel Deaconess Medical Center (BIDMC) in an informative news article which appeared on the *Phys.Org* website ("Relaxation Response Can Influence Expression of Stress-related Genes," 2008).

Another suggestion is to engage with stressors differently. For example, when you're stuck in traffic, breathe. Breathe in slowly and breathe out slowly. Slow breaths, taken from your lower abdomen, calm your central nervous system. Try it, it works. Also, concentrate on *worry-free* things, like enjoying the scenery or listening to the radio. Be mindful. Enjoy the ride.

The relaxation response may back our appetite (stress diverts blood from digestion) so we can digest/absorb our food, giving us the opportunity to harness our natural healing powers. Simply by repeating slow breaths, thoughts, movements, song, or more, we can literally channel our ability to heal. We can slow down and relax our way back into vibrant health.* I believe this is how the placebo effect may work. If one believes one will heal, one may relax, and then the body may harness its natural healing powers.

---

*This is not a simplistic solution. Rather, it is harnessing the power of the body and nature. One can be engaged in life and work, and still relaxed. It is about cultivating calm energy, so one can heal and thrive.

Deep breathing tells the vagus nerve to send a calming message to your nervous system. Here are some ways to cultivate deep breathing: meditation, mindfulness, walking, yoga, Tai Chi, Qi Gong, biofeedback (Heart Math), massage, warm baths, exercise, sex, being creative, nature, pets, prayer, counseling, coaching, essential oils, candles, connection with others, etc.

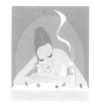

Need some physical help in addition? Try Rescue Remedy, L-Theanine, GABA, passionflower, kava, or valerian. Plus, I can't recommend yoga or Heart Math enough. You can calm yourself by being aware of what stimulates you (biofeedback) and consciously slow your heart rate through deep breathing. Likewise, yoga stimulates your parasympathetic nervous system through *pranayama* (breath work) and/or *vinyasa*, which connects breath with movement. You can move but stay calm, which is a lifesaver for anyone with ME/CFS.

Yoga helps to activate your vagus nerve, which can *help you to self-regulate* (and may influence your microbiome as well). **Self-regulation may be the key between illness and wellness.** Try cat and cow asanas and cultivating ujjayi breath (D. Chopra, personal communication, 2015).

Brain Chemistry

We've been talking about *stimulants* and the *power of the mind*. Relevant to both of those topics is the subject of brain chemistry. You cannot have good health without balanced brain chemistry. Your brain needs first-rate nutrition, glucose, healthy fats, exercise, and sleep. Since I believe that ME/CFS may be at least in part a neurally-mediated condition, brain health is vitally important for those of us with M.E./CFS, MS, etc. Balanced brain chemistry is crucial to well-being.

A hint about the cruciality of balanced brain chemistry is given to us by the number of prescription drugs* designed to affect our neurotransmitter systems, in an attempt to stabilize brain chemistry. This is how important brain chemistry is for your overall health and well-being. And, while I no longer avoid stimulants (*I use them strategically in very small amounts*), an overly stimulated brain may spell trouble (see Chapter Three on glutamate excitotoxicity in *Focus on Neurotransmitters*). Why are so many of us addicted to stimulants such as caffeine? *The answer may lay in our brain chemistry.* As we discussed in Chapter Three, some of us may have been born with deficiencies in certain neurotransmitters or may have weak links.

*I know several people whose lives have been saved by prescription drugs. If there were a prescription drug I could tolerate that took away all my symptoms, I might take it. But, wellness is a lifestyle too.

For example, it could be that those of us who are naturally low in dopamine may use stimulants to pick us up and normalize our brain chemistry. In fact, taking caffeine stimulates dopamine production because the caffeine occupies adenosine receptors. Why is this important? Because normally adenosine is what makes us sleepy. Yet instead of slowing down and resting, our body is told to get up and get going by caffeine occupying a receptor site that doesn't differentiate between adenosine and caffeine.

The point is: you may be self-medicating to balance brain chemistry. But, there are alternatives in addition to stimulants that may also support you in your quest for more energy, while bringing your brain chemistry into balance.

First, eat well, exercise, and really do try to get the sleep your body needs. Secondly, try spirulina or natural Vitamin C to produce norepinephrine in your brain. Another avenue is to take DL-Phenylalanine (DLPA), which is used by the brain to make norepinephrine. DLPA also might lift your mood.

You can try L-Tyrosine to help boost your dopamine levels. However, using amino acids such as L-Tyrosine is very specific for different people. You will have to experiment to see which, if any, amino acid supplementation works best for your brain chemistry. Remember, amino acid therapy is not recommended for long-term use. Check with a natural healthcare practitioner to see what is recommended.

The bottom line is to be aware of what you consume and how you interpret stressors, because you are most definitely affecting your brain chemistry. As I mentioned, during my first bout with fatigue, I avoided chocolate, as I suspected it made me more tired. The sugar was definitely one of the culprits, as *refined sugar wreaks havoc on delicate brain chemistry*. I have to be careful of overstimulating myself, and I also avoid coffee, wheat, and alcohol.

These days, I have found a dynamic balance between nutritional and lifestyle support and **very small amounts of strategic stimulation**. I use small amounts of stimulation from acai, Korean Ginseng, etc. (we're taking **trace amounts** in supplements, primarily) almost as *kindling,* as well as a way to find the *sweet spot between active rest and eustress*. I give myself the *choice* to do whatever will make me feel the best every day. This strategy has worked very well for me along with mind-body fitness and reinterpreting stressors.

I also use Fo Ti, Gota Kola, raw vitamins, ginseng, homeopathic arnica, and superfoods. I love organic protein shakes, or making my own organic protein smoothies with Hawaiian spirulina, an organic banana, spirulina, Cellfood, and vanilla stevia to brighten up my day and wake up my energy naturally. There are so many healthy options these days!

If I do use chocolate, I go for the healthy versions Greens Plus energy bars, etc. *I use just a very small amount.* But I also try to choose what will *lift up and support my energy levels naturally,* without stimulation, like Fo Ti. *I also focus on liver support/ health for energy.* Most importantly, *I trust myself* to make the best decisions for my body each and every day.

As I mentioned, I avoid coffee. Did you know caffeine may interfere with the signals your body is sending to you? You need to be able to read your body's signals in order to heal. ☺ Consider monitoring your caffeine intake so you can *hear your body* talking to you about its needs. Caffeine also raises cortisol levels and that can be a major problem!*

If you are a poor methylator, like I am, caffeine* may metabolize very slowly in your liver. This may have serious side effects on your heart, kidneys and central nervous system. Use with caution. Know and respect your body's needs, strengths, and challenges. It's okay.

Your brain and your body need essential fatty acids (EFAs) to thrive and operate properly. Your brain especially needs EPA and DHA. Look for flax, borage, hemp, vegetarian DHA algae oil, and evening 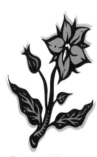 primrose oil to assist your brain health and function, reduce inflammation (which may be contributing to fatigue symptoms), balance out hormones, give you energy, and make your skin and hair beautiful! There are supplements that may help the function of your brain performance including Fo Ti, ginkgo, spirulina, lavender, L-Theanine, acetyl-choline, DMAE, choline, gota kola, phosphatidylserine, and Siberian ginseng, to name a few of my favorites.

Borage Flower

Also, when we yield to the yin side of our brain - our creative brain - we actually may be able to restore balance to our brain chemistry. When we do this, it may kick in our natural mind-body connection that may lead to a more healing state of being. See Chapter Three.

For me, being present is the real high, vs. being overstimulated (by fear)

Exercise also raises energy levels by creating numerous feel-good chemicals in the brain like *beta-endorphins, dopamine, and serotonin.*

*Cardamom oil or seed may help with detoxing caffeine. Reversed cortisol levels are implicated in fatigue.

Exercise: Just Do It, If You Can
If You Can't, Don't Sweat It

We generate fears while we sit; we overcome them by action.
Fear is nature's warning signal to get busy. ~ Henry Link

If health practitioners could bottle exercise or encapsulate it in pill form, it would be the *number one* prescribed remedy of all time.

Why? Because movement is fundamental, not only for our overall well-being, but for controlling stress levels as well. It also enhances our immune system and keeps our lymph system fine-tuned.

For people with pain, low energy, ME/CFS, or with other conditions which make it challenging to move, try **restorative exercise** such as slow walking to build up your chi levels. Other types of restorative movement include Tai Chi, Qi Gong, yoga (try yin or restorative), etc.

Do what you can within your pain and **energy envelope.**

Even if you can only walk around your couch, try to move. Even if you are in a chair or in bed, try to find a way to move exactly where you are. Keep your life and *chi* moving in some way. Keep building up your energy, and therefore your well-being, and even your health.

Action is the law of well-being. ~ Dr. Bob Delmonteque

Take baby steps. Eventually, baby steps will get you where you want to go. Actually where you may want to go is right where you currently are, *only operating out of love instead of fear, which may reduce cortisol levels.*

Trust and love yourself to take all the baby steps necessary to gradually move toward your health and wellness goals.

A flower grows where it was planted or where the seed took root. Then it blossoms into its full expression of being. You can bloom too.

*I can't recommend the DVD's by Freedom2Move enough. They are home and exercise videos customized to you. If you have a chronic condition, check them out! Whether you are an athlete or have MS/CFS, etc. try to keep moving!

http://freedom2move.org/

I am a huge fan of walking and mind-body fitness. You might find you can do it as well - even at a very slow pace - and gradually build up your *chi* over the course of the walk or yoga/tai chi/Qi Gong practice. Time is on your side. See if you can find mental energy/time to move.

Those who think they have no time for bodily exercise
will sooner or later have to find time for illness. ~Edward Stanley

Let air and breath, love and sex, water and food, nature and even connection to the universe be your energy, your medicine ... get in touch with your *chi*, your life-force. Your mind, body and soul are inextricably linked. Affect one, and you affect the others. Don't think about what you've lost. Think about everything you stand to gain.

If you can't exercise much or at all, consider listening to music. It may sound strange, but I believe hearing music can be a sort of workout. Faster music may increase your heart rate. Slower music can calm you down and turn on The Relaxation Response. Who knows, you may even feel like dancing a bit. Whatever you can or can't do, just love and accept yourself as you are. There is nothing you have to do or be.

Exercise and Your Immune System

Even more so than nutrition, exercise has the capacity to protect and enhance the immune response. *How does it do this?*

Experimental studies show that a regular exercise program of brisk walking, five times per week at around 30 minutes each time can bolster many defenses of the immune system, including the antibody response and the natural killer (T cell) response.

> There are actually physiological changes in the immune system that happen when a person exercises. Cells that promote immunity circulate through the system more rapidly, and they're capable of killing both viruses and bacteria. After exercising, the body returns to normal within a few hours, but a regular exercise routine appears to extend periods of immunity. (Brown, 2013)

This may be important for someone with ME/CFS who often has an altered immune function. Please refer to the section in Chapter Three on *Th1 to Th2 Shift*. Of course, exercise can be a challenge due to low energy, which is why I recommend mind-body fitness* instead.

*Mind-body fitness can keep you in the parasympathetic state, where healing happens. Try restorative exercise too, like a yin yoga class, to help your body gain ground. Qi-Gong helps to build energy too.

Exercise raises your glutathione levels, and adjusts your cortisol levels, depending on what your body needs. Talk about a built-in adaptogen! And, as we've noted, **exercise raises your energy levels** by creating numerous *feel-good* chemicals in your brain like beta-endorphins, dopamine, and serotonin. Feeling good may strengthen immunity as well. ~ **I am a big believer in doing what feels good to be well.** ~

Movement also creates energy because of the oxygen you bring to your system. Remember, disease cannot exist in a well-oxygenated environment. Also, do what you can to protect your **emotional heart** and **heart muscle**. Your heart has more neurons than your brain!

Wellness is about realizing one's value, as well as the value of the life and well-being of the planet. Even if you're very sick, do what you can to make healthy choices for yourself. **Remember that you matter.**

Restorative Movement

I don't mean to undermine those of you who literally can't move at all. Remember, I was in bed for six months. I get it. I know what it's like to feel zero energy. I also know the word *exercise* can feel intimidating and even boring or frustrating. That's why I like the words *movement* and *restorative*, because *movement is restorative*. So, anything you can do to move - anything at all - may help support your return to health. I believe this. If you can find a rhythm - some kind of rhythmic pattern with movement - even better. This will engage and maybe even recondition your nervous system and facilitate new positive pathways of health, relaxation, and well-being.

Energy: What It Is and How to Create More of It

The windmill never strays in search of the wind. ~ *Andy J. Sklivis*

When we let go of fear and doubt, a world of pure energy opens up to us, and comes directly from within us. We also may have to pro-actively seek ways to increase energy within us. Ultimately, since the body is an energy system, two things are always happening: we move energy in, i.e., we create energy, and we move unwanted energy out.

This is yoga, FLOW, and union too.

Within our overall energy system, here are five energy areas as well as ways to take care of/be aware of the energy within each one:

Care Tactics for Our Five Energy Areas	
Physical Energy	Nutrition and stress management
Mental Energy	Our thoughts - conscious and subconscious - our beliefs about others, the world, and ourselves
Emotional Energy	Self-care, being authentic, setting boundaries, and seeking *joy*
Spiritual Energy	Trust in the world at large, getting into the flow of life, faith in life & one's self
Communal or Social Energy	Fitting in, connecting with others: exchanging energy with others may greatly influence personal energy levels

You might be wondering about your own personal energy in each of the five areas that you interact with every day. Let me ask you: *What is your natural energy or energetic signature?* By that I mean: What is that **frequency of everyday life** you can tune into where your energy flows naturally and spontaneously? Where and when is your energy effortless, and under what circumstances? In Chapter Five you can explore your natural signature musical note as well. Mine is C. The C note grounds me and resonates with me.

I've thought a lot about my personal energy. I know I'm sensitive to energy, whether it's my own energy, or external energy, such as from another person. Even environmental energy, artificial or natural, affects me. And it's perfectly okay that I have these sensitivities.

I had a few practitioners along the way tell me I was sensitive, not sick. I appreciate their well-meaning intentions. Being sensitive* is a gift, and makes me more "sensitive" to energies. This is the good news about creating more energy. If you are sensitive to it, i.e. *aware of it*, you can harness it and *live from passion and purpose*. Living from passion/purpose is a whole different kind of energy. You are then connected to the universe, and can channel infinite energy, which is what energy is: *infinite...it cannot be created nor destroyed...it just flows and changes form... *I am sensitive. I am an HSP, and easily stimulated (see pg. 204)*

The key is to not obsess over low energy. It's about *focusing on raising your vitality*, and finding a positive way to engage with *life* that is meaningful, purposeful, and joyful. This way of *engaging with infinite energy* then *helps you to harness eustress* (positive stress), and find ways to calmly yet actively and positively engage with life. I am not belittling your condition at all. These are hard-won tips, as I have said before.

The biggest thing I've learned about energy is that it's not about trying to control my energy levels. This took me forever to figure out. I used to think that if I manipulated my low energy I could function normally, and be like others. *But, it's about supporting your body/mind, not controlling it.* It's about support, balance, and getting into *flow*. Find a new, dynamic balance where you can *flow with the natural energy of life...*

When you put your energy into raising your *chi* levels - your level of natural vitality - through diet, positive mindset, restorative exercise, faith, connection, community - you naturally raise your energy levels. When you take care of yourself, you build *ener-chi*. You build life-force. You learn how to re-condition your nervous system to handle more stress (through self-care/nutrition) and reinterpret stress as a positive.

The definition of suffering is *resisting what is*. When we resist being tired, guess what persists? Instead of fighting low energy, I encourage you to put your power into raising your vibration, your natural vitality.

Your body doesn't know the difference between different types of stressors. Whether they are physical, mental, emotional, spiritual, social, or environmental, your body reads them as being the same and responds to them similarly. Try to cultivate *joy* - because feeling joyful is one of the quickest and best ways to heal – and *purpose* to find the energy to live. Go for *joy* and *purpose* to awaken your energy/potential.

Energy Envelope

If you keep your expended energy within the limits of your available energy, you have a chance to reduce symptoms, and over time may be able to expand your limits. (Bruce Campbell, 2005)

Are you living within your energy envelope? You are if the energy you *have* and the energy you *use*, on either side of the fence, are in balance. The idea is to *make the best use of the energy that inhabits your body at any given point-in-time* and to build your reserves through self-care: yoga, walking, tai chi, good food, great company, deep sleep, and so on.

> *[Sleep is the] magical time*
> *when **the healing vibration of night***
> *sweeps the earth.* ~ Caroline Sutherland

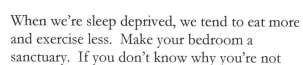

Don't you love this quote? The nighttime is for resting, relaxing, and healing. It is sacred time to reboot before you start another day. It is just as important as any other part of your routine.

When we're sleep deprived, we tend to eat more and exercise less. Make your bedroom a sanctuary. If you don't know why you're not sleeping well, seek professional help. This is your time to recuperate and recharge so you can take on the next day energized and focused.

Sleep is a big issue for people with ME/CFS since many sufferers may not get the kind of rest that feels refreshing. *Do people with ME/CFS have low melatonin levels because they have low serotonin stores due to severe stress? Remember, stress depletes serotonin levels and raises cortisol levels.*

If so, what is the solution? As I have described, I use 5-HTP to help restore the balance of my serotonin and melatonin levels. I also use deep, slow breathing to engage the vagus nerve, combined with not thinking about anything important when I'm falling asleep. GABA also helps with slowing down my brain waves, so I think less.

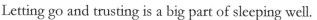

Letting go and trusting is a big part of sleeping well. Trust in the healing process of sleep. Trust your body. Trust the skies. Trust in the healing energy of the night. Trust in the poetry of the night. It is dark, mellow, relaxing, and enveloping feminine energy. Let the night take you where it will. Believe that you can and will get the sleep you need so you return again in the morning for a new day, refreshed, full of hope, light, energy, and increased trust in your own power. Listen to the words of *Miranda J. Barrett:*

"Every time you make a commitment to your own self-care, self-love and self-respect and then follow through, you build trust in yourself" (2014).

Tools for De-stressing

We've already talked in detail about some of these tools for destressing, and we'll talk about a few more of them, coming up. But for now, here's a list of self-care ideas for reducing and/or reinterpreting stress in your life.

- Yoga — Move, breathe, relax, activate your vagus nerve to self-regulate

- Meditation — Do it your way, e.g., repeat prayers, thoughts, sounds

- Music — Listen, play, sing, let music be a source of medicine & harmony*

- Nature — Get into rhythm with nature, relax into well-being

- Exercise — Do what you can as regularly as you can

- Journaling — Write a diary, poems, letters

- Biofeedback - HeartMath Story — Connect your mind and heart

- Massage — Relax, even allow yourself to fall asleep

- Acupuncture — Manage stress and pain naturally

- Friends/Family — Connection is the currency of wellness

- Deep Breathing — slowly, deeply, and from the abdomen

- Moderation — The key is to be moderate in all choices

- Quit Smoking — See your last smoke ring float away

- Inspiration w/passion — Look up, listen, imagine, create, live

- Slow Down — Smell the flowers, be PRESENT for your life

*The Chinese word for medicine comes from the character that means music (and herbs and happiness) ☺

Music ~ Don't forget about music's ability to calm and soothe your body and soul. Music connects the right and left brain hemispheres, and literally helps our bodies to heal. If you have forgotten to play music lately, load up your car with your favorite cds and listen while you're stuck in rush hour traffic. Get connected to what inspires you. Inspiration is a great way to relieve acute and on-going stress.

Bodywork - Massage and Acupuncture ~ It's amazing what a *massage* can do to restore your body and it's great to keep your fascia healthy too. *Acupuncture* is another method to manage stress. It's one of the best ways to manage chronic pain as well, which can be a source of stress. Massage and acupuncture shouldn't be viewed as *extras* or *pampering*. They're viable tools to reduce and manage stress levels. Do whatever it takes to refocus and manage your stressful feelings. It can make a huge difference in the quality of your life - on all levels. Don't be afraid to seek other types of somatic therapy or counseling as well if you need it. We're all in this together. People really can and do help.

Small Goals/Moderation ~ You know the old saying, *everything in moderation.* Whether it's stimulants, cortisol levels, or eating fresh food, amounts matter and affect how you *feel.* Too much of a good thing, may be just too much. The reverse is true for too little of a good thing, like eating fresh produce, for instance. Even if you think you don't like veggies, there are usually a few that you can think of - if you try hard - that you can tolerate, or even enjoy eating. How about brussel sprouts, snow peas, red potatoes, pumpkin, or butternut squash? Superfoods are another way to get high doses of the nutrients we need, and a good dose of chlorophyll. Superfoods include wheat grass, acai, chlorella, spirulina, and mangosteen. Set a goal to start with small amounts of fresh food/healthy food. Setting small goals helps you integrate them. *And, no, you can't just have a salad once or twice a year and expect results. Greens are so good for you and can make you feel great!* ☺

Inspiration ~ What inspires you? Inspiration is life force and has everything to do with being healthy and stress-free. If volunteering inspires you, do it on a regular basis. If listening to and/or playing music inspires you, join a group or invest in a sound system. Take a yoga class, rent favorite movies, read a new-release novel, surround yourself with people you admire. You can't be stressed and inspired in the same breath. Well, maybe you can, but it's much more difficult, and inspiration, not always, but usually, wins out.

Quit Smoking! ~ Easier said than done, I know. Perhaps you smoke to lessen stress. Instead, you may be increasing your anxiety. That alone is a *stressful* fact. Tobacco use remains the single largest preventable cause of death and disease in the United States (CDC, 2015). Maybe now is your chance to rethink why you choose to do something that carries such a *huge price tag*. Can you afford it? There are many ways to kick the smoking habit. For example, you can try good nutrition, counseling, neuro-linguistic programming (NLP), and hypnosis. Remember, change happens in stages. In fact a book written on *how* change happens – *Changing for Good* - was, in large part, based on the study of people who quit smoking on their own, in little increments (Prochaska, Norcross, & DiClemente, 2007). People smoke now than less than they used to. People quit every day. You can change. Don't ever give up on yourself. Keep in mind that there are even *positive habits* that can replace smoking overtime: meditation, and exercise. Living well/well-being is a habit, too. You can condition your mind and yourself to cultivate it.

Slow Down ~ It's a cliché, but don't forget to stop and smell the flowers. There's a reason people do this. It makes you feel pretty darn great. If you don't like flowers, slow down and watch the game, cook a meal with someone you love, or read a book. Take time to appreciate where you are in life, wherever that may be. Notice the details. *This is your precious life.* Feeling stressed means you may be missing out on how it really feels to be alive. So slow down, breathe, look around you, look up at the sky. Ask how someone else is doing, and listen to their answer. Experience your life *now* while you can. Never lose your sense of wonder with this amazing world we live in.

Tension is who you think you should be. Relaxation is who you are. ~ *Chinese Proverb*

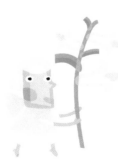

Just be your awesome, amazing, authentic self!

Note: The main tactics that have helped me are practicing mindfulness and finding balance – that sweet spot – between support (rest or downtime, nutrition, yoga, connection) and eustress or positive stress. I used to try to stimulate my body for energy. Now, I support my body, and address immunity and inflammation first to reduce fatigue.

My Wellness Tools

*Yoga, mindfulness, positive thinking, staying connected with people

Real Food Diet ~ avoiding refined sugar and refined flour, some raw foods, live and cultured foods, fresh foods, alkaline foods, superfoods like wheat grass and Hawaiian spirulina, sprouted foods like brown rice, veggies like brussel sprouts, foods high in glutathione like sweet potatoes and avocadoes, leafy greens (make them the base of your meals), small amounts of organic whole fruit alone or in smoothies, cage-free eggs, gluten-free oatmeal and non-GMO cereals; organic, high-quality protein shakes. I honor healthy cravings and *emphasize fresh fruits, vegetables, herbs, and supplements to support my liver/body.*

Supplements ~ *Raw & food-based vitamins, superfoods, EFA's, herbs, etc.*

Deep sleep ~ *5-HTP, food-based minerals, Black Cohosh, Theanine-Serene*

Cultivating eustress (positive stress) ~ interpreting life as positive

Home ~ Make my home a safe, happy, healthy, loving, holistic haven

Restorative exercise ~ yoga, walking, hiking, Qi Gong, Tai Chi

Love & Boundaries ~ Respecting my *energy envelope/staying connected*

A Snapshot of My Life

I wake up between 6:30 - 8:30 a.m. My body likes 6 ½ - 8 hours of sleep. The more balanced I am the day before, the less sleep I need. Occasionally I wake up earlier or later, say 4:30 a.m. if I have gone to bed early. I try to go to sleep when I am first feeling tired, whenever that may be. It is so worth it to catch that first wave of healing sleep.

A shower is my spa/self-care time. I love natural HABA care products that are ethical, organic, and natural*. Afterwards, I put on essential oil blends. They help my energy levels, especially cocoa & citrus. I may do yoga poses while there's heat and humidity in the bathroom, or a short time later I do a concentrated yoga practice to set the day's tone.

*This term, natural, is essentially meaningless, which is why you have to read labels and do your research.

First thing in the a.m., I have fresh citrus juice or some kind of protein shake. I have an Orgain protein shake, drink hemp milk, or I make a protein shake with hemp milk, stevia, and superfoods. I often add Cellfood to help my body make extra oxygen and energy. In colder months, I love to make herbal tea – like Roobios – or I make a carob powder drink, which is high in magnesium. Hemp Milk is my go-to base. I use Pacific Vanilla. I love Trader Joe's soy creamer for hot tea, or I often just use straight hemp milk.

I often steep Tazo's Wild Sweet Orange herbal tea in cold water for 5-10 minutes. It has mint* for inflammation and licorice, which has phytosterols. *Some days I juice a fresh, organic lime, lemon, or orange*, add Truvia, and a few drops of liquid vanilla *stevia*. Sometimes I combine the tea and juice for homemade herbal lemonade. Either formula *gives me tons of energy* and a good dose of live enzymes and vitamin C complex. I make stevia and hemp milk for a sweet, consistent energy pick-me-up, often later in the day, around 4 pm.

For the first hour or two of the day, I answer and send emails, write, edit, or study. Contemporary music boosts my concentration. I *love* music. For breakfast, my body likes protein, carbs, healthy oils, a touch of sweetness, and nutritious, high-quality organic foods in the morning. In cooler months, I have organic, gluten-free cereal, and buckwheat or oatmeal in cold months - with, bananas, hemp milk, cashew butter, or yogurt. Organic eggs, sea salt, and organic avocadoes are a powerful combo for me with carbs. I use spirulina powder, VitaMineralGreen, and real Vitamin C powder in shakes.

~ I use herbal supplements and raw/food-based vitamins for real energy ~
~ I don't "fight fatigue: I support my body and reduce inflammation levels ~

After breakfast, I work on my business, attend meetings, teach yoga, work out, make phone calls, etc. I try to do the most important things first.

I often have a protein shake mid-morning to mid-afternoon. I'll have an Orgain or CalNaturale shake. I snack on grapes, apple slices, or healthy nuts.

I prefer to exercise earlier in the day rather than later. But anytime is better than no time. I do yoga often, walk, hike, Pilates, or get on the treadmill if it's raining. Of course, I built up to and do this within my *energy envelope*.

I emphasize mindfulness, self-care and stress management, and deep support with a small amount of strategic stimulation when necessary. Support can be food, self-care, mindfulness, etc. and stimulation can be food/supplements, positive stress, passion, purpose, people, positivity, positive interaction, etc.

Join my site ConnektWell.com to learn how to live mindfully and live a healthy lifestyle. Come and join our community! *I notice mint seems to really help my neuro-inflammation as well as my energy levels. Does this point to a brain's activated immune system?

After walking/hiking, I stretch or do yoga. Staying active is win-win. Exercise increases energy, oxygen, and immune levels. I realize this doesn't work for those who are exhausted. Start where you are. Sit by a sunny window and do breathwork, or listen to uplifting music.

To keep my blood sugar steady, I snack on grapes, strawberries, apple slices with peanut butter, and Yum Nuts (I like their flavor-roasted cashews with honey) or Sahale Nuts. Raw, organic cashews or tamari almonds are also easy and healthy. *I take Nature's Plus vitamins, Raw/Food-Based Vitamins, Spirulina, Acai (non-standardized) with me* when I'm on the road, running errands, traveling, etc. *I plan ahead to stay well.* ~I carry small bottles of DMAE, L-Theanine, and vitamins in my purse~ I take various supplements throughout the day, depending on what my body needs, *like raw/food-based supplements, ginkgo, gota kola, 5HTP, etc.* I love Aveda's Comforting Tea during the day or early evening. It has a perfect mix of herbals to heal and tone the nervous system.

If I am feeling stressed or excitable at any point in the day, I take Mood Up, Stress Down, Busy Brain, L-Theanine, or milky oats. Rescue Remedy works well, but I'm sensitive to alcohol, so I actually take Rescue Remedy for Pets, as it has a glycerin base. I love to take L-Theanine to have calm, focused energy especially when working. *Toward the evening, I use Fo Ti, DMAE, raw or food-based minerals (I love MegaFood's Calcium, Magnesium & Potassium formula), real vitamin C, or Pacific's hemp milk with stevia as natural energy boosters.* I try to honor my body's innate bio-rhythms, and wind down naturally as evening approaches. There is always time to make the choice to take care of yourself. Self-care is a choice and an orientation to life and well-being!

~Pause for Meditation~

Take five deep, slow breaths - starting from your abdomen - do some yoga, or take a walk to activate your parasympathetic nervous system and the Relaxation Response. The aroma of Lavender lavender also helps with relaxation (Lehrner et al., 2005).

I eat dinner between 6 - 8 p.m. If there's time, I make a healthy meal and I try to keep it varied. If I'm on a tight schedule, I make a *go-to* healthy dinner option – some are listed under *Recipes.* (Join us on ConnektWell.com for many more recipes!) *I base my meals on fresh, live, yummy food.* The synergy of the meal makes it healthful, not to mention delicious! Living well feels good and has synergistic benefits!

In the early stages of recovery - if I could drum up the energy to work or write at all, and that energy only came in brief spurts - I was done for the day even before dark. Sometimes I was so tired I was ready for bed as early as 5:30 p.m. Fast forward to my life now. My usual pattern is to finish working around 5 or 6 p.m., although that's not always possible. But I'm usually done by 7 p.m. in terms of being *"on."* After dinner, it's time to relax, watch a movie, read, or whatever.

Travel Well! I plan ahead to travel successfully and stay well on the road:
~ I carry DMAE, L-Theanine, and raw/food-based vitamins in my purse ~

Every day, as I move through my schedule, I remind myself that *well-being is about dynamic balance.* Balance is one of the primary foundations of well-being and it is how one achieves self-regulation of daily stressors. That's why I'm big on time for self-care, even during the day, to allow my body, mind, and soul to rest, relax, reboot, and recover (at night). *See Chapter Five, Riding the Wave of Health/Well-Being.* Another major foundation of well-being is connection with other people (and pets too!). I make sure to interact *face-to-face* with people during the week. I see more people when I teach yoga and through my work (even Skype). And I try to socialize just to have fun. ☺

I try to go to bed around 10 p.m. I may take 5-HTP either an hour before I turn off the lights, or right before sleep. On occasion, I take valerian or GABA to relax my whole body. GABA receptors are produced in both brains, meaning your head and your gut. GABA calms me, and it also slows down my brain waves, so I don't do as much random thinking, i.e. worry. I take Wishgarden's Serious Relaxer and/or Target's black cohosh for extra support, when stressed, or L-Theanine Serene, standardized valerian, etc. Valerian is a natural, cool adaptogen and L-Theanine Serene has adaptogens in it as well.

Do what you have to do in order to recover. It's okay.

And finally, paying attention to symptoms is a huge part of feeling better! *I pay attention to symptoms.* Symptoms can be my best friends if I listen to them. They can also be my worst enemies if I ignore them indefinitely. I'm a creature of habit. So are you. Learn to develop and refine the habit of listening to your symptoms and taking action on them. Symptoms are what I call *instinctive healing energies.* You can read much more about instinctive health in Chapter Five's section titled *Symptoms and Instinctive Health.* ~ *Do what it takes to feel good and be well. It makes all the difference. Give yourself a fighting chance to heal and be well.* ~

The Practice of Well-Being

The Art of Self Care and Practicing Boundaries

~ Whatever's right for you is always right. Take care of yourself first ~

I have deferred taking care of myself far too often. Perhaps it was because I was trying to meet other people's needs first. *Oh, I should do this for myself, but I need to help this person first.* Or maybe I couldn't *feel or acknowledge* my own needs for any number of reasons. Or I may have recognized that there were things to do for myself, but I was caught up in the rush of the moment. *I'm busy. I'll do that later.* The problem is that *later* becomes *never.*

When is the right time to take care of yourself? Right now. This is the only time there is anyway, ever. There may not be a *later.* You are worth the time. You *need* to be taken care of…by yourself. Your body needs you, *now.* This is your road back to well-being: *self-care.*

Sustainable health is a practice, like yoga. And if you practice on a regular basis, it becomes an integral, built-in part of your daily life. *In fact, I now practice self-care in a spiritual way.* Doing so gives me new insights every day into my own self-worth, my purpose and mission here and now, my part in the larger scheme of things.

Figure out how to value yourself.

As you learn to value yourself, you will achieve more and more balance in your life. It's all about balance, about creating a healthy, pattern of sustainable living … and, most importantly, it's about letting go of what you can't control … which, believe me, is most things.

Life is meant to be enjoyed. That's the bottom line. Stress does not have to control your life. If it is, then it may be time to overhaul and reprioritize what is truly important to you. Having low stress or responding to stress in a positive way is a *huge* factor in getting well and staying well. Live well, be well, and don't take life too seriously. Remember: *Don't stress, progress! Allow stress to be your growth edge …*

Does everyone have a right to be healthy and happy? Yes. And that means you too. Whatever your health or life challenges, consider making well-being one of your *highest priorities. It can change your life.*

Use whatever resources you have. For example, my imagination has shielded me through many a painful hour. Also, memories of good times have lightened my thoughts. My mom collects and memorizes poems to use in stressful times. Use what is at your fingertips and try it all. You never know what will work and ultimately save you. Also, reach out and stay connected. Seek and build community.

But don't discount the reality that illness and/or unhappiness may be part of your life at this time. If you *disown* what has happened to you, believe it or not, it makes it harder to heal. Put another way, if you don't acknowledge what you've been through, you can't move ahead. Accept and embrace all parts of your life, the ups and downs, good and bad. You have to move through your pain. So, be grateful for the lessons and downtime illness has brought you. But then find out what works for you and do it consistently to gain ground.

Also, know that you are not to blame for your illness or condition. Despite all the things you may have lost: health, time, friends, family, jobs, self-esteem … it doesn't mean it was your fault or that you deserved it. Don't let any lack of support keep you from progressing on your journey. Instead, if you receive criticism, use it to build a tunnel around yourself as you head toward the light of healing. No matter how painful it may be to feel misunderstood, choose to use this to your advantage. The paradox of judgment is that the more it is piled on you, the more you can use the heaviness of it as a shield to protect yourself. Focus on all the positive progress you're making, and that *YOU ARE WHOLE* just as you are…right now, here, forever…

As we have acknowledged, one of the most central steps you can take in your healing process is to *realize your inherent value*. Realizing your own self-worth is so crucial that I would put it #1 on your list of priority *thoughts to hold* - along with the focus and intention to heal. Your well-being is your best investment of your time and energy.

And don't be ashamed of wondering why you maybe don't have positive self-image yet, or that you can't figure out how to think positively about yourself. We all struggle with these issues. They may be part of the most defining battles of humankind. Once you realize that *your life matters* - that you have something unique and wonderful to contribute to this amazing world - then everything else falls into place.

*He who has a **why** to live for, can bear almost any **how**. ~ Friedrich Nietzsche*

The meaning of Nietzsche's quote has carried me through one of my biggest challenges of all: the combination of trauma and illness. My core sense of self-worth was deeply affected and it felt like my entire being descended into a dark hole. Finding a way to climb out of that hole was the *how* in Nietzsche's quote. My valuable purpose for living was the *why*. I realized that I was inherently worthy. You are too.

Healing and releasing the trauma attached to my soul was and still is a huge part of the on-going process for me. Think of it this way: Yes, we have physical bodies that need real, unprocessed, untainted nutrition in order to be well or get well. But we also have souls, or whatever you wish to call that mysterious part of ourselves, that must be awakened by joy, nourished regularly with unconditional love, and sustained by light. Please see Chapter Five for both practical and more in-depth tips and tools to consider on your journey toward well-being.

Keep in mind that your body is you, but *you are more than your body*. Much, much more. Your body may be at the mercy of illness at this time, but *your spirit is not*. You have a beautiful soul and that will never, ever change.

Perhaps part of your journey to well-being may be to understand that the universe is made up of energy, and you are part of this infinite source of energy. Unblock and mobilize your own energy. Use this wisdom to ease through wherever your mind may be currently stuck.

Be beautiful on the inside. You *do* have control over your feelings, attitude, and mindset, no matter how out-of-control your body seems to be. However, keep in mind that your body *may not be out of control*. It may be doing what it can under current circumstances. It may be trying to protect you or be seeking stabilization. Your body may be asking for change in your inner and/or outer environments.

Of course, I'm not referring to conditions which may go beyond exposure to environmental toxins, inadequate nutrition, negative energy, etc. Genetics do play a role, even though genetic influence plays a role in around 2% of diseases. However, remember, even genetics can be influenced by lifestyle. YOU play the biggest role in determining the quality of your life and well-being.

It takes hard work to lead a healthy lifestyle. A routine of devotion, dedication, focus, and determination is necessary to provide your life with long-term wellbeing. This progression can be intimidating, confusing and can lead to frustration unless you are given the right tools, like having enough information, to make good decisions for sustainable health. (unknown)

Do you agree with this quote? I don't totally agree. It *can* take conscious effort, at first, to reach what is your most healthy state of being for you. **Focus is needed to create new habits,** *which* **takes concentrated energy.** But your own personal level of optimal health should come naturally and effortlessly, once you establish healthy pathways. *You can reach a place of cruise control, your flying altitude. This is when being healthy feels effortless.* What is required is to establish new pathways in your brain. These new, healthy pathways will become your focal point. Healing should be a state of instinctual ease. The path of least resistance really does lead you to yourself. **Tip: focus on new, healthy habits instead of your old ones!**

You might be thinking: *You've told me how **you** got better. How do **I** get better? What will work for me? And what if it's not as simple as following my body's symptoms, eating super well, and keeping my stress levels down? What if I have other obstacles in my way such as abuse, trauma, or fear? What if I can't change my health habits even if I know I need to in order to save my life? What if I can't get well, due to genetics, no matter what I do? What then?*

Putting It All Together:
How to Give Yourself the Best Chance to Heal

In order to answer your questions, let's start with one basic premise:

The big and little choices you make each and every day - every hour and even every powerful moment, really - greatly impact your ability to heal and be well.

Why is this premise true? It's true because we have learned from recent research that we have more control over our genes and genetic expression than previously believed (epigenetics – which means above and beyond genetic expression – factors like mindset, lifestyle, etc.).

In order to talk about how we have a certain amount of control over genetic expression, let's review what we know about *telomeres*.

Remember our discussion of *telomeres* in Chapter Three? If not, you can review these sections:

Stress and Depression

A New Theoretical Model of Depression

Potential Treatments and Interventions for Depression

A Connection between Depression and CFS

Early Stress and Chronic Illness

Childhood Trauma and Risk for CFS

Maybe you recall Zeb, the cartoon zebra, and the little drawing of him showing his stripes unraveling. We said that our chromosomes can unravel like Zeb's stripes. But telomere cells can help keep our chromosome structures intact. Why? Because telomere cells act like the tip of a shoelace. They're cap-like assemblies found at the end of each chromosome. Thus, telomeres protect our genetic information. However, we also know telomeres can get shorter overtime, resulting in possible negative health outcomes.

> A telomere is a repeating sequence of DNA at the end of a chromosome. Each time a cell replicates and divides the telomere loses some of its length. Eventually the telomere runs out, and the cell can no longer divide and rejuvenate, triggering a poor state of cell health that contributes to disease risk and eventual cell death. (Richards, 2013)

> Telomeres are the protective caps on the ends of chromosomes that affect how quickly cells age. They are combinations of DNA and protein that protect the ends of chromosomes and help them remain stable. As they become shorter, and as their structural integrity weakens, the cells age and die quicker. (Fernandez, 2013)

The good news is that telomere length and telomerase - the enzyme that causes telomeres to lengthen - are both largely in your control when you make the big and little daily and hourly choices we mentioned at the beginning of this section: what you choose to put into your body, how you decide to move your body and on what schedule, how you allow yourself to react to stressful events, how you interact with others and well as the frequency of interaction, etc.

> A small pilot study shows for the first time that changes in diet, exercise, stress management and social support may result in longer telomeres, the parts of chromosomes that affect aging. (Fernandez, 2013)

> Telomere length is epigenetically regulated, meaning it is influenced by nutritional status, and the healthy function of telomeres requires adequate methylation. (Richards, 2013)

We have at least some control over our genetic potential: genetic expression and even telomere length and the telomerase enzyme.

Another major point we discussed in Chapter Three was methylation, one of the body's most important chemical processes.

Healthy function of telomeres requires adequate methylation. The primary methyl donor for this purpose is called SAMe, which uses nutrients like methionine, MSM sulfur, choline, and trimethylglycine as building blocks. Forming SAMe from these building blocks requires vitamin B12, folic acid, and vitamin B6. Folic acid and B12 actually play multiple roles in supporting telomere genomic stability. The most important basic supplement for telomere support is a good quality multiple vitamin, along with adequate dietary protein, especially sulfur-rich proteins. Examples include whey protein, eggs, cottage cheese, dairy, red meat, chicken, legumes, duck, nuts, and seeds. Eggs contain the highest source of choline in the diet, with others such as red meat, chicken, dairy, nuts, and seeds containing moderate amounts. Your brain also requires a large supply of methyl donors to maintain a good mood. Chronic stress and depression typically indicate a lack of methyl donors, meaning telomeres are undernourished and prone to accelerated aging. This is a major reason why stress ages people. (Richards, 2013)

We're also realizing more and more how crucial Vitamin D is to our overall health:

Vitamin D determines how much inflammatory heat the immune system generates. With a lack of vitamin D, it is easy to overheat, generate a ton of free radicals and damage your telomeres. Your ability to tolerate stress successfully is based in no small part on your vitamin D status, including your ability to fight infection. (Richards, 2013)

Protect yourself from the sun, yes. But, put on your mineral-based sunscreen and protective clothing, and get out there, especially before and after 10-3 pm and also when UVB rays are dominant. And, consider vitamin D3 supplementation, as well as eating sources of Vitamin D like sustainably-sourced salmon and free-range eggs.

Even more so, telomeres are not only influenced *by* epigenetics, but **specifically** by exercise, social support, and nutrition.

Nutrition can be defined for this purpose as the very specific nutrients that may contribute to enhanced telomerase activity as well as glutathione production.

Some crucial nutrients for telomerase lengthening may be vitamin E and zinc. Also, reservetrol and turmeric may mitigate inflammation, which can jeopardize telomere length (Richards, 2013).

Another such nutrient is magnesium, which I strongly suspect to be a pre-cursor to both glutathione production (Ewis, Abdel-Rahman, 1995) and epigenetic potential, i.e., lengthening of telomeres: "Magnesium is necessary for many enzymes involved with DNA replication and repair" (Richards, 2013).

So you may imagine that magnesium could be important to our health overall. Indeed it is. Magnesium is implicated in energy production, and heart health. It is involved in these conditions as well:

> Certain medical conditions, however, can upset the body's magnesium balance. For example, an intestinal virus that causes vomiting or diarrhea can cause temporary magnesium deficiencies. Some gastrointestinal diseases (such as irritable bowel syndrome (IBS) and ulcerative colitis), diabetes, pancreatitis, hyperthyroidism (high thyroid hormone levels), kidney disease, and taking diuretics can lead to deficiencies. Too much coffee, soda, salt, or alcohol, as well as heavy menstrual periods, excessive sweating, and prolonged stress can also lower magnesium levels.

> Symptoms of magnesium deficiency may include agitation and anxiety, restless leg syndrome (RLS), sleep disorders, irritability, nausea and vomiting, abnormal heart rhythms, low blood pressure, confusion, muscle spasm and weakness, hyperventilation, insomnia, poor nail growth, and even seizures. (University of Maryland Medical Center, 2013)

Also, magnesium deficiency* may contribute to low serotonin levels. You remember that serotonin is one of our neurotransmitters that affects our mood, emotions, sleep, and appetite.

> Inadequate magnesium appears to reduce serotonin levels, and antidepressants have been shown to raise brain magnesium. A 2008 study found that magnesium was as effective as the tricyclic antidepressants in treating depression among people with diabetes. (University of Maryland Medical Center, 2013)

Low magnesium may be indicated in fibromyalgia symptoms (not to mention ME/CFS) and supplementation may help:

> A small preliminary clinical study of 24 people with fibromyalgia found that a proprietary tablet containing both malic acid and magnesium improved pain and tenderness associated with fibromyalgia when taken for at least 2 months. Other studies suggest the combination of calcium and magnesium may be helpful for some people with fibromyalgia. (University of Maryland Medical Center, 2013)

In addition, I wonder if very low levels of Vitamin C play a factor in chronic fatigue and pain. I also believe low electrolytes – which produce an electrical charge in your body – may be implicated in symptoms of pain and fatigue.

*Our top-soil is so depleted that quality supplementation is ideal. I choose raw and food-based vitamins. I love Megafood's Daily C-Protect and Planetary Herbals True To Nature C™ as real Vitamin C sources.

Could the answer really be as simple as deep, real nutrition and "avoiding or minimizing irritants" (T.Malterre, personal communication, 2015)? If you are like me, you're not going to roll the dice. You realize the bottom line is that anything you can do to keep your nutritional levels up and stress levels down may play a major role in unlocking your body's full potential to heal and thrive. Look inside, live in the moment, and *pay attention to what feels good* to you. Try to focus on love instead of fear to move out of the stress response. *Do what Feels Good* to *Be Well* ...

One cannot think well, love well, sleep well, if one has not dined well.

~ Virginia Woolf

When I first developed fatigue, I told myself the way to get energy was through stimulants, and I couldn't take them (to function) as I was sensitive to them. Later, I rebelled and used chocolate for energy. But, the original belief stayed with me about where I thought energy came from, and this belief directly influenced my subconscious mind, i.e. my body. Until I changed my thoughts (my belief) about where energy came from – i.e. that energy doesn't just come from stimulants, but rather comes from an infinite source that cannot be created nor destroyed, and rather just changes forms – I was able to **manifest energy in holistic ways**. I manifest energy through love, faith, breath, inspiration, motivation, nutrition (which is electrical energy), earthing (which is magnetic energy), and, yes, sometimes, small amounts of stimulants (which raises cortisol levels so you can access more of your body's natural energy stores). Change your thoughts to change your body. Your body believes and manifests what your mind believes. It is your subconscious mind.

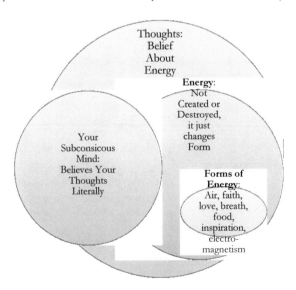

Steps Toward Well-Being: Small Changes (*Can =*) Big Results

1. Know & love yourself. Choose to be positive. Live and radiate love.

2. Rev up your *nutritional status*. **Find your upper antioxidant edge.** Take EFA's and consider taking a raw or food-based multi-vitamin. Most importantly, **eat real food!** This alone can make a huge difference! For ex: *avocadoes have B vitamins my body recognizes & loves!*

3. Create a **diverse** microbiome: *eat real fruits and lots of vegetables & greens (choose organic and non-gmo whenever possible).* Talk to your practitioner about supplementation with probiotics, or experiment with brands.

4. Get enough **sun exposure for Vitamin D** (but protect your skin!). Practitioners recommend D3 as well, but I find there is nothing like getting Vit. D from the sun. It plays a critical role in mood & well-being! It is critical for serotonin production and immune function!

5. Become a *conscious consumer.* Read labels. Ask questions. Read research. Learn about traceability and sustainability.

6. *Titration* - Ease your nervous system back into well-being. *Small amounts of stimulation (positive stressors) activate your body's healing mechanisms.*

7. *Remember to consider synchronicity when building a healing plan. Foods, herbs, etc. work in synergy together. Life & well-being are an orchestra, not a solo song.*

8. Check your *mindset* and be *mindful* of your choices. More important than anything else are mindset and mindfulness. *Mindset* is the state of mind that influences your life and well-being. *Mindfulness* is the true memory of health and what it is like to be "well." Be mindful of inhabiting true well-being and **choose a positive, healthy outlook** on life! Join us on ConnektWell.com to learn about mindful living…

Memory in its deepest form is mindfulness and mindful living. Your journey - if you choose - is to believe that it is possible to move from chronic illness to mindful living and inhabit the endless possibilities …

Make the conscious choice to live mindfully. Believe it, Inhabit it, Live it.

Chapter Five - The Memory of Health:
Your Journey to Well-Being

Healing is about waking up to the bright light of awareness. You have to vibrate at a higher frequency than when you are sick in order to be in a state of well-being.

You have to find a way to wake up and evolve your awareness and head into the light, and then stay there no matter what. You have to become infinitely, indefinitely brave...

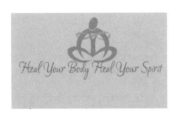

Heal Your Body Heal Your Spirit

> **Health is Holistic**
> ~ it is mind, body, and spirit
> ~ it is the joy of being alive
> ~it is *your* Memory of Health

Note: It's not my intention to say you will or should heal. My primary focus in this chapter is on well-being. That being said, you may find what you need or even inspiration or motivation in these pages for manifesting *your* most optimum level of well-being. You may find you can begin to reinhabit your home: your body, mind, and even spirit. In any light or circumstance, mindset is a major factor in achieving well-being. And memory in its truest spirit is being mindful of being alive.

Your Memory of Health

Your cells and your soul have a memory of health.

Nourish, cleanse, and protect your precious cells.

Awaken, remember, and rejoice in your infinite spirit.

Be mindful of your life, as you live it right now, each hour.

Remember what it means and how it feels to be truly alive.

Heal Your Body, Heal Your Spirit

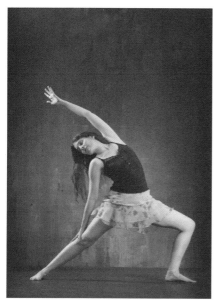

Reverse Warrior Yoga Pose: Dance-Inspired

Dear Friend,

This, the final chapter, may be the most important one of this book.

Theories aside, what matters is that you make peace with yourself - your body, your mind, and your spirit. You may find ways to do those things in this chapter because it is not like the others. This chapter is like your soul, the way it's already free. It's like the river that flows because it knows no other way. It's like a bird that has a song it cannot help but sing.

Your body knows how to be well. Healing is a state of instinctual ease. It is getting back into flow: the moving dream, the moving stream of life.

Even if you can't be well the way others view health, you can still embody health with your spirit, and you can experience well-being.

Believe it, dream it, and surrender to it, no matter where you find yourself in the ever present, electric moment.

Well-being is like a beautiful, flowing river. It's full of ease. It's bliss and flow. Flow is the merging of conscious feminine and masculine energy.

Masculine energy is bright, powerful, positive, and active. Feminine energy is gentle, flowing energy that surrenders to mystery. United, these energies uplift, strengthen, and rejuvenate your inner sense of well-being.

The perfect flow of well-being is instinctive, embodied energy that rides the wave of health. More on this concept in a bit, but first, let's get you grounded in health.

You can't heal - or feel better - if you aren't in your body because *health resides in your body.*

Beyond the two to five per cent of illnesses that are purely genetic, chronic illness, for most of us, involves some kind of disconnect from being in our bodies. Is this the only reason we can't get well?

Of course not. There are multitudes of reasons. For example, we still don't understand auto-immunity well, or the immune system in general, and therefore we don't understand how to truly influence it, although diet, chronic inflammation, and the microbiome are probably factors to consider.

But, tracking, listening to, and following your symptoms is a big part of well-being too, along with never, ever giving up on your beautiful self.

Just please consider this…

~Not feeling well may be disconnection from your authentic self ~

Your *authentic self* includes your physical body. Why is this? Because *our minds and our bodies are, in fact, one and the same.* There seems to be little differentiation at this point, if any. The field of psychoneuroimmunology, and mind-body practices like yoga illuminate this concept of a dynamic mind-body (even spirit) field. Your mind is everywhere in your body. It's in every cell. It's your job and privilege to experience and honor your mind and body as one living entity.

It's your job to express and experience your emotions *through* your body. For the most part, you can't think your way out of a situation, including poor health. You must feel your way through it - with and *in* your body. *Your feelings are literally in your body. You have to feel good to feel good…*

You have to feel good emotionally to feel good physically … Some would say you have to feel good spiritually – whatever that means for you – in order to be well.

If you can *stay present long enough to feel what your body feels,* you can truly change. You can also literally build new neural pathways that will strengthen your mind and body. You will also *become* **embodied.**

Many of us have abandoned our home, and by that I mean our physical bodies as well as our hearts. We have turned our back on ourselves. The problem is, you cannot heal if you are not present in your body. This is your first step: get back into your body and stay there. It bears repeating: *health resides in your body.*

> *My body became like a house I no longer inhabited.*
> ~ Marianne Williamson, <u>A Course in Weight Loss</u>

Coming to grips with your embodiment is one of the most profound philosophical tasks you will ever face ... unmask [your] dream of pure thought ... [we can only] think and imagine ... through our bodies.
~ Mark Johnson, <u>The Meaning of the Body: Aesthetics of Human Understanding</u>

Have you ever noticed how if you get a massage, or take a dance or martial arts class, or get some kind of bodywork done, all of a sudden

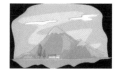

you feel a rush of unexpected emotion rising to the surface?

Your memories and emotions are experienced through and stored in your body.

This is why mind-body fitness is so important. It's not just your body you are working out. *You are working out your emotions and thoughts so you can stay well. In order to get or stay well, you must keep releasing stored energy ...*

Any emotion, if it is sincere, is involuntary. ~ Mark Twain

Your body knows more than you consciously understand or are aware of.
~ Daniel Staite

We must allow our primal emotions to be processed and released through conscious practices such as mindfulness and yoga, etc.

I believe the entire universe is mirrored in your precious body. How could you disown yourself from this most ancient connection?

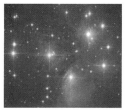

When we are present, truly present, we go deep into experience, and the world opens up into a billion galaxies

Remember when we discussed how research has shown that many people who have CFS have also experienced childhood trauma?

Trauma is no small thing these days. We have all experienced it now with the current state of the world. We live in uncertain times. Guess what trauma does? It takes you out of your body. It may also numb you so you can't feel what's going on in your body, which may make it more challenging to follow your symptoms in order to heal.

We may start to run on a *short-circuited feedback loop of fear*. What makes matters worse, is that we may not be present in our body to recognize the possibility of other potential challenges. It's not your fault either.

Hypervigilance is a hallmark symptom of many people with ME/CFS, FM, PTSD, and trauma. Hypervigilance may keep you stuck in primitive response, and/or stuck in your *head*, making it harder to heal.

You might wonder: Which comes first? Being ungrounded and then getting sick, or vice versa? It may be both ways, depending on circumstances. For instance, someone may have developed PTSD first due to an extreme incident such as war or violence, but also may experience health problems later as a result of chronic vigilance.

Even in uncertain times, I try to stay grounded and try not to worry too much about the origins of things. *Worry keeps you in your head.* These days, I just wish to *feel well*. Feeling well is rooted in your body.

The first step may be to take control of fear and replace it with the feeling of being grounded. Find a way to get yourself and your body grounded in dynamic change (e.g. yoga). *Then you can do and be anything.*

To become grounded, embrace love, change, impermanence, and resilience (G. Wu et al., 2013) and the inherent wisdom of your body:

> *There is more wisdom in your body than in your deepest philosophies.*
> ~ *Friedrich Nietzsche*

> *Harmonious self-regulation is the body's **ground state**.*
> ~ *Deepak Chopra*

> *The fully **integrated** body may be a body that is entirely free of restrictions to the flow of signals.* ~ *Dawson Church, The Genie in Your Genes*

One of the basic elements you may need in the mix of feeling grounded in your body is the element of loving yourself and feeling *love for your body exactly as it is right now*. We are here to love, not be perfect.

~ This is your anchor to well-being: being grounded in love ~

When we turn ego into self-love, the love of your body, *no matter what condition it is in,* we can become reconnected to our body. The gift of illness is an opportunity to be released from our ego, which is a blessing in disguise. *Accept yourself and your body just as you are and it is.*

When you really "get" something, you embody it. You embrace it. It becomes second nature. It becomes your body's nature. All there is to *get* is that you are love. Equally true is that you deserve to be loved.

~ Let your body experience what it wants to experience, which is the experience of love on this plane ~

When you truly love yourself, you become your authentic self.
~ Blake D. Bauer, You Were Not Born to Suffer

I believe the path to freedom - physical, emotional, spiritual - is through the body, not despite it. Love what IS.

Yes, we live in an imperfect world. But that is exactly why it is so beautiful here, because it is imperfect. Its beauty is transient but hauntingly effective, as we are deeply affected by senses and emotion.

Embrace your body in all its forms and conditions. It is only when you accept your body exactly as it is - in its current state, whatever that may be - that you fully sink into it, love it, and embody it ... and your life.

I accept and love my body, just as it is.

This may also be the path to transcendence: *through the body.*

We may have to go through the physical to get to the spiritual. But, oh, how good it feels to be in the physical form here on this plane. We have such an opportunity here to experience conscious love.

Disconnection from your authentic self may, at least in part, contribute to the experience of chronic illness.* Here is what is important:

~ Your power lies in being yourself ~

What are some qualities opposite to disconnection and exhaustion?

Joy
Power
Courage
Presence
Being Well in Mind

What does *well-being* really mean anyway? Perhaps it means some of these qualities: inhabiting joy, love, presence, personal power, courage, resiliency, and allowing the free flow of energy/signals in your body.

What may influence us getting or staying chronically ill is because we are *disconnected from the experience of being in our bodies* - whether it's physically, mentally, emotionally, and/or spiritually - or maybe we're even disconnected from the world or universe at large.

What do you say to yourself over and over again? What would you like or need to hear instead? How would it feel to *feel perfectly whole* just as you are, and to *feel good* just as you are in your body and in your life?

What would reconnect you to this vision of how you experience yourself and your life? Where do you feel disconnected in your body? Where are you disconnected from your authentic self? What interfered in your stream of well-being? Was it fear? Trauma? Loneliness? Abuse? Worry? Self-Esteem? *What disconnected you?*

How do you reconnect with your body so that you can be well? What is there to love and appreciate about your body *right now* even if you're not feeling well? Being honest about where we truly are, allows us to shift and inhabit well-being. Change occurs through authenticity plus courage. *This is your launching pad...wherever you are right now, in the present, electric, powerful, magnetic moment.* By reconnecting with love of yourself, you may be able to reconnect with the love of your body.

*I believe the onset of chronic conditions can be influenced by genetic vulnerabilities, activated by epigenetic factors like diet, lifestyle, mindset, and even the history of your ancestors (Hurley, 2015).

Being present is how you get and stay *well*. Many of us are afraid to be really present, perhaps due to abuse or trauma. *But being present is how you can access your instincts and intuition.* Remember these truths:

Presence is Power
The Present Moment Equals Possibility

Cultivate a lucid state of awareness, where your perception of the world is crystal clear and you feel a deep sense of knowing.

When you check out, you close down opportunities. Which would you rather have? Do you want to be checked out or do you want to have opportunities to re-claim your well-being?

Being present is the *real high*, the real excitement. You get to navigate the roads you go down, and how you handle and experience life, including other people. Being present is everything. Deep presence is where possibility unfolds. It is where infinite potential resides.

Being present is also the safest place to be in this world.

Along with being present, is feeling at peace within your body. This is crucial. No matter what your condition or conditions, please *make peace with your body. It's your best friend.*

The sun is on your side, the moon is on your side, your body is on your side...

You only have to let the soft animal of your body love what it loves. ~
Mary Oliver

Health and True Well-Being

When health is absent, wisdom cannot reveal itself, art cannot manifest, strength cannot fight, wealth becomes useless, and intelligence cannot be applied.
~Herophilus

First and foremost, well-being is about being present, showing up for yourself and your life. It's about loving yourself. A cliché? Hardly. Being present and loving yourself are not clichés. They are what enable you to experience what it means to be alive, to fully embrace and be embraced by the loving, energetic awareness within you.

So, is there really a loving, energetic awareness within me? Hmmm … What is this awareness and energy? Is it me? Is it God? Consciousness? What is consciousness anyway? Science still cannot explain it …

Getting curious is the first step in any journey toward self-discovery. In wellness coaching, being curious can help you move out of where you're *stuck*. Are you curious about feeling good again, what it would feel like to be in your body and embrace yourself for all that you magically and beautifully are? Loving yourself is one potent way you can mobilize the healing process.

Dear Self

*You can't force yourself to love yourself. It's not something you **do**.*

It's a revelation, an innate knowing, an intuitive understanding of your true, incredible nature, and behaving/acting accordingly. It also comes from being able to see yourself from the outside, like others do who love you.

That's one reason connection with others is important. They're mirrors of ourselves; they mirror back to us our true nature. Sometimes that gets lost in translation if they mirror back what we don't love about ourselves.

*But if you can get a **flash of insight** of the **unique spark that animates your being** as to how your loved by other loving people, then the realization is instantaneous: you are a **luminous, beautiful soul** with unlimited capacity for expression of wonder, joy, and love. Wow. Now those are traits to adore, respect, and take care of, no matter what the outcome, eh?*

Letter from My Body

Dear Self (Mind),

I wish you would listen to me when I talk to you. I don't speak in words, but I speak in feelings and sensations. I tell you what I need, if only you would listen.

*My wisdom is deep and primordial. I am telling you everything you need to know so that we might raise **our** well-being. Because I am You, and You are Me.*

Can you slow down enough to hear the happy voice of the stream as it flows? Can you feel the deep currents of well-being that are aching to rise up in you and me?

There is a place we can go together where there is nothing but peace …

*Let your **mind** travel here to meet me, once and for all. Realize that you and I are one and the same. Come, let's merge: I AM.*

How to Reconnect with Your Body

Any activity that combines mind, body, and spirit will help you foster reconnection, like tai chi, dance, or yoga. Please refer to the section *Yoga: Mind, Body, and Spirit* in this chapter. These practices and healing arts *open* your natural pathways to physical and emotional healing.

But, perhaps even more immediate than these practices is anything you can do or think about that opens your heart ♥ and reconnects you to the *feeling of well-being*. Here are some suggestions: doing something new or creative, hiking or walking in nature, singing, meditation, visiting with friends, calling someone, taking care of others, having pets, etc. Whatever opens your heart lands you straight back into your instantly grounded body and can be the quickest route. Go for the joy factor.

Joy inside of your heart can heal any moment. ~ Santana

Reconnecting with your body can be just a joyful heartbeat away.

I have wondered lately if exhaustion, or at the very least, anxiety - which can contribute to depleted energy - could really be unexpressed joy. *Think about it:* we have so much anxiety about what will be or what was or wasn't, that we have no place to put our joy. Anxiety can lead to a chronic fear state – *and fear can lead to depleted energy via chronic activation of the fight or flight* response - **or** it could be manifested into a state of indefinite, genuine joy.

In the same vein, I've speculated that CFS is not a lack of energy, but rather the *blocked free flow of energy*.

Perhaps joy and well-being are the free flow of energy. Re-connecting with the joy of being alive - no matter the current state of your body – may be a key to improved well-being. Seek joy and what feels good. Seek and be love.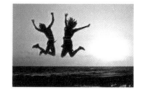

I will love the sun for it warms my bones; yet I will love the rain for it cleanses my spirit. I will love the light for it shows me the way; yet I will love the darkness for it shows me the stars. I will welcome happiness for it enlarges my heart; yet I will endure sadness for it opens my soul. I will greet this day with love in my heart."
~Og Mandino, The Greatest Salesman in the World

Coming Home to Your Heart 🖤 and Using Your Energy (Life) Currency

Many of us have abandoned our homes, and by that I mean our physical bodies as well as our hearts. We've turned our backs on ourselves, especially if we've been through any kind of trauma, including being diagnosed and/or living with a chronic condition.

Your *Energy Currency* Pathway Home: Reconnecting with your body is about coming home to your heart. What does this mean exactly? I like to describe it as a process of connecting with your *energy currency*. You must connect with whatever brings you well-being, as much as possible, right here and now. It's how you can show up for yourself, and *take care of yourself* and your body *right now*.

Your energy currency could be in any form. Is it music, healthy food, good company, work, inspiration, nature, family?

When we connect with life - with ourselves, our bodies, and others – health, or at least well-being, is often a natural byproduct.

It's that recognition of **Oh, here I am**. *I'm home now*

The Circle

Hands who listened to silence
and spoke to darkness only a whisper.
Or was it, to the lost wraith, water mumbling underground?
Same thing. No. Don't move. No sound,
but a spark in closed eyes
sun burning, sky reeling in a long forgotten land.
No sound but the heartbeat of a buried sea calling: listen
Listen. Someone breaks the lost name.
Then, clearly, in the mossy stillness, sings
dear heart, come home.   ~Diana Rowan 🖤

Your *New Energy/Direction* Pathway Home: *Try a new perspective. Free your energy: s h i f t … What opens your heart over and over?*

Connect to something bigger than yourself. Try volunteering, caring for another living being, coming from love … feel the shift in energy.

Your *Core Values* Pathway Home: What are your *core values*? What are your highest *ideals and beliefs*? When you identify and can verbalize your belief system, you will have a clear shot to mobilize your energy and get back in touch the energetic field of your living bodymind.

Your core values might include concepts like love, faith, nature, integrity, creativity, passion, excellence, kindness, compassion, spirituality, honesty, service, connection to others, authenticity, community, etc. What values, beliefs, and ideals do you hold dear? What brings you home to your heart? What energizes you?

The more you lose yourself in something bigger than yourself, the more energy you will have. ~ Norman Vincent Peale

Passion is energy. Feel that power that comes from focusing on what excites you. ~ Oprah Winfrey

Your *Needs* Pathway Home: Another pathway home is what you *need*. What do you most need in this very moment? Is it health, peace, safety, joy, play, courage, connection, or something else? What do you need in order to be truly well in this living moment?

Your *Love* Pathway Home: Your well-being is nourished and *blossoms* when you *let love live inside of you*. It's about loving and accepting yourself, *just as you are*, here in this precious, once-in-a-lifetime, priceless, never-to-be-experienced again moment. *You are enough …*

~Keep the light of love lit within you~

I tell you, deep inside you is a fountain of bliss, a fountain of joy. Deep inside your center core is truth, light, love. There is no guilt there, there is no fear there. Psychologists have never looked deep enough. ~Sri Sri Ravi Shankar

You, yourself, as much as anybody in the entire universe, deserve your love and affection. ~ Buddha

Keep the light of love lit within you

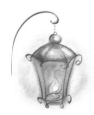

Connection with Self and Others

Why does connection with Self and others and the universe work? Because everything is inevitably, inextricably interconnected.

How does a lamp burn energy? Because it is plugged in. A loose wire cannot produce light. We're all linked in someway to someone or something. Remember the Web of Life? We thrive when we connect with our own life and with the lives of others, as well as the world and universe around us.

Connection is the currency of wellness. ~ John Travis

I believe this quote 100 %. Solitude has it purposes, but we are social creatures and we're meant to connect. Loneliness has plagued me since my teens. I've spent long periods either living alone or feeling alone. In the past, I isolated myself due to traumatic incidents. When one is alone, one is safe. Except that is not true. When we're alone, we tend to hurt ourselves emotionally, sometimes, especially if we've been exposed to violence, trauma, etc. Remember: safety lies not only in the present moment, but in the warm light of the presence of others. My friends teased me that I needed to get out more. Loneliness is no laughing matter, especially when it comes to the state of your health. I urge you to connect.

Connection and Feedback Loops of Energy

When we're in a state of health or well-being, we often don't notice our bodies much at all, unless we are in a state of bliss or pain.

There is a stream of well-being that just keeps bubbling up with or without us doing anything about it. It's supposed to be a state of bliss that we are constantly in: subtle bliss ... even a state of subtle ecstasy

It's when we don't feel well that we notice our bodies more often than not. This is your gift – that you notice your body and current health. Ironically, this is also what reconnects you to your body:

the fact that you don't feel well

Symptoms help us heal by alerting us to natural feedback loops of communication. What kind of information are your symptoms communicating to you? What areas of your body need your attention? Where do you need to reconnect with yourself and your body?

Have you ever heard of *Norbert Wiener*, a child prodigy who lived on this earth from 1894 to 1964? If not, he's an inspiration and worth looking up. In his productive lifetime, he developed the theory of *cybernetics*, which is the study of communication and control, primarily with automatic control systems like our nervous system (Wiener, 1965).

Wiener's work, first published in 1948, is central to our discussion. We learn that messages from our body are communicating either positive or negative feedback to you. Negative feedback as a symptom is not a *bad* thing. It's just a message. It means you need to make an adjustment of some kind in order to re-establish equilibrium or a sense of coherence again in your system.

Stress is one of the biggest feedback signals and information to your brain, and this may also be why the brain is so affected by stress.

~ Stress alters the structure of your brain ~

But remember that we previously discussed the fact that we also have the ability and power to change our brain structure through creating new neural pathways. We do have a large amount of control in how our minds and bodies function (Begley, 2007).

~ We can change the structure of our brain and how adaptable and flexible we are through neuroplasticity ~

At the same time, it's *how we perceive stress* that affects the feedback loops in our body, including how smoothly they run. If we can perceive stress as positive, we can stay in the zone and heal. However, if we perceive events as stressful - or our body gets worn down, probably from stress - and we may have trouble healing or staying vibrantly well.

Our well-being is set up on feedback loops, like the circle of life and energy in the body. When you pay deep attention - become aware, cultivate mindfulness - of your body and its signals/symptoms, you have a much better chance to reconnect with your health and vitality.

When you become *aware*, you can become embodied again. You *become love* and you are able to *show love for yourself*. *Awareness* is what **connects** all the feedback loops. The loops involve your *body, mind, and spirit*. These three entities are inextricably and inevitably linked. If one is out of balance - out of harmony - so will the others be. Your body wishes to be in effortless (i.e. self-regulated) balance. Just like the brilliantly interconnected universe *(one song)*, all is connected through harmony.

Health, wholeness and holiness ... all three share the same root word and all three share the same state of harmony or disharmony. ~ Deepak Chopra

Healing is a process of becoming whole. Even the words heal, and whole, and holy come from the same root. ~ Dean Ornish, Love and Survival

Your Body as Your Guide to Well-Being

Your body is much wiser than you may realize. In fact, your body is designed to be your guide, your best friend, and your best ally when it comes to your health. *Symptoms* are your body's way of talking to you, telling you what it needs and what is out of balance. Symptoms are part of your body's *voice*.

When I was sick, I felt my body was trying to talk to me, but I wasn't yet fluent in the language. The more I paid attention to my body's symptoms, the more I became fluent in my body's language. It was a matter of staying present, staying mindful. Of course it is hard to stay present when you've been abused on top of being sick. This is the rub. Abused people tend to disassociate. But checking out makes suffering worse, ultimately.

I learned that being present - *being mindful* - is where I could address both my current physical challenges as well as my emotional and psychic wounds.

What is your body communicating to you right now? What does it need? How can you learn to better listen to your body?

Here is one way I learned to understand my body's language better: by taking calculus. I'm not a math person by nature – *although I love math and feel it is connected to music* - and I wasn't sure I could pass the class. But, I did pass, and in addition to the confidence this gave me, I also learned more about the nature of presence and maybe even well-being.

The Calculus Method for Manifesting Well-Being

- Picture yourself being well, several times.
- Then, focus just on the present moment and the goal at hand.
- Listen to what your body needs or wants you to do in the present moment. Don't think about the end goal anymore.
- Stay focused, relaxed, and present. Follow your body's cues.
- All of your "energy" is needed to manifest your final outcome.
- This is where the magic of change lies: The Power of Presence

When I took calculus, I found out that:

*~ Total change happens at the **integral of instantaneous change** ~*

In other words: *integrating well-being* happens when you *picture yourself being well,* believe it, practice it, and then *sink deeply and peacefully into the present moment and stay there* as the end goal is realized/integrated. *Visualize being well then just be in the present moment* where you have the *best chance to integrate change,* and heal from physical and psychic wounding.

The Solution Is In the Problem

There is no such thing as a problem without a gift for you in its hands.
~Richard Bach

You might be wondering: What could the solution possibly be in this continuous problem of not feeling well that causes so much suffering?

With any chronic condition – this may be one of the gifts: the chance to *practice more self-care.* Of course, self-care would include rest, nutrition, and stress management, as we have covered in this book. The other gift may be realizing self-acceptance and having the opportunity to be with love and life on a slower and deeper level.

You may have to do some meditating on what your solutions may be, and how they are wrapped up in the gift of your current condition.

Oftentimes, the solution may be the opposite of what you're thinking or doing. But, only you and your body will know for sure. This does not mean faith, hope, and love don't assist you as well, for they do. But your body is talking to you all the time. *Your body is your best guide.*

Symptoms and Instinctive Health

Instinct is a visceral *knowing* which is sometimes interpreted as an inner voice. Instinct is in your bones, your DNA. It's awareness, coherence, mindfulness, connection, … it's *your* **~Memory of Health~**

*Instinctive health is where intuition becomes **instinctive healing action**.*

Instinct is part of intuition, but different too. Instinct is automatic. It is what *you can only access in the present moment*, which is where health *and well-being* reside as well.

Instinct and health (as well-being) are both situated in the *present moment.* This is where you must be as well: living in the present moment: deeply, fully, surrendering to what is …

When you live in the present, you will be able to listen to, pay attention to, and *respond and adjust to the messages of your own feedback loop systems of communication, including optimal conditions for well-being.* Then you can respond intuitively - at the level of instinct - and hopefully gain ground.

When you are truly present and pay attention to your symptoms - *in the moment* - this is where your power to change resides as well.

Story, Symptoms, Metaphor

When we listen to our body's voice and ourselves at the deepest level, we can *get to the heart of our stories,* which is where freedom lies. Deep, elemental feelings are the heart of stories (think of your aha! moments), and stories are where we pinpoint feelings (including stuck emotions).

We often access or understand stories – have those lightbulb moments – through metaphors that light up our minds, spirits, and imagination.

Metaphors unite mind and body. Another way to access our deepest feelings and get at the heart of our own storylines is through metaphor.

Reach for the moon and you will land among the stars.
~Norman Vincent Peale

Try this: *imagine your most positive state of wellbeing.* Imagine yourself in a state of dynamic well-being. Even if you aren't sure *how* you will get there, *imagine it anyway*. Make the imagined result into a tangible metaphor, a new storyline you can step into that enlivens you.

Turn your deepest feeling into metaphor. Then let metaphor move naturally through your body and *encourage you toward instinctive healing actions* so you can achieve the awakened and dynamic well-being you desire.

Feeling ◄► Metaphor ◄► Instinctive Healing Actions ◄► Well-Being

Using metaphor, here's one way well-being feels like, looks like, and sounds like for me: *Well-being is like a cool, mountain brook in an alpine setting: serene and beautiful with a flowing sense of peace in mind, body, and soul.*

Another powerful metaphor for me is connected to *the sound of a flock of wild geese flying overhead.* There are, perhaps, few sounds more thrilling to me. *It's the sound of freedom.* To me, well-being is being and feeling free.

What does well-being look like, feel like, and sound like for you?

Feelings are a direct experience, yet we often access them through stories and metaphors. While direct experience (being in the *Now* is ideal, and not being attached) we are hardwired for stories, in how they help us to understand and process life. Here's how one person turned her feeling of grief into a release by naming what she was feeling, but in a language she could recognize (hint: it's a metaphor):

The winter of my grief is turning forward and I feel fall approaching. In normal time, fall doesn't follow winter, and I very much feel myself slipping into real time. Here in Maine, the sweltering days of summer are folding into crisp days of fall and I want to be in that time frame also. So I'm allowing myself to be there. When winter comes in a few months, however, I won't call it grief. I'll call it beautiful. ~Joan Gordon (on coming to terms with the death of her husband)

The greatest thing by far is to be master of metaphor. ~Aristotle

Just like music, metaphors unite the left and right sides of our brains, and therefore *metaphors unite our minds and bodies* as well. They are both *creative and logical* in nature, just like us. They also reside in *stories.*

Our next exploration will be into your body's story, the one it is telling to you ... or the one you are telling yourself about your body ...

Our biography becomes our biology. ~ Carolyn Myss

We love stories because we love the process, the journey itself. We want to know the entire plot, how it starts, how it ends. We want to see the hero or heroine overcome their challenges and emerge on top.

In our own life story, we are the heroes and heroines, whether or not we are aware of this fact. You are a hero/heroine. You are brave.

Sometimes, when we don't like the way our story is developing, we tell ourselves and even others a different story about ourselves. We adjust details, maybe lie, omit, or adjust the plotline. *Yet, every story you tell others about who you are or how you're feeling shows up verbatim in your body.* Just create awareness of how you tell your story to yourself and others.

You may be able to lie to yourself or even other people about who you are or how you feel, but you can't lie to your body…and it is *impossible* for your body to lie to you. So if the story you're telling yourself or the world is different from the story your body is telling, it's your body's story and symptoms that hold the essence of the truth of who you are.

Your body's story is the one *you* should listen to, especially if you're on a healing path. It's the path of healing that leads you to your authentic self. It is a true gift - to tell your truth - and a direct path to your *Self*.

Studies show that people with multiple personality disorders also have different stories and bodies. Some of the manifested personalities may be *"sick"* and some may be *"well."* What if you had a different personality? Would you still be sick? Again, I am separating health and well-being. I would never tell you how your body feels. Only you know that: how you feel and what makes you feel sick or well. I am not saying what you are experiencing isn't real. But, consider this:

~ Rewrite the story you tell yourself and others about your body ~

Inhabit & Tell **The Story of Well-Being**

Some people advocate not being attached to your story at all. While, I believe you get to choose if you are attached to your storyline or not, we can stay in the *Now* and in the *Flow* by naming what we truly feel …

What is your secret story? What are you afraid to tell about yourself?

Telling your whole, true story sets you free. It can literally heal you if told to a witness, i.e. someone who holds space for you: readers, friends, family, professionals like therapists or counselors, pastors, etc.

I believe, that in order to truly inhabit well-being, you must find the courage to embrace fully who you are, no matter what the condition your body or life, in addition to adopting a positive way of thinking.

Track your joys and your sorrows. Speak your heart. Find your voice.

You may find it hard to tell your whole story. If so, where are you possibly *stuck* in your storyline? Does your body manifest recurring symptoms? There is no judgment here. Just consider:

> ~ *Recurring symptoms may be unresolved storylines* ~

Where are you (maybe) STUCK in your storyline?*

Believe me, I have been stuck, several times. It is nothing to be ashamed of…it is just a pattern with which to bring *awareness* to…

When we are chronically sick, we often pull ourselves out of the game…we step out of the collective story and onto the banks of the river. Perhaps we don't believe we are worthy because we are sick, or for some other reason. *Whatever story you tell yourself*, step back into the game, the river…*step back into your storyline*. But this time, step back into a story you wish to believe about yourself. Keep going, keep moving.

Let go of your old fears, insecurities, doubts about who you are and what you *have to be*. Let go of what you cannot control, which is just about everything. T*rust life*, trust *yourself*, let go, surrender, and let the stream, the moving dream of life, carry you safely down the river …

Your only job is to show up, by loving your life and yourself exactly as you are right now, in the moment. Show up for yourself and this world each day by *loving what is*. Focus on creating a positive storyline.

Writing your story not only helps you and heals you in ways you can only imagine, but it also heals others and gives them permission to tell their story, too!
~ Sarina Baptista, A Bridge to Healing: J.T.'s Story

*Note: Keep your "storyline" flowing, but don't attach to it or the outcome. Just be joyful and present.

As you inhabit your body's authentic storyline, you will learn how to dwell in new metaphors and archetypes, all of which will reveal the path of your journey toward well-being. What's a new metaphor, story, or archetype within which you can now reside? Here are a few:

*~I am **well** on my way~*

~ My body is a river, my body is an ecosystem ~

When you do things from your soul, you feel a river moving in you, a joy. ~ Rumi

The sun shines not on us, but in us. The rivers flow not past, but through us, thrilling, tingling, vibrating every fiber and cell of the substance of our bodies, making them glide and sing. ~ John Muir

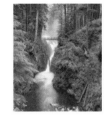

Have you ever noticed how water runs? When a stream is healthy, the water runs freely, bubbling and moving along. When the water gets stuck in the stream and stands still, stagnation occurs.

Your body heals like water runs. Your body enters into well-being on the path of least resistance, like the way water flows downstream.

In fact, your body is a river. If you flow along with the river, you tend to stay well, both physically and emotionally. If you stop and hold onto a rock (fear, stagnation) you will be affected by the currents and experience *resistance*, a feeling of blockage. Illness may *blocked energy or stagnant energy*. Disease grows where there is stagnant energy, just as a river becomes stagnant when it stands still. It's the same principle.

Hint: *Try living from Divine Mind instead of from your ego (more on ego coming up soon in this chapter). When you flow with life and live from Divine Mind, and follow a positive path, your enter the realm of soul.*

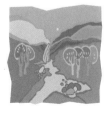

Most of us get sidelined on the bank of the stream now and then. Regardless of the cards dealt, get back into the stream of life: the moving stream, the moving dream of life. I love the sound of flowing and even falling water. Water is life-force and is meant to be in motion, just like your body and life.

Being Present and the Metaphor of the River

Picture yourself on a raft, floating down a river. The present moment is represented by you on the raft. Time is the flowing river.

You don't have to worry about being present for each point in time. Your job is to stay on the raft and notice the scenery as you float by it.

This is what it means to be present. Presence is witnessing the flow of time (however relative "time" is...) and the ever-changing river of life.

Being present doesn't mean breaking time apart second by second. It means witnessing what is going on around you, each wave, rock, tree.

If you stay on the raft as you float through time, that is your presence. Presence is not static, it is a state of f...l...o...w. Change is what happens in the present moment. Healing can happen when you step off of the static riverbank, jump back onto the raft, and ride the waves.

Life unfolds as it will. Your job is to be present and show up for yourself and your life consistently. *This is how you enter into the realm of well-being, of mindful living.* Do it until it becomes effortless, until you don't have to think about it. Stay on the raft, in the ever-moving river.

Get in Touch with Nature, Relaxation, and Feminine Energy

Another pathway to healing begins when you get into rhythm with Nature. You can reduce the *stress response* and boost immunity. I believe nature is one of the best stress relievers ever. Additionally, nature may help you activate *The Relaxation Response - or the RR for short -* which is closely associated with healing and well-being in the body.

The RR is the opposite of the stress response. The RR may be in synch with *feminine healing energy* and the habit of *going with the flow.* Release your worries. Instead *get into flow with the RR. Allow the free flow of energy in your body...no matter the state of your health.* Trust life, trust yourself, and trust your body's *natural healing energy. Imagine well-being...*

The quality of the imagination is to flow and not to freeze.
~Ralph Waldo Emerson

Feminine healing energy is connected with nature and the divine. It's the natural order of things, the flow of life and well-being. It may be the heart of the RR, which is an ideal setting where healing can occur. Positive stress (eustress) is masculine, but when either feminine or masculine energy is out-of-balance, one can enter into an acute or chronic stress response, a state that can impair healing over time.

Activate the RR in your body in order to have a fighting chance at healing. How do you do this? Again, try biofeedback, meditation, music, yoga, walking in nature, *whatever elicits the RR in you*. Not only do these activities move your body out of the fight or flight response (the sympathetic nervous system) and into RR (the parasympathetic nervous system) *but they encourage brain plasticity*. This is doubly beneficial: cultivating The Relaxation Response and building brain plasticity to gain the upper edge is what builds vitality and wellness.

Also, practice *trusting life*. It may be that, on a primal level, your body has learned not to trust, and may be in a constant state of fight, flight, or freeze. When we live in a state of unconscious fear, we can burn ourselves out. *Practice positive thinking, pacing and titration to ease your mind and body back into a natural flow and trust with Life. Seek help if you need it.*

Also, trust your body. Listen to your body's cues. Conventional medicine has its place, but is has also lassoed in our natural healing energy, which is a combination of both the masculine and feminine principles. You can't sit back, take a pill, and expect to get better.

If you do get better, more power to you. But for most of us, we have to *actively* participate in the healing process, as well as trust and surrender to our bodies' cues.

Be proactive is masculine, going with the flow is feminine.

Spontaneous healing does happen, and the *placebo effect* is a real phenomenon. How do these both occur? My guess is the placebo effect is the result of dropping into The Relaxation Response. When we take a pill (sugar or not) and are told we have the possibility to heal, our bodies may relax, and then spontaneous healing may occur as our natural healing defense mechanisms kick in.

Flow & Self-Determination

I respect science, but remember: *medicine is 50% science and 50% art.* We have a responsibility to empower ourselves and to do everything we can to champion our own health and well-being. The internet is the perfect medium for connecting with others and for initiating research. Just be discerning and weed out misinformation, which is everywhere.

An example would be "adrenal fatigue" which is really, technically hypocortisolism. Self-inquiry (and connection, of course) allow us to grow and become empowered. True knowledge can be life-altering.

Feminine healing energy is greatly underutilized, along with our own volition to self-determine our quality of being. Modern medicine has its place and it saves lives. But, we have ignored an entire spectrum and resource of health and well-being: the self-determination of masculine energy and the intuitive, healing nature of feminine energy.

Masculine energy is proactive, and feminine energy is mystical, magical, supportive, intuitive, and instinctual. It trusts the body's ability to heal itself in due time and assume a state of *dynamic equilibrium:*

...there is time to **allow the body to participate, to choose just what it** **needs.** *As it slowly heals, it can develop a new balance; a dynamic equilibrium that helps it cope with stress in the future.*

~ *Dr. Andrew Weil (on using whole plant medicine vs. isolated, synthetic drugs)*

I am not anti-drug, nor supplement. But, actively participating in one's life and health is the *masculine principle*, which is powerful and necessary. The *feminine principle* is the natural flow of life. *Life flows toward active, dynamic well-being, if we surrender. It's a paradox and a new paradigm:*

> The mind gets over-worked, trying to solve, fix, process and analyze. The intuitive, creative and artistic nature, when in balance with this, allows a higher flow of Consciousness to enter, without risk of error or poor judgment. The right and the left brain merging - awakens the expression of Unity; in every moment it can restore [repair] the divorce of Science & Spirituality, Masculine & Feminine, Nature & Humanity. (Robbins, 2013)

Seek unification of masculine and feminine energies. Healing energy is creative, unified energy, which is from where life force originates.

We are creative beings, and the unification of masculine and feminine energies is a state of ecstatic F...L...O...W...

Harness the masculine power of action, of taking responsibility and seeking to change that which is within your power. Surrender to the feminine principle of release, and allowing for and receiving healing, intuitive energy.

*Acknowledge yourself, Know when to rest, Let go of expectations, Stay in gratitude, FEEL Your feelings, Do not compare yourself to others, Embrace your humanity, Maintain perspective, Speak positive to yourself, **Smile** as you move toward a goal, Remember to balance, Go with the flow, Allow for many paths, Breathe through, **Giggle** and laugh, Create solutions for your excuses, Practice patience, be grateful... ~Tiana Meckel*

Finally, do your best to stay in the present moment. Say to yourself, when you can: *I am alive.* By saying those words silently in your mind, you can drop into the *here in the now.* Just by seeking to be conscious, you become conscious. Simply *focus on your breath in the present moment.* This is mindfulness and mindfulness practice. Over time, it will get easier and you will get better at it. Use this practice to replace fear and anxiety, or any stray thoughts that do not serve you or your body. Harness this *mindful energy* instead, and allow joy, presence, and courage to fortify your life and well-being.

Let go, let go of feeling helpless, let go of worry. Healing is a spiritual practice, an exercise in confidence, strength, and love. ~Unknown

We focus so much on having the Next Best Year (this will be your best year yet!) or Best Thing, yet we fail to realize that the path to get to your best year, life ever is to first cultivate This Moment: practice being deeply in the moment, practice being mindfully present for whatever unfolds, and the rest of your life will follow. It will all fall into place effortlessly.

~ Surrender to This Divine Moment ~

All good and fine, you say, but I'm having trouble letting go of fear and anxiety. What if it's not as easy as flowing down the river, cultivating Chi, and embracing and embodying The Relaxation Response? What then?

I can tell you this: When you *operate from a place of love instead of fear*, the whole world changes, your whole world opens up. Healing is made out of love. Live from Divine Mind and see what unfolds for you ...

Wake Up to Your Suffering

Your pain is the breaking of the shell that encloses your understanding.
~ Khalil Gibran

The Fear/Pain Body: Your Shadow Self

I looked into the waters and what did I see? A sleeping/shadow lotus of me. The lotus sleeps under the water at night. In the day, the lotus rises up out of the water and opens exquisitely to meet the sun.

Wake up to your fear, pain, and suffering. Understand that they are nothing but a lotus floating underneath the water.

Your shadow is your fear, pain, and suffering. It is also your unexpressed beauty. There is no need to hide from your shadow...let it flower as it opens up to meet and grow toward the light.

Let your shadow be a lotus, and let it blossom...

Let what is dark within you - all of your fear, all of your pain, all of your suffering - open to rays of warmth and brilliance. Let the unexpressed beauty in you open up to meet the sun and blossom in its exquisite light.

When you let go of resisting what is- your suffering - your shadow self becomes experience...and this is what gives you roots and strength. The depths you rise from is what holds you, and gives you context for the light.

Our shadow self, or our fear/pain body, is composed of dense, dark energy. But it is not to be judged. It is to be loved.

Recall...remember the meaning of the word health. The root of the word health comes from the word holy which means, among other things, sacredness, salvation, forgiveness, happiness, wellness, wholeness. The word health means freedom from pain. When you are free from the shadow of suffering – free from the fear of your pain body - you are truly free to inhabit your awake body in a state of joy, trust, and health. Your awake body is the opposite of your shadow body. Yet, your awake body is supported by the water it rests in. Rest well and shine well...

Avoiding the dark energy of your shadow self only delays your emergence into well-being. There is nothing to fear. It is all you. Check out these profound pieces of advice from experts:

Negative emotions are a signal of our growth edge...one's negative emotions are messengers... avoiding one's suffering brings disconnection and isolation.
~ Margaret Moore, founder of Wellcoaches

We are healed by suffering only by experiencing it fully. ~ Marcel Proust

Out of suffering have emerged the strongest souls;
the most massive characters are seared with scars. ~ Kahlil Gibran

May you feel joyously and completely alive and savor this feeling without any fear or hesitation. I wish for you the thrill of truly living deeply in the present moment where *lucid awareness* leads to ripe, endless possibility.

When we surrender to the present moment, life opens up and blossoms like a shining lotus upon the water.

When we move beyond the ego of being addicted to our fear and suffering, there is just pure life. We can capture this *moment of feeling alive* at any given moment in time when we choose to *harness our courage* to just be our pure, shining selves.

Blog from Smashon.com

Addiction to Ego: Wake Up To Your Suffering

"So many of us check out. It often seems like the easiest option in this challenging world. But what is on the other side of checking out and using our addictions as a way of supposedly shielding us from pain?

Addiction is a heavy word. I'm not talking about chemical addiction either, or addiction that is a disorder of the brain. If you're suffering from a chemical addiction or addiction diagnosis, check out my interview with Darren Littlejohn, and make sure you get the help you need:

http://www.blogtalkradio.com/thewellnesscoach/2013/09/06/healing-with-buddhism-the-power-of-vow-darren-littlejohn

I'm talking about addiction to our egos. This kind of addiction can also cause us great pain and suffering.

The thing is: our pain and suffering can set us free too - when we move beyond the shadow of what is consuming us.

On the other side of pain and suffering is the NOW, present, waiting for us patiently like a lotus on the water, awakening in the presence of the sun.

On the other side of pain and suffering is the POWER OF THE PRESENT MOMENT, beyond our egos, and beyond who we think we are supposed to be.

When we surrender to the present and release our egoic addiction to suffering, we find there is a whole universe of possibility right in front of us.

When we step outside of our own shadow, we find our purity of self, power or non-egoic presence, and brilliance of soul."

*~ When you are free from your pain body **literally and figuratively**, you are free to inhabit true well-being no matter your circumstances or cards dealt ~*

"Between the dreams of night and day, there is not so great a difference."

~ Carl Jung

The Shadow-Self: Unexpressed/Repressed Emotions

What remains unexpressed or repressed in you?

On the energetic level, it may be helpful to look at your blocks to joy and true well-being. In order to survive, *what have you repressed, or what are you potentially repressing?* For me, it was not expressing joy, courage, love, romantic love, my feminine self. What interfered with the expression of these in me? *Abuse, trauma, chronic illness, and probably mostly: loneliness.* Also, I wasn't allowing myself to receive love. I was stuck in a fear cycle (potentially PTSD), and my unexpressed joy and courage was manifesting as fear, anxiety, and chronic worry.

Regardless of the deck you were dealt – regardless of your circumstances, what might you be repressing in yourself? Chronic illness can be isolating, even devastating. Regardless of the cards you were dealt, or what unfolds, could an antidote to anxiety, worry, illness, or overwhelm be unexpressed joy or even courage? What about other possible antidotes such as power, presence, awareness, and purpose?

Expressing our truest needs, feelings, and fears takes *courage*. What exactly is courage, anyway? *Courage is telling the true story about who you are and standing up for what you believe.* It's *being* who you are, and being okay with who you are and how you feel. *It's about shining a light on your fears.*

Courage is *warrior energy*, located and accessed in your third chakra, where the adrenals and liver are located, vs. *victim energy*, which is in the same chakra. For an explanation of chakras, please see the sub-section *Chakras and Your Health* in the section *Energetics vs. Genetics* coming up in this chapter. These sections are meant to help you perceive differently.

Filling the conscious mind with ideal conceptions is a characteristic of Western theosophy, but not the **confrontation with the shadow and the world of darkness**. *One does not become enlightened by imagining figures of light, but by making the darkness conscious.*
~ Carl Jung

Listed in this chart's first column are examples of *unexpressed emotions or experiences*. In the second column are *possible results** from these experiences being unexpressed, and in the third are some suggested *corresponding antidotes*. The chart is inspired by the work of by Binnie A. Dansby (2015) and is just meant to help you see things in a new light:

Unexpressed Experience	Possible Result	Corresponding Antidote
Empathy	Suffering	Compassion
Love	Anxiety	Joy/Love
Power	Pain/Fatigue	Courage, Trust
Fear/Grief	Addictions	Joy/Presence
Anger	Depression	Power
Fear	Victim Mentality	Love

*These are simply suggestions, and I am in no way labeling, diagnosing, or pigeonholing you. There may be multiple emotions or experiences for each result, and multiple antidotes/archetypal energies.

Blocked Energy/Interference

~ Unblock the corresponding spiritual and/or physical energy ~
*You can either get bitter, or get better. ~ Carolyn Myss**
Fear, worry, and anxiety can interfere with our *gifts*. Fear can block your true *voice*, along with your power, and your energetic signature.

What is your *energetic signature?* It's who you are, naturally, without fear. It is who you are authentically. It is your entire essence and it aligns your soul, mind, emotions, and body. It is your vibrational frequency.

For me, *my gift* is the ability to *see, speak, write about, and weave together* what I see in *patterns of human nature and in the world of nature*. It is also my ability to dwell in pure love. What are your rare and special gifts?

*This quote used to drive me crazy, as I resented the insinuation that my illness was all in my head, and that just changing focus could "heal" me. What I realized, however, is that it is not about healing, it is about getting better, whatever that looks and feels, like, and being well in mind, no matter the cards dealt.

My interferences were: fear, anxiety, abuse, trauma, loneliness, synthetic chemicals, and chronic illness. For others, interferences may be obstacles like viruses, bacteria, neglect, addiction, isolation, etc.

You can use your gifts, and even your faith in life, love, or yourself, to break free from your blocks. Here's another tool: Remember your energy currency? *Combine your energy currencies with your energetic signature, and the interferences in the stream of well-being can be removed.* You can release the free flow of energy, which may result in better health or well-being.

For me, I also had to re-learn how to trust: life, others, and myself. I had to step into my courage, my truth, and back into my body. It was hard for me, and I didn't do it on the first try. But new experiences, along with renewed courage, allowed me to trust life again and build resiliency and neuroplasticity.

Dear friend, I say to you, shine your light so brightly you can't help but illuminate and catch the world on fire. In the process, you may *burn fat off your soul*, which will make you a stronger, healthier person. You know what I mean by *fat on the soul?* I mean things like focusing on the negative, *which never works*. When you focus on the positive, the negative will dissipate on its own, as it loses its hold on you, its power.

Make use of your fears too, while you still experience them. The path to your peak potential is often straight through your greatest fear.

The only way out is through. ~ Krisin Neff, Ph.D.

Fear and worry only take away from your bliss. Surrender to life, and fear dissipates. Release fear, and merge into who you truly are, which is love. Stay true to your path and treasure those you meet along the way too. They are your support system. You need people because being loved gives you strength. Loving someone gives you courage…

Addiction

What is addiction* anyway? There is a physical component for sure, documented by significant research, which cannot be discounted.

But, to me, energetic addiction is checking out from suffering.
We all check out now and then. But it's how much we check in that matters.

~

*Process or behavioral addictions, sometimes called "soft" addictions, are what I call energetic addictions.

Substance addiction is a brain disorder and requires treatment. Please seek help, and there is help out there: therapy, counseling, detox, etc.

Energetic addiction, to me, is avoidance of fear and suffering, or being addicted to suffering itself. Checking out from pain and suffering just creates more pain and isolation, which is actually the real suffering.

When we ride our emotions like waves, we can travel higher and higher. This way, we can reach the next plane of living and existence, instead of going in emotional circles or staying frozen in perpetual fear.

Remember, fear is dark, dense energy. It is contracted. Breathe into life and your fear. Release your stuck, contracted energy, and find a way to get in and stay in perpetual motion. It is the key to joy in life.

When you try to check out from or escape your suffering, you only delay the inevitable. What you can do is *look at it, hold it, feel it...and then graciously and with love and compassion let it go...*

Whatever your *addiction* is - fear, abuse, drama, trauma, co-dependency that sucks your energy - *your power is in being sober*, in being mindfully present. Look at it with sober eyes, and see it for what it is.

What's more exciting than addiction? Transformation ... when your addiction loses it mystique and power and you mindfully move to the next level.

> *It takes tremendous courage to go into the dark depths of the human Ego and shine your little God flashlight in there. ~ Princess Superstar*

Labels and Blocked Energy

What exactly is a label? A label can be a trap. A label can be limiting. On the medical front, I never truly believed I had CFS until long after I was labeled as so. I knew something was wrong, but I was still well.

A label can be a description of something about us, such as a medical condition, a personality quirk, a weakness, a habit. If the label is negative in nature, or perceived as negative, then it may be interpreted as *a caricature of one facet on the diamond of who we truly are.* I've been labeled various things in my time, as I'm sure you have. I'm not a fan of labels. What labels do you need to drop and release about yourself?

Funny thing is, as cultural creatures, we love positive labels: superman, princess, savior, wizard, hero, heroine, star, supergirl, etc.

Just keep in mind, if you *label* someone, you may miss the chance of knowing them.

If you judge people you have no time to love them. ~Mother Teresa

You may run into *trial by fire*: the jury of your peers, culture, family, etc. Sometimes, when people don't understand, or they're looking into your life from a distance, labels can be harsh, for example: crazy, lazy, addict...

I even labeled myself by thinking: *all my soul mates are addicts.* I used to believe this and I said it to myself, almost like a joke. I was going to write a book about it, with that title. That's how much I focused on it, like it was my *badge.*

What did this label do to my psyche when I repeated it to myself? What does it do to our psyches when we label each other, even with well-intentioned diagnoses? CFS, ME, diabetes, autism, MS, cancer, depression, sick, disabled?

In my personal life, I kept attracting men with varied blocked energies. Because I labeled myself and didn't value myself enough, I chose partners who didn't value me, nor themselves.

People with limited visions of themselves can't possibly have a large vision of you.
~ unknown

How was I going to break free from this pattern? This was the lesson I had to learn in love: how to value and love myself first.

After my experience with my first boyfriend, I promised myself I would walk away from red flags in behavior, especially regarding alcoholism or chemical addiction. I did listen to my instincts with my future husband, initially. But, for some reason, I later ignored them. He was very persuasive. As I've recounted in this book, we married, and in our marriage, our life was ruled by the glass walls of addiction.

As *Beth Hart* sings in <u>Setting Me Free</u> *(2006)* "this house made of glass, is shattering."

I felt like I had to *side-step around everything* for fear my marriage, or I, would break wide open. As it was, I should have broken down those walls much earlier. I was only delaying the inevitable pain I had to move through to be free.

We argued about money. He complained about my purchases of *health food* and supplements. I finally realized he was spending much more on alcohol and cigarettes. It's ironic that I spent money on health, and he spent it on feeding his illness. *Addiction is costly in more ways than one.*

We had different core values. I valued health and well-being. He valued getting high, on whatever was available, or not available. When we first hung out, there was already red flag behavior, and I actually got up to leave. But, he persuaded me to stay open to him. I should have known his first behavior was a sign of things to come. He pursued me with fervor and passion. *I was his new addiction of choice. I was his new high.*

I bought into the fantasy of living happily ever after and being *craved.* It also wasn't long before I discovered I had married a stranger with hard-core addictive energy. In the beginning, he was addicted to me, until the day he was done with me and informed me so. It literally felt like he threw me away, as if I were disposable, even though we took vows and swore covenants that were supposed to last a lifetime.

It's taken me a long time to pinpoint that horrible sense of feeling like I was *disposable.* Pinpointing feelings is one of the major keys to resolving issues related to well-being, I believe, like we discussed.

In somatic wellness coaching, it can be helpful to identify where your feelings are in your body, what they feel like physically, and, of course, allow yourself to experience them. So here's what I articulated:

*I felt like I had been thrown in the trash, a junkie's discarded needle. I had served my purpose. I was no longer his immediate **fix**.*

Problem was, he got it all wrong and didn't have the faintest idea who or what he was leaving behind. He was asleep, perhaps, or consumed by dark, addictive energy. I was painfully awake. Exhausted, but awake. I am not a victim, however, of these events. These painful experiences ultimately made me strong. It turned me into a Warrior.

That is the dark side of addiction: whatever you use to fuel your high or your escape is often there afterwards to remind you of what you feel you cannot face in yourself. *Remember to seek help for a substance addiction.*

What you love, you feel you need to get you high, is the very thing that may torture you when you come back down to earth.

And, if the vehicle you use to get high is another person, it's usually too late that you realize *their love is the natural high, the reward itself.*

Be careful to whom you give your *heart and body.* Some people may take all they can, no matter what the cost to you.

And yet, what in me was addictive behavior? Turns out, plenty. I can't point the finger at anyone without looking at myself as well. And, ultimately, all I can do is forgive them and myself ... and move on.

I still believe in happy endings, but *not at the price* of the quality of my life, health, peace of mind, or value of well-being. Nothing is worth losing your well-being over, not even the fear of being alone.

You have the whole world and its subtle, ecstatic energy to keep you company.

The world breaks everyone, and afterward, some are strong at the broken places.
~Ernest Hemingway

How does one move out of an energetically addictive (even shameful) place where fear, labels, and blocks are everywhere? It doesn't matter whether you are the one with the addiction, or whether you are involved with an energetic, addicted personality.

How do you move out of the equation? How do you set yourself free?

You must find the courage to inhabit your own mythologies, your own archetypes, and your own *landscape for healing and well-being.* You must find the joy, purpose and courage to *discover what wakes you up*, and to pursue that to pure *transformation.* You must find the courage to move to the next level. You must step into your power to become a Warrior.

The present, whether painful or perfectly imperfect, is where magic, electric, ecstatic life resides. It is the real high. It is heaven…nirvana.

Embody Your Archetypal Energy

Archetypes are energies that inhabit our bodies, souls, psyches. We choose which ones are allowed to inhabit us.

According to Carolyn Myss, archetypes are ancient, universal patterns of behavior that are embedded in what Carl Jung called our *"collective unconscious."*

I believe there are both *positive and negative* expressions of archetypes. Whichever way (*positive or negative*) you focus on an archetype, may be the path you will go down.

It's interesting how in the Gnostic Gospels, all negative archetypes - one of which is The Addict - is that which is unexpressed. In my previous marriage, there used to be *so much energy* around my former husband's addiction - chaos, violent feelings and actions - that I used to think that all sorts of emotions, feelings, etc. were being expressed. *But energetic addiction is ultimately feelings that are unexpressed* and left hidden in the dark recesses of our bodies, minds, and souls.

Ultimately, it's about whether we express the positive or negative version of our signature energies and archetypes.
This is what we are: *spiritual / energetic patterns.*
Relax into yours, nurture your unique patterns.
For they are the keys to your bliss, freedom, and
wellness of mind, body, and spirit…

Heal Your Body Heal Your Spirit

> From an awakened perspective, life is a play of patterns, the patterns of trees, the movement of the stars, the patterns of the seasons and the patterns of human life in every form…**These basic patterns, these stories, the universal archetypes through which all life appears, can be seen and heard when we are still, centered, and awakened.**
>
> ~ Jack Kornfield

It's up to you how you want to express and experience life. What positive archetypes or mythologies do you wish to bring forward into your conscious life: Warrior, Hero, Heroine, Lover, Creator, Caregiver, Ruler, Seeker, Teacher, or Sage? What energy will you be?

Where Is Your Focus? The Parable of the Two Wolves

Here is a popular metaphor that may help you to see how there are different facets of yourself. Have you heard this *parable* of the two wolves? While we are light and darkness, which wolf deserves your focus? Which energy do you wish to express on a regular basis?

> Everyone has two wolves living inside of their person. One wolf is evil - he is fear, anger, envy, sorrow, greed, regret, arrogance, self-pity, guilt, resentment, inferiority, lies, false pride, competition, superiority and ego. The other wolf is good - he is love, peace, benevolence, joy, generosity, hope, humility, serenity, kindness, friendship, empathy, truth, sharing, compassion and faith. These wolves are constantly fighting one another - it's a terrible fight; a fight to the death, and the prize is that the victor will claim your soul. Which wolf will win? The one that you feed.
>
> ~Author unknown

Whether or not you believe we have souls, or believe in good and evil, which wolf keeps you up at 3 a.m.? *The wolf of fear or the wolf of deep and abiding peace?* Where are you putting your focus on a regular basis?

Protect Your Precious Energy

Recall that we discussed highly sensitive people in Chapter Three. Whatever energy you manage and express, you may have more of a challenge if you are a HSP (Aron, 1996). I am an HSP, and I found that *coping with an addictive personality in an intimate relationship was exhausting.* I needed someone who gave, as I already gave so much.

Carl Jung believed that highly sensitive people (HSP) have a deep connection to the unconscious mind, as well as to archetypal dreams.

HSP's may naturally *invest high amounts of precious energy* into relationships. In turn, there may be more relationship boundaries to set, and establishing boundaries may require more of your energy.

People who are *coming from a place of ego or addiction* may take more than they give, and may only suck up your precious, cultivated energy.

Your energy is to be cultivated and protected, yet not contracted. You can do this by accessing your *warrior energy*, and *carry yourself with courage, charisma, and conviction*. No one can truly affect you if you come from this stance.

When you are awake and present, you are strong and able to fend off any energy that is not yours or not welcome. Block it with your *light saber*, and don't ever doubt yourself, even for a second.

This is *warrior energy*. You have to step into your inexhaustible Power.

There are infinite ways to access your authentic self and *warrior energy* and explore which *archetypal energies* empowers you. Art is a great way to explore your true energy, including dance, acting, music, writing, etc.

~ *Step into the role you were born to play, not the role handed to you by others.* ~

Imagine the role you are destined to play: *be it, feel it, live it.* Instead of inhabiting a label slapped on you, *flip the label.* Flip it to a positive image of who you know you are, just like flipping a coin.

Ego, Power, & Boundaries

What keeps us prisoner to our addictions? The false belief that we're *powerless.* Believe it or not, this belief is due to the ego.

I now see that everything I thought was *supposed to happen in my life* - the things I thought had to happen in order for me to be happy - were all ego-based.

Transcending, or moving beyond my ego and changing my focus and my energy saved my life and preserved my sense of peace. **There is nothing I could want more than what is currently happening in my life at this present moment.** *My life is blessed …*

~*I have made peace with my life, my choices, and my actions.* ~

My life is blessed, even after having experienced trauma and chronic illness. How can you find your own sense of peace of mind and body?

The opportunity that illness affords is to be released from your ego. This release is a blessing in disguise. How so? Because it temporarily dissolves all sense of boundaries between you and the Divine.

Don't get me wrong. Boundaries, in general, are essential. When navigating life, we're constantly testing and developing boundaries with others. We test the integrity of those boundaries. We do that by establishing and maintaining better boundaries through interaction with others, and sometimes through conflict with others.

Establishing and enforcing boundaries with others is paramount. But the ego can get stuck in boundaries and *egoic boundaries may keep you feeling separatated from others.* Be mindful of your ego, especially during upset/as what causes upset. In my experience, conflict and drama are often about ego and addiction. As I mentioned, I had to step back to see where I was addicted in my life: to sadness, loneliness, not being treated well by men, trauma, *victim energy.* Oh, yes, and to chocolate!

The most challenging teachers are those who confront our egos. They are also the hardest people to forgive. Yet, instead of reacting to what we perceive has hurt us, we can let go, evolve, transform, even elevate. Showing kindness and compassion go a long way too.

The most important lesson I learned about ego, though, was that holding on to memories of abuse and trauma - *and the way they can make you feel so bad* - is a part of ego as well. Even holding on to my own regrets and mistakes, was a mistake!

If you hold on to feeling bad, you are stuck in Ego, you are not in the flow of life and well-being. When I first learned this concept, it blew me away. It was wild to wrap my brain around the fact that feeling troubled over the past, present, or future was part of my egoic identity, and causing me harm, not to mention keeping me stuck in one spot on my path to true well-being.

> *You can carry a burden of guilt (self-identification with mistakes)*
> *vs. The Power of Presence.*
> *~ Eckart Tolle*

The future, too, needs to be honored, without making it more important in your mind than the present. But the power for creating a better future is contained in the present moment: **You create a good future by creating a good present.** How do you do that? By recognizing the goodness that is already inherent in the present moment, **even in the midst of challenges.** Discontent, blaming, complaining, self-pity cannot serve as a foundation for a good future, no matter how much effort you make. *~Eckart Tolle*

Sigh. *Darn it*, right? The present moment is such an easy place to not be, isn't it? ☺

How do you move out of ego and also the feeling of powerlessness?

Feel. Don't analyze, just feel. Don't worry. Just be.

You are worthy just by being here, just by being born. Stand in your power and goodness, not your ego. Stand in your own light and shine, like the sun.

> *The sun shines on you...it doesn't ask you 'how did I do?' It just shines.*
> ~ Gary Zukav

So what is powerlessness? It is *fear*: not being in the present moment, interference, the feeling that you're flawed, unlovable; the feeling that you have no value.

With my history of abuse and trauma, I had a distorted sense of self. I had falsely learned about myself that I had no value.

> *So much of being healthy is being aware of, and honoring your inherent worth, your inherent value.*

If you remember nothing else, please remember this: You have *value* just by being alive, just by being here.

Your power lies in the present moment. However, addiction by nature, takes you out (sometimes far out) of the calm, loving, present.

What do you think? *Where does your power lie?*

> *The secret of health for both mind and body is not to mourn for the past, not to worry about the future...but to live in the present moment wisely and earnestly.*
> ~ Siddhartha Gautama Buddha

Can you tell, yet, that I find quotes inspirational? Yet, the most inspiring thing to me is when people step into their own power...

> *~Presence is Power~*

> *In the Light of calm and steady self-awareness, inner energies wake up and work miracles without any effort on your part.*

> *~Sri Nisargadatte Maharshi*

Personal Power

None of us is really safe except for those who summon unreasonable courage and dare to stretch their limits by doing the hardest work which is not impossible.
~ Yeats

What is personal power? Personal power is about your integrity and congruency. Are you congruent with who you are on the inside and the outside? So much of inhabiting true well-being is, about becoming empowered. And a big part of being empowered is being who you really are, 100% of the time, inside and outside. When who you are on the inside matches who you are on the outside, guess what? You manifest well-being because you have integrity, you're congruent, and you radiate authenticity. This genuine energy gives your body strength.

~ When you are authentic and congruent about who you are,
you step into your power, and become a warrior ~

Warrior Energy vs. Victim Energy

If you bring forth that which is within you,
Then that which is within you
Will be your salvation.
If you do not bring forth that
Which is within you,
Then that which is within you
Will destroy you.
~ The Gnostic Gospels

We talked about trust in Chapter Three. It's about stepping into your "heroic, instinctive energies," as Peter Levine says.

You want to re-establish the trust between your body and the world. This takes monumental courage. It takes *warrior energy.*

There is no room in your life for feeling like a victim of abuse, trauma, or chronic illness. Since *victim and warrior* occupy the same chakra (see *Chakras and Your Health* in the section *Energetics vs. Genetics* in this chapter) but are opposite archetypes (*victim energy* is the shadow archetype) it's either one or the other.

You can do this. Warrior energy is your shield. Trust, faith, courage, love, joy, and self-compassion are your energy currencies.

Trust is Healing

Trust allows you to give. Giving is abundant.
Trust allows the experience of bliss. Bliss is awakefulness.
Trust allows you to laugh. Laugh at the richness, the beauty,
and the playfulness of the universe.
Apply consciousness to this process and all roads will lead to home.
~ Gary Zukav

Here are some more tools to move through fear, powerlessness, and, traumatic stress. First, conquering fear is about re-establishing physical, emotional, and spiritual trust. The most important kind of trust is to *trust yourself and life itself.*

For trauma victims, saying *"I trust, I trust in Life"* is a powerful way to get instantly grounded. Try it. Allow yourself to sink into the RR, (The Relaxation Response), and *stay there...*

Markings in dry clay disappear, only when the clay is soft again.
Scars upon the self disappear, Only when one becomes soft within.
~Deng Ming-Dao

The seashells do not fear the velvet crashing of the tides. ~unknown

Another tool is to create a safe haven, ideally where you live, to re-establish physical trust so you can relax, reboot, and heal.

Another tool is to seek to establish trust with other people, which does involve boundaries. Therapy or counseling may assist as well.

From my experience, re-establishing trust is a process that involves time, a safe place and safe people, and good experiences and possibly a retraining of your unconscious and subconscious. I prefer to use yoga to work through my subconscious mind patterns and belief systems.

The way *Peter Levine* says to re-establish trust is to rely on your **heroic, instinctive energies** that can only be found in the present moment. But, trauma can thwart your instinctive energies as well. So I would add that your body's *instinctive voice* will let you know when it is safe to re-establish trust with the world. But you have to listen to your voice and also find the courage to be present so you can allow others in. There is compassion out there. Trust in at least that, my friend.

~ Presence is everything ~

Presence is Power

Not being present, that is, living in the past or future - or living more or less *unconsciously* - is when you may have a greater tendency to lose vitality. *While not always true of course,* this is what happened for me.

Surrendering to the present moment is your greatest chance to heal and inhabit true well-being. Your body talks to you all the time, telling you via feedback loops of communication what you need to do to be well. Staying present – no matter how challenging your current story - is where you have the greatest power to change and harness well-being.

> *"…the rapt observation of the present moment as opposed to a plot-driven preoccupation with what will happen next…"*
> *~Maximilian Le Cain*

Ironically, as we have said, being sick also can put you straight into your body. Remember, this is a gift in disguise. It gives you an opportunity to be present. Likewise, one of the worst things that comes with the experience of abuse is *losing trust*. What's so vital is that you do *not* allow the energy of that trauma or abuse to linger in your body. *Don't embody someone else's dark energy. It's not yours.* Release what's not yours and take back your own energy. Got it? That's all you need to know. Allow only vital, positive energy into your living space.

I ask myself: who would I be if I didn't have the scar of abuse in my soul? Am I who I am, despite of, or in light of, all that happened? Maybe I'm a better version of myself. Maybe this *is* the best version of myself: my warrior self, emerged from the shadows. I feel compassionate and kind, brave and real *because of what I have experienced.* All I must do is focus on being confident *as my authentic self* who has clear boundaries, as opposed to feeling like a victim of my life's events.

In healing, I've learned that whenever you *move something out,* you must replace it with something else. *So I replace victim energy with warrior energy.* The best warrior is peaceful and strong, calm, focused, and not easily affected by slings to the ego.

> *The two most powerful warriors are patience and time. ~Leo Tolstoy*

I also felt my body had betrayed me. I felt I couldn't trust my body or life anymore. But, did I betray myself by not listening to my body's voice before my ski accident, when I failed to check my skis' binders?

At this point, it doesn't matter. I can't live in or analyze the past. I was young. I was still learning. I forgive myself. I crave only the *power of presence* now. I just do my best to be in my body and live in the present moment with mindfulness. *I do know this: working toward a higher state of well-being requires infinite bravery.* Using my own personal power, I release grief and replace attachment to the past with joys of the present. That doesn't mean I dishonor my past, for it has shaped me.

Grief and longing ... give shape and texture to the contours of the heart ...
~ Flynn Johnson - Journey to the Sacred Mountains

The most important decision we make is whether we believe we live in a friendly or hostile universe. ~Albert Einstein

Physical and Spiritual Strength

Heal Your Body Heal Your Spirit

Power and strength. We all want these. The truth is, we have them already: inside. The human spirit is indomitable and limitless, and keeping or getting back your strength is necessary for healing and true well-being.

For sensitive people, or people who tend to get sick easily, establishing clear boundaries has everything to do with keeping both physical and spiritual strength, and staying well. This might seem like a strange concept, but it's real and absolutely crucial to your health and the quality of your life. And this is actually the one area in your life you have complete control over: *your personal power.*

> *Many people who get sick easily sometimes have boundary issues, meaning they often let people with negative and/or toxic energy into their worlds, and energy fields. It's no surprise that they then get sick.*
>
> *We are all sponges for better or worse. Our energy fields expand or contract depending on with whom or what we interact. Energy fields are the electromagnetic part of our bodies. As much as this sounds like science fiction, it is real and a crucial part of your health.*
>
> *Your energy field is represented by your aura and meridian points on your body. The concept is like a four-dimensional information superhighway connecting you physically, mentally, emotionally, and spiritually. It takes into account things like your food, friends, state of mind, beliefs, genetics, and emotional heritage. Your energy field encompasses both your physical and spiritual strength.*

Do the impossible, stay true to yourself.
Your destiny is no further than your heart. ~ Lori St Jon

My friend, *your energetic body is holographic.* In fact, it is a *GPS map of the current state of your life and health.* This is why it's crucial to allow only *positive energy* into *your* field of energy, including thoughts, people, and even food. If negative energy gets through, and we're human so it does, then you must move that energy out again to re-balance.

By allowing into your world *energy demons that have unresolved issues,* such as substance abuse, anger, or negativity, you're playing roulette with your health. Creating boundaries will help you get and/or stay well. This includes relationships *and* life in general. *Don't take on any more than you can handle.* People's lives won't fall apart if you can't take on a task. Many of us, especially those with boundary issues, tend to say *yes* too easily. Create a safe zone for your physical and spiritual energy.

The energy you have is precious. Use it to build your physical and spiritual health first, then reach out to others. Doing something for someone else can give you energy, but be sure you have the energetic resources for the commitment. People will respect you when you come from a place of authenticity. It will do wonders for your health.

I had a dream where my mom - whom I love dearly - told me I had been elected to lead a book club meeting. The book was gargantuan and I had never read it. I was already overwhelmed, but the prospect of telling my mom, in a room full of women, that I couldn't do it seemed impossible. But I said *no,* emphatically, over and over in my dream, despite objections from the group until they finally got it. I was so relieved and it was profoundly liberating for me.

If you feel immobilized or exhausted, take deep breaths. Breathing deeply makes you feel better. It transforms fear into action, excitement, and potential. It grounds you back in your body too. It is the essence of yoga. If you're too tired to even breathe, *think a positive thought.* Being positive is a *decision* and its consequences are life-altering. Find out what works for you and do it. Your precious life is waiting.

Healing may not be so much about getting better, as about letting go of everything that isn't you - all of the expectations, all of the beliefs - and becoming who you are. ~ Rachel Naomi Remen

Keys to Authentic Health

Here are a few key points to real, authentic health.

+ *Slow down*: We've been far too rushed for far too long. Authentic health is about slowing it down to real time, where your body lives, breathes, and heals in the present moment. Take time to take care of *you*. Make time for being lazy. Make time for being mellow. Make time for others. Make time for love. Make time for making love. Slowing down is deliberate.

+ *Tell stories*: Be mindful of the texts and emails you write. Set aside an hour, gather a group and re-kindle the joy of hearing and telling stories. Stories are where and how we heal.

+ *Align yourself*: Forget about branding your persona. Drop disparities between your public and private selves, or merge them. Congruency is when who you are on the outside matches who you are on the inside, and that's when your life and health align.

+ *Be honest*: Your body tells the absolute *truth* of what's going on in your life. When *you* tell the *truth* about your health habits and your life - what you eat, do, feel, how your exercise, or don't, etc. - you and your body will align, match up, be in perfect synch, and be unified in real, authentic health.

+ *Express your feelings*: Say what you truly feel, whatever it is, and whether it is positive, negative, or neutral. Be honest in expressing your emotions.

+ *Be where you are:* Health resides in the present moment. Accept your body just as it is. Acknowledge your life and who you are just as you are, *right now*! You can only begin from where you are. And where you are is perfect for you right now. You get to where you are going from where you are!

*If you're out of shape, be okay with it *right now*
*If you're addicted to sugar, be okay with it *right now*
*If you hate exercise, be okay with it *right now*
*If you're depressed, be okay with it *right now*

+ _Do what feels good:_ Health feels good! It's not meant to feel like torture or taste like cardboard. The bottom line is: _health as well-being_ and pleasure are intimately linked! Do something that feels good to you each and every day. Whatever it is, do it, buy it, listen to it, watch it, connect with it, experience it now.

*Read that book you bought last year
*Go to that class you've heard about
*Make that call – Invite someone for tea
*Dine in that new restaurant
*Take that trip you've been dreaming about!

+ _Be fearless and impress yourself:_ The liberating truth is that the only person usually paying close attention to you is _you_. So forget what others think and impress yourself. Just be fearless and _step into your personal power_. When you step into your power, you stand grounded in well-being. Have faith in your ability to be grounded in health as an expression of fearless well-being.

+ _Be assured that you matter:_ Remember Don Miguel Ruiz and _The Four Agreements_ (Ruiz, 1997)?

> _Do your best, say only what you mean, don't take anything personally, and express what you truly want..._

Why do these tenets work? Because when you come from an authentic place, life lines up and everything flows out of that place. When you know, in your heart, that what you say, feel, believe, and think matter - if only to you - then that's all that counts, ultimately. Why is this?

> _Because you and your life matter,_
> _more than you could possibly know,_
> _All you have to do is believe it is so._

+ _Keep watch and be mindful:_ Abide by these words of guidance from Patrick Overton:

Watch your thoughts, they become words.
Watch your words, they become actions.
Watch your actions, they become habits.
Watch your habits, they become character.
Watch your character, it becomes your destiny.
> ~Patrick Overton

The Journey to Well-Being and Change

Change, but start slowly, because direction is more important than speed.
~ Paulo Coelho

You never change things by fighting the existing reality.
To change something, build a new model that makes the existing model obsolete.
~ Buckminster Fuller

When you want – really want – answers, they are there.
When you are ready – really ready – to change, the opportunities abound.
When you are willing to listen and to learn, even the stones speak.
~ Lazarus

Yard by yard life is mighty hard,
But inch by inch life is a cinch.
~ unknown

You must find the place inside yourself where nothing is impossible.
~Deepak Chopra

~ The most important things you can do is change the lens you're looking through
and keep pulling those weeds from your head. ~

Choice, Focus, and Change

Inhabiting and living from a place of well-being is a choice. Health may not always be a choice, but you can *choose to be well* in mind.

Conversely, when exercising willpower is an option, there is something automatically to rebel against. It's only human nature. When we are faced with decisions that may affect the course of our health, we don't always choose wisely. Ultimately, it's about which lens you're using and what you choose to focus on every day. Where is your focus?

~ What you focus on takes focus ~

How *will* you choose your focus? Wherever you decide to focus largely determines the energy or *chi* you have flowing throughout your body. Your focus may influence how much *energy currency* you possess. These ideas are connected to two concepts known as *li and chi*,* or rather *energy and consciousness. Li is consciousness and chi is energy.*

The more *li* you connect with - *the greater your understanding of the natural patterns of the universe* - the more you can live a fulfilling life within these patterns. Additionally, the more *chi* you create, the more likely it is you will be in the state of and the in the flow of effortless well-being.

*Please see page 404 in this chapter for a more detailed discussion of li and chi.

The reality tends to be however, that we tend to focus on states of mind that are dramatic, traumatic, or on substances that artificially modify our state of mind, like sugar, or drugs. Just bear in mind, the higher you go, the further you must fall, like a sugar crash, for instance.

Instead, focus on naturally sustainable, even-flowing states of mind that create an ecstatic, easeful flow of *li* (organizing principle) and *chi* (energy) in all your systems. And be equally mindful of what you put into your body. There is more on li and chi coming up here soon.

When you're injured, your body freezes the part that's injured until it has healed.

I wrote this sentence in Chapter One when telling my story and it is one of the themes in this book. When - or maybe because - you are sick, *your body freezes*, or shuts down, at least so it seems. The logical antithesis to this statement is that *change and movement* are what unlock your body's healing potential and *frees your body again.* Free yourself:

~ Change FREEZE into FREE ~

The quality of the imagination is to flow and not to freeze.

~Ralph Waldo Emerson

The secret is to keep moving. Keep changing. Move into action. You may spark transformation within yourself. *Move in thought, if nothing else:*

All wrong-doing arises because of mind. If mind is transformed can wrong-doing remain? ~ Siddhartha Gautama Buddha

The secret of health for both mind and body is not to mourn for the past, not to worry about the future...but to live in the present moment wisely and earnestly.

~ Siddhartha Gautama Buddha

Take your time, keep moving forward, and in good time, vibrant health will be yours.

~Dr. David S. Dyer

One of the mysteries of how people recover - not only from CFS - but from any chronic illness, is that not one approach works for everyone. One supplement or diet works great for someone and a completely different protocol helps someone else who has the same condition. While some of this is biochemistry and genetics, *change itself works too.**

*A little bit of stress can kick in the innate healing response. So keep changing it up to stimulate healing.

Why is there such disparity in healing pathways for the same illness? It may be that *change* itself is the answer. It's not so much what you do as it is that you *do something, try anything*. Small stress itself yields results.

Even more relevant perhaps, is that it's the nervous system we are affecting when we try something new. This may be why "new" tactics help for a bit, and also perhaps why our sensitive nervous systems vacillate so much...because our nervous systems are hypersensitized.

Because our nervous systems are more sensitive (whether due to early childhood trauma, illness, abuse, poverty, or because we are HSP's), they may be more volatile. However, this also may be why "change" works so well. I believe you can strengthen your nervous system over time. Keep trying new tactics. Figure out what works! Whatever you do, above all else, keep trying, and do what works for *you*.

Change now, while you still can. Change now because you can, change now because it is the right thing to do. Change now because there is no right, no left, no time left, no space left. Only you. Change. ~Richard Bartlett

> Change happens in the present moment.
> Change makes change happen (mix it up).
> What does that feel like to you, look like to you?
> What feels good to you?
> Hint: use your intuition/bodymind.
> Either you'll make progress or you won't,
> but the most important energy is that
> you tried.

Begin doing what you want to do now. We are not living in eternity. We have only this moment, sparkling like a star in our hand – and melting like a snow flake. Let us use it before it is too late. ~ Marie Beynon Ray

*Until one is committed, there is hesitancy, the chance to draw back... . Concerning all acts of initiative (and creation), there is one elementary truth the ignorance of which kills countless ideas and splendid plans: that the moment one definitely commits oneself, then providence moves too. A whole stream of events from the decision, raising in one's favor all manner of unforeseen incidents, meetings and material assistance, which no man could have dreamt would have come his way. I learned a deep respect for one of Goethe's couplets: **Whatever you can do, or dream you can, begin it. Boldness has genius, power and magic in it!** [supposed translation of Goethe's Faust, lines. 214-30].*
(W. H. Murray, 1951)

Joe Dispenza, who was featured in the movie <u>What the Bleep Do We Know?</u>, says that change is uncomfortable because chemically the body feels threatened by unfamiliar firing of peptides and neurons in the brain: **'If you remember one thing about change, remember that it causes the "self" and the body to go into complete chaos because the self no longer has any feelings to relate to in order to define itself. If we stop having the same thoughts, feelings, or reactions, we stop making the same chemicals, which sends the body into a state of homeostatic imbalance. ... Therefore when internal order is altered by our change in thinking, we do not "feel" like the same person. As a result, our identity wants to return to the feelings of the familiar, and our body is trying to influence our brain to return to a recognizable state of being, so that the body can recalibrate itself with past feelings.'** *I think the degree of willingness to experience this uncomfortability/unfamiliarity is the degree to which you can grow as a person. And also the degree to which you can experience true joy and true bliss, which- as Sharon Gannon says- is our true nature. ~ <u>www.princesssuperstar.com</u>*

When you stop changing, you stop evolving. ~ Unknown

I can change. I can live out my imagination instead of my memory. I can tie myself to my limitless potential instead of my limiting past. ~Stephen Covey

As you pursue your own healing path, focus on your strengths:
Choose a positive stance in life. Lean positively into your future. Choose Life.

Focus on what you can do, not on what you can't do.
~ Rachelle Friedman

Your life is important. Honor it. Fight for your highest possibilities.
~ Nathaniel Branden

We cannot change the cards we are dealt, just how we play the hand.
~Randy Pausch

Well-being is first and foremost a *state of mind*. As Deepak Chopra points out, when we change the way we experience life, our biochemistry literally changes. We produce dopamine, serotonin, oxytocin and opiates vs. cortisol and adrenaline (Miles, 2015). When we focus on what is positive, our neurochemistry and brains literally change (Broderick & Blewitt, 2010). Allow yourself to relax and trust Life. Ultimately, well-being is not about your will power, it's about your spiritual power. *Harness your positive energy …*

Positive Psychology and Your Health

Positive psychology is a new and exciting branch of psychology that focuses on, you guessed it, positivity. For example: What is *going right* in your life? What are your strengths you can focus on, instead of dwelling on your perceived weaknesses, such as having a chronic condition? Focusing on my strengths and experiencing life as loving and positive was a game changer for me. It can be for you too. Choose to see and experience life as positive!

Focusing on what you can do, as opposed to what you can't do, as Rachelle Friedman says, can change your over-all well-being. Our attitude is positively powerful. The mind is so powerful and you can use this along with your innate strengths to gain ground. S(he) who leans positively into the future, creates just that - a positive future. Give yourself a fighting chance: Think positively!

What matters are two things:

> ➤ First, how you *react* to events will sway outcomes. Hint: stay positive, hopeful, and most importantly, *resilient.*
> ➤ Second, when we take our *ego* out of the equation, life is modified. Things that were essential, hardly seem relevant.

Most everything we view as having gone wrong is because of *ego.* When you step back from your ego, you're left with your luminous soul, or the part of you that just *is*, and only wishes to express and receive love. It's a beautiful, easeful, stress-free place to be and live. Life looks a lot different from this perspective.

Tenets of Positive Psychology: More Tools for Your Tool Belt

Pleasure - What do you enjoy?

Meaning - What gives your life meaning? What are your core values? How would you describe your spiritual energy?

Engagement - What plugs you into life?

Creativity - How can you create meaning, purpose, and enjoyment?

Flexibility - Can you adapt to change? So much of what comprises the process of *changing for good* is the complementary process of *outgrowing our problems.* Instead of our problems just *going away*, things that are more important to us take precedence. *We see the bigger picture.* We become more *flexible.*

What's Going Right? - Are you able to focus on what's going right, as opposed to what you perceive to be going wrong?

Resiliency - The most crucial hand you play may be when you get up and try again. Resiliency is turning adversity into strength.

> *No matter how hard the past, you can always begin again. ~ Buddha*

> *Your present circumstances don't determine where you can go;*
> *they merely determine where you start. ~ Nido Qubein*

> *Never give up. Too many people lose the light from their eyes. Don't ever give up.*
> *~ Ronald S. Gordon - my dad*

Love & Infinite Creative Potential Energy

Your mojo is your magic. ~ Melani Ward

As you love, you attract. ~ James Allen

In my opinion, life is quite magical. Yes, hard stuff happens, but there is this subtle, pervasive energy that is blissful – even magical - if you are open to feeling and experiencing it. Be open to life:

Be Open (Be in the vibration of Love)

Commit 100%...

Then...

Act

when the intuitive nudge is felt

Receive

with joy, enthusiasm, and passion

Acting on your intuition utilizes your instinctive healing energy. This is not only magical, it can change the landscape of your life and body, which is the whole point of the power of intuition. It's your GPS. Go to your intuition first in your mind.

If you've been there in the mind, you'll go there in the body. ~unknown

This is especially true when you are seeking to recover your lost energy. When you reconnect with your intuitive, emotional, and healing energy, your physical energy has a better chance of returning.

Notice the power of tapping into your healing intuitive energy, along with focusing on positivity, power, purpose, and passion:

The mind has 40,000 to 50,000 thoughts a day. When 1,000 to 2,000 of these daily thoughts are directed to a goal, it will come rapidly.
~Orin in <u>Personal Power Through Awareness</u>

Finally, add *gratitude* into the recipe for manifesting true well-being. Remember this: gratitude is a *receiving energy*. Practicing gratitude may be one the biggest shifts you can make in general, and especially for manifesting results in your life. Gratitude changes the quality of your thoughts, which changes the quality of what you attract and manifest.

In summary, here is a simple formula you can try for manifesting:

<u>Build a Base of Positive, Passionate Purpose</u>

Be Open, Commit, Act, Receive, Be Grateful, Repeat

Most of us attract by default. But you can change that statistic for yourself. How? Try to keep your ratio of positive to negative thoughts at a 5:1 ratio. *Try to set thinking positively as your default way of thinking to achieve results.* You will start to rewire your brain and this affects not only your internal outcomes, but also how you interact with the world.

By focusing on positive thinking, you can literally change your neural pathways, which can lead to different outcomes and real results.

Gratitude and positive thoughts raised your natural vibration. You feel stronger, even healthier, and the universe will correspond with your focus. What you think, what you feel will always manifest in some form or another. The universe is unlimited creative energy potential. When we live from a place of infinite creative potential, life opens up. When you live from a positive P.O.V. your potential is unlimited.

l enjoyed _The Secret_ (Bell, Bloomfield, Byrne, Goldenfein, Harrington, McAvoy & Heriot, 2006), but one of the best motivational/self-development movies I've seen is _The Compass_ (Ellis, Greenlee, & Stone, 2009). Check it out here: **http://www.thecompass.tv/**

Another way to look at attraction is to realize that you often attract what you *are (Wayne Dyer)*. So strive to be your highest self and see who and what shows up in your already beautiful life.

What you are seeking is also seeking you. ~ Rumi

Spiritual Power

When you examine the lives of the most influential people who have ever walked among us, you discover one thread that winds through them all. They have been aligned first with their spiritual nature and only then with their physical selves. ~ Albert Einstein

If we truly want to create a life that is grounded in basic well-being, we must decide to commit ourselves to learning what it takes to thrive instead of merely survive. ~ Susan Velasquez

We've talked about spiritual power off and on in this book and now we'll study it more closely. What is spiritual power?* Faith, love, etc. We have the capacity to harness our love and live mindfully at any time. You have so much love and are braver than you ever thought.

*I believe spiritual power can be faith, love, light, courage, knowledge, mindfulness, trust, wisdom, etc.

In the light of living in our modern, unpredictable world, let love be your legacy. *Let it shroud you in safety and shine a light in the darkness....*

Fear and anxiety can twist our thinking and short-circuit our spiritual power. Right before my dad passed away, he expressed the fear that, in the final analysis, he was a failure. Nothing could have been further from the truth. In life, my dad was respected as a scientist, professor, department chairman, dean, and businessman. He was a beloved son, husband, father, and *pappy*. Colleagues, friends and family alike valued his intelligence, passion, and dry wit. My dad had a passion for living.

So what was going on in my dad's mind that would lead him to think he had a failed life? All of the years I knew him, he dealt with anxiety, sometimes extreme. It's hard to say what factors might have fed his anxiety. It could have been a combination of genetics and nutrition, extreme stress at work, the strain of my divorce, or the effects of chemotherapy. But I do believe it was possibly his intense anxiety that started him on the road to becoming ill and caused him to fear he had failed to meet his life goals. *Yet, in fact, his life fed the life of his family...*

Anxiety takes you out of the present moment. It creates an acute, unbalanced amount of stress hormones in the body. Unrelenting stress combined with genetic factors, poor nutrition choices, etc. may set the stage for chronic illness. Yet, we have epigenetics on our side.

My dad did go into remission for a while, but then the cancer returned. After his second round of chemotherapy, he felt apprehensive that he had made a poor decision to receive further treatment. Indeed, it may have been the tipping point for his greatly weakened body.

For you, dear friend, it is crucial to listen to your body's cues - your instincts - no matter who says what in your outer world. Your body knows best even if you can't explain it. Trust yourself and your body.

So, while my dad had great anxiety that plagued his physical person, he also had remarkable *spiritual character.* He was an honest, hardworking man. *He had honor. He also had passion and lived to serve those he loved.*

What have you done when your passion was greater than your fear? How can you live from a place of spiritual power no matter the cards?

There is so much spiritual power in honor. I believe if my dad could have tapped into that part of himself, or been more aware of his power on that level, he may have at least gained some time.

Either way, let me share a humorous and powerful story, as well as lesson from my father. It's about one of his last days here on earth.

He was working on his book, as usual, sitting in his therapy chair, typing on his laptop, when all of a sudden he became agitated and said, "Where's that file?" Bear in mind that at this point in his illness, he used a walker when he moved about, because of his vigorous pain. However, he was so *focused on finding the file* he thought he had misplaced that he *spontaneously* got up from his chair - ignored his walker - and started *booking it around the room*, from one stack of papers to another, looking with, great purpose, for that file! ☺

When we are truly present, mindful, and passionate about something, not only does the whole world open up, but our minds, bodies and spirits can do things we previously thought we couldn't. Our bodies, minds, and souls are intrinsically linked. It is because of this intimate, inscrutable, and powerful connection between mind, body, and spirit that we are able to *manifest spiritual energy* with all of its inherent power.

My father had no memory of this event, or at least of not using his walker. He was so focused on his book - his passion - he momentarily forgot his body was sick. His passion and purpose over-rode his pain.

Energetics vs. Genetics

We don't see things as they are, we see them as we are. ~Anaïs Nin

So, what does the story of my father and his walker mean? It means that *ultimately, our well-being is not so much about genetics alone, it's also about energetics.* When you understand this principle, your well-being may shift for the better. Harness your spiritual power to shift awareness.

What does this mean exactly? **When your belief system intersects with your biology, the landscape of your body can literally change.** It was my father's passion versus his perception of his condition that propelled him to walk freely. *Clearly his energy had temporarily shifted.* Who knows what could have come to pass if he'd stayed in that state - or if any of us could stay in that *state of being connected to love* indefinitely.

In his book *The Biology of Belief* (2008), Bruce Lipton explains in detail how this phenomenon of energetics vs. genetics can occur. He describes the field of *epigenetics*, which is the study of how your choices and your environment can influence your genetic expression. He also describes how our thoughts, whether positive or negative, have *the most influence* on gene expression. In other words, the *energetics of our thoughts* may influence our genetic potential more than our actual genetics.*

Remember The Relaxation Response or the RR? The RR *turns off* gene expression. This discovery was made by the research of Herbert Benson (1975), who also coined the term *The Relaxation Response.*

Why is this big news? First, it points to the powerful mind/body connection. Second, it also underlines the fact that what we think and how we act can affect immune function, as discovered in studies conducted by research specialists in the field of *psychoneuroimmunology.*

Any way you look at it, the *power of the mind* is undeniable. And your mind is *everywhere* in your body. So, your mind has a profound influence and expression on and in your body. In fact, when you have *peace of mind you peace of body*, and that state-of-being invokes the RR.

>   *~The Relaxation Response also turns off the gene expression of cells*
>   *which produce inflammation~*

This is critical, as chronic inflammation is an enormous problem and may have an affect or even lead to chronic conditions like heart disease, Type II diabetes, stroke, and possibly even MS, CFS, or at least exacerbate them. Remember, chronic inflammation is *one of the main biomarkers* of chronic disease. When Herbert Benson was interviewed by Lauren Ware for an article on Protomag.com, here's what he had to say about the RR and its positive influence to reduce inflammation:

> We compared 19 people who had regularly evoked the relaxation response for an average of nine years with 19 people who had never done so. In a scan of each subject's 50,000 or so genes, we found that the activity of about 2,000 genes differed between the two groups.
>
> Among those in the relaxation response group, roughly 2,000 genes active in various stress-related physiological pathways, genes that trigger inflammation and genes that prompt cell death, had been deactivated. There is no evidence that the deactivations are permanent. [But] **we believe that daily practice of the relaxation response is necessary to sustain the changes.** (Ware, 2010)

*Very important to understand is also that your genetic expression can change in the moment, e.g. think of my dad who got up out of his chair without his walker. His passion allowed him to move without pain.

An example of energetics vs. genetics, may be chronic stress that has such an effect on our well-being and genetic expression, even immunity/auto-immunity. But I believe your spirit can inform and influence the immune system as well. *Remember the power of divine mind:*

The soul always knows what to do to heal itself. The challenge is to silence [monkey]* mind. ~ Carolyn Myss

How do we set ourselves and our well-being up for success? Recall, we are just now learning how the *mind, microbiome, brain, and gemome can act as a single system* (Ornish, 2015). Some strategies may include diet, faith, positive thinking, restorative exercise like yoga, meditation, and mindful living. Between all of our choices in what we do, eat, and think, we have much more power than we currently realize.

For every action in the universe there is an equal and opposite reaction. This can be a comforting law and a frustrating one as well. When you don't feel well it can seem as if the laws don't apply to you.

Like we touched upon earlier, there are ways the body breaks down that seem to go against patterns of well-being. Some diseases seem to fly in the face of patterns like cancer and AIDS. But there are also ways the body recovers that seem to defy the design of nature.

Then again, what is the design of nature? She seems to be built on both order and chaos. Scientists talk about entropy and the tendency of all things toward disorder. Yet nature clearly also has structure and works according to an *order of patterns* and has the organizing principle of Li. See *Riding the Wave of Health/Well-Being* in this chapter.

Either way, the point is to realize the power of your thoughts and your *energetic nature.* You have way more power than you realize. Your response to life/stress is key. What does this potentially mean for you?

It means everything: it can change your well-being and maybe even your health.

Make the best use of the energy that inhabits your body at any given point in time.

Believe in the potential of your body, when you combine it with the powerful forces of your divine mind and your infinite spirit.

*"Monkey mind" is the primitive part of our brain. While it is instinctive, it can be fearful and reactive. Divine mind is that part of us that is connected to Source. Creative mind is the part of us that is divine that is connected to the Earth. However you view Life, connect to that within you that is divine/creative.

When you become self-aware, great things can happen:

The world is made up of energy and awareness. ~ *Deepak Chopra*

Well-being – *and perhaps even health* - are the *free flow of energy and the free flow of communication* in the body. At any moment in time you can set yourself *free*. You can give yourself permission to be *free*.

Spiritual Power and Your Energy Body

So many of us get caught up in other people's energy. But true power, energy, and freedom come when you realize *you* have all the energy and power you need right *inside of you*. It is like in the movies when the heroine steps into her power and all of sudden the world lights up. Your body is an *energy system and you are connected to its Source.*

Let go of fear and doubt, and a world of pure energy will open up to you, and come directly from within you (which is connected to Source). Remember, our bodies have the power to light up the whole United States for a week. Can you imagine what your soul can do?

Light tomorrow with today. ~ *Elizabeth Barrett Browning*

Unblock the corresponding spiritual and/or physical energies and your well-being may shift. Our bodies, minds, and spirits are intertwined.

Give yourself permission to step into your power, and invoke the archetypes that move you into action. For me, it's warrior energy. For you it might be different, just as you may need different foods, relationships, types of movement, and experiences to be well.

Work to unblock your emotional and spiritual energies first to release corresponding blocks in your physical energy. There is a source from which we all originate. The energy from which you originate is eternal. *You, as energy, are eternal.* Harness this *eternal, creative* part of yourself to elicit change in your physical landscape.

As you explore your spiritual energy, still be aware of where you experience your emotions on the physical and visceral levels. When you are *not feeling well*, you know it in your gut. When your heart breaks…*you feel it in your body. Still listen to the visceral voice of your body.*

What creates well-being in your body? Your (divine or creative) mind, as well as the natural instincts of your body, connected to natural flow.

Honor, trust, and respect what your body needs for unified well-being. When you do your best to respect your body's needs, this is part of what makes you emotionally, mentally, and spiritually healthy.

How do you set your soul free? By acknowledging that you have a body. How do you set your body free? By letting your soul inhabit it. Your (divine) mind is in your body and your body is your mind:

The body is solidified mind and the mind is rarified body. ~ *Ancient Yogis*

Nothing can cure the soul but the senses, just as nothing can cure the senses but the soul. ~ *Oscar Wilde*

So, what do you do first? How do you free up your emotional and spiritual energy? You can unblock your emotional and spiritual energy by finding and following your energy currency. Sound familiar?

Your authentic nature is your body's nature. True well-being is first and foremost a state of mind. ~ Be your *real self* and *live in the now.* ~

In order to be well, you can't be chained to the past. For me, my past felt like the heavy weight regret and trauma. I could feel it pulling me down. My shadow-self said I had no value. I was literally weighed down by stress, grief, and fear.

The strength of your spirit greatly influences well-being. I make the choice to do my best to be strong and resilient. This is a form of mindfulness. I raise my vibration through positive thoughts and behavior. This influences my biology and allows me to produce a biological landscape of dynamic well-being. The beautiful message is that you have the freedom to choose how you feel in mind and body.

No matter the condition of your body, your mind is more powerful.

This is the mindset that has allowed me to gain ground and feel better:

On some level of reality, some dimension, I am well.

This is the reality I choose to live in. I am well, no matter what

Balancing/Raising Your Vibrations and Shining Your Light

I relax into the perfect spiritual pattern for my body. ~Orin

*If we truly want to create a life that is grounded in basic well-being,
we must decide to commit ourselves to learning what it takes
to thrive instead of merely survive. ~ Susan Velasquez*

We've mentioned the concept of vibration and now we will explore more of what it is and how you may be able to find *balance and/or raise your vibration.* We will also talk about the importance of radiating your love, i.e. the powerful light of your spirit.

I'm not a scientist so I'll give a simple explanation of vibration and what it means to our health. As I understand it, our bodies possess *electromagnetic energy.* This energy is known as electromagnetic radiation or EMR. We recognize environmental forms of EMR such as light, heat, and sound. Various forms of EMR have a wave-like character. EMR also can be made up of minute photon particles. Or, EMR may be formed as string-like structures. Whatever the character of EMR, it

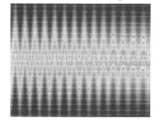 appears to cause atoms to vibrate. The vibration phenomenon occurs all over the environment around us and in every part of the human body. I'm indebted to Patricia Spadaro for the following description:

Our cells, organs and tissues vibrate. Billions upon billions of frequencies interact with each other and resonate within us. Just as importantly, those vibrations constantly interact with what's happening in our environment.

In short, in a world where vibration reigns supreme, the sounds and vibrations that fill the world outside of us can influence and change the vibrations inside of us, affecting our health and well being for better or for worse. The converse would also be true ... (Patricia R. Spadaro, The Body's Symphony of Sound and Vibration, Part 1) http://www.practicalspirituality.info/bodys-symphony-of-sound-and-vibration.html

You can raise your vibration by connecting to your spiritual energy, through the thoughts that you think (*or don't think – just focus on your breath when negative thoughts arise – trust me, it gets easier over time*) and the foods you eat, such as raw foods, live foods, and superfoods. Also try mind-body fitness such as yoga, Tai Chi, and QiGong, quality essential oils, music, and surrounding yourself with positive energy and people.

Remember to focus on what is positive in your life. This powerful practice will literally change your biochemistry, and influence your well-being tremendously, by influencing gene expression. Practice peace, compassion, forgiveness, gratitude, and try connecting with spiritual energy in some way, perhaps through prayer or meditation.

When you are in vibrational harmony,
your body produces whatever it needs to remain in perfect balance.
~ Abraham

Crystals, which have a high vibration, and may help to raise your well-being. I also use Himalayan Salt Crystal Lamps for energy when it rains. They produce negative ions to offset positive ions and it works!

Light is another example of electromagnetic energy. Our environment is full of light and so are we. Our bodies and minds radiate light. Just as the vibrational sounds of our bodies are silent to our ears, the light radiated by our bodies is invisible to our eyes, but nonetheless, it exists.

You, my friend, are made up light. Your body is a river of light. You are captured light, a projection of ancient light.

We do not see the light. We are the aperture through which the light breaks.
~ Gabriel Marcel

I dwell in all that is light and leave the shadows to the shadows.
~ unknown

There is a lantern in your soul which makes your solitude luminous.
~ John O'Donohue

Faith is the strength by which a shattered world shall emerge into the light.
~ Helen Keller

I wish I could show you,
When you are lonely or in darkness,
The astonishing light of your own being.
~ Hafiz

If light is in your heart you will find your way home.
~ Rumi

What feeds your light? You do. This is why taking care of your body is vital. You are a vehicle for light. Your body is a bio-energetic system. Use positive energy to focus on being well and feeling good:

I will use all of my positive energy today to focus on being & feeling well.

It's not about feeling better – it's about getting better at feeling. ~Michael Brown

Meridians/Energy Lines and Well-Being

Each one of us, as a human being, is essentially an *energetic matrix*. Within the matrix there is a natural intersection between divine mind and body. When we become aware of the intersection, we can change the dynamics of the interplay between these two dimensions.

I am going to share with you some of the techniques that have helped me to build energy and vitality working with my energy body. One example is QiGong, which works with a map of our energetic matrix.* This mapping includes what are known as meridians, which are like rivers of energy, like the many "rivers" that run throughout your body.

Meridians are lines of energy that connect our body, mind, and spirit. Qi Gong, which precedes yoga, means *energy cultivation*, and works with your *dantiens (energy centers)* to build energy and raise your vibration. Meridians are energy channels fed by your *energy centers*, i.e., your *three dantiens: lower, middle, and upper*. The *Lower Dantien* is the power center, i.e. your lifeforce energy, represented by a white ball of light. It is located below your navel. The *Middle Dantien* is golden light, your emotional body, located at your heart center. The *Upper Dantien* is your spirit. It's violet and fed by grace, light, and universal energy. It's located at your third eye, or sixth chakra (more on chakras coming up).

Your meridian lines are energy channels. One way you can raise both your vibration and your energy levels is to work with your meridians and energy centers. Try QiGong to do acupuncture on yourself, working with your meridian lines. You can also do Reiki this way. Even if you have little energy, QiGong can be a great tool to raise your vibration. You can even do QiGong sitting in a chair. Even subtle changes in energy bring relief.

Another example of meridians might be chill-bumps/activated energy points. There are some of the 10,000 energy points (*Thai massage uses this principle of working on your energy points*) on your body being activated by *emotion, etc.* Feeling our emotions is crucial to well-being. However, emotions are to be felt and then released, not stored in your body.

> *Practitioners know that each of us will experience one of the meridians as particularly relevant - holding our constitutional weaknesses and potential for brilliance. We often have a sense of which is our meridian (and corresponding archetype) of change and destiny.* The Atlas of Mind, Body & Spirit
>
> ~Paul Hougham

*This mapping of energy is also used in Chinese acupuncture. Acupuncture is great for pain relief, building vitality, etc. Acupuncture is routinely offered in CAM and preventative care now.

Stones, Metals, Oils For Energy

I have found that quality essential oils, semi-precious stones, and precious metals can open up or clear meridian lines and also raise my energy, vibration, and contribute to my overall feeling of well-being.

I love amethyst, moonstone, crystals, and turquoise, along with citrus oils like wild orange, lemon and tangerine, as well as cocoa, ylang ylang, sandalwood & peppermint essential oils. Try opening up a bottle of quality peppermint essential oil for a boost of energy! I also love white gold, diamonds (*conflict-free*) and sterling silver to uplift both my mood and energy levels. Stones and metals can connect loops of energy in your body. These levels of reality can expand your experience of well-being. Be open to new ideas and to expanding your conscious energy!

Chakras and Your Well-Being

Chakras are another part of our energetic matrix, as well as another topic to explore for holistic and unified well-being. Generally speaking, the chakra system is based on the practice of tantric yoga and Hindu tradition. Note: the various components of our energetic matrix complement one another and act in synergy and coherence.

The seven main chakras correspond with the endocrine system, and are centers and sources of energy found along the spine of the body. They are *part of the same network where your body, mind and spirit interact as one unified system* (recall: just like your mind, brain, genome, and microbiome). They're part of your *light and energetic body. Your light body is your subtle body, your energetic blueprint for health and holistic well-being.*

Let's focus on two chakras: the first and the last. The *first chakra* correlates with your *adrenals*. One of its shadows is insecurity. Its strengths include feeling secure and grounded. The *seventh chakra* correlates with your *central nervous system*. Its shadows include grief and isolation. Its strengths include self-awareness and interdependence.

> *The HPA axis may serve to connect your first and seventh chakras, making a connected loop of energy and creating well-being. It may create a circle of connection via electromagnetic energy and power on the physical level via enzymes, mitochondria, minerals, etc. and via the cultivation of mindfulness and awareness with your spiritual Self.*

We have so much more power than we realize ...

Try creating a circle of connected/continuous energy by *cultivating your awareness*. *Be mindful*, eat *real food*, spend time in *nature and* reconnect to the *circle of life*, try earthing *(for magnetic energy and negative ions)*, practice yoga, meditation, Tai Chi, QiGong, peace, anything that connects you.

Connecting to my subtle body helped me heal tremendously. In fact, it was one of the first ways I began to heal. I was able to recognize how I could work with my spiritual energy to affect my physical energy in subtle and even significant ways. I cannot tell you what your path is, but I have learned that when we connect to energy that is greater than just ourselves, we have the best chance to step into true well-being.

Interconnection and Universal Mind

~This may be how you heal: through synergy and coherence ~

Connect back to yourself, your soul, your body, and the circle of life and the circle of energy on all levels of being and existence.

Heal Your Body Heal Your Spirit

Transpersonal Well-Being

What do I mean by *universal mind* and *transpersonal well-being*? We're all connected, including animals, stones, rocks, stars, planets, and all that exists in the universe.

In psychology, there's a field known as *transpersonal psychology*. When we're able to see and *step beyond our own egoic fields*, we can feel and understand this very deep connection we all share.

Transpersonal means to *go beyond your ego, to go beyond what is personal to you*. I also believe that we're all part of a *universal mind*. Whether that mind is God or a field of unified energy, I don't know for sure.

But when you plug into life on this level – *the level where all of matter is connected in a unified energy field* - energy and consciousness can shift in a positive way. This is what I wish for you: to not only connect deeply to your true Self, but to connect to creative, timeless, universal energy.

When I came up with the title for this book, *The Memory of Health*, I was thinking literally about my memory of being well, earlier in life. This memory is a part of my story and history, and that is worth remembering.

Through research, I also learned how *memory* on the deepest level means to be *mindful*, and the deep lucidity that comes with living in the ever present moment. More than anything, *recall what makes you whole...*

Similarly, we all have a shared history: **the story of the universe**. This is how we are all connected.

The story of the universe holds the memory of all of our origins, and therefore includes all of us, and all of time, energy, and life.

It is not just our story, it is the story of every living being and non-living entity. We are all united through the story of time and space.

Nature is our storyboard.

The goal is to honor the path we have all walked upon, and respect our common bonds of a unified origin:

"*Time does not change us, it just unfolds us.*"~*Max Frisch*

Nature knows and goes her own way...

Want to know see what healing energy looks like? Look no further than Nature...or your pets.

~ *Every time my cat got out of balance, she used to disappear into my closet, sometimes for a week or more at a time. She would come out to eat usually, unless she was really sick, but beyond that she would stay in there resting and healing. She had no timetable but her own.* ~

Nature goes her own way and all that to us seems an exception is really according to order. ~ *Johann Wolfgang von Goethe*

Again, I now see that everything I thought was *supposed* to happen in my life - the things I wanted to happen or thought must happen in order for me to be happy - *were ego-based.* They only existed in my mind because of my ego. Transcending the ego and moving into a place of *transpersonal well-being,* saved my life, and my peace of mind ...

Moving into a more transpersonal way of living and being has been a factor in harnessing my own personal well-being. *Recollect these thoughts:*

> *I know there is nothing I could want more or hope for more than what is currently happening in my life at this present moment. This is my reality. I know I am not alone. I feel intimately connected to all living Beings and all of Life. This is my Memory of Health and mindful living.*

Even more than moving beyond ego, is the realization that we are all in this together. If one of us is suffering, we all are. In fact, we can move even *beyond transpersonal* into *transbeing*. *If one sentient being is suffering, we all ultimately suffer. Whatever is felt reverberates throughout the whole web of life.*

> *Come forth into the light of things. Let Nature be your teacher.*
> *~William Wordsworth*

Where does despair fit in? Why is our pain for the world so important? Because these responses manifest our interconnectedness. Our feelings of social and planetary distress serve as a doorway to systemic social consciousness. To use another metaphor, they are like a "shadow limb." Just as an amputee continues to feel twinges in the severed limb, so in a sense do we experience, in anguish for homeless people or hunted whales, pain that belongs to a separated part of our body - a larger body than we thought we had, unbounded by our skin.

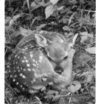

*Through the systemic currents of knowing that interweave our world, each of us can be the catalyst or "tipping point" by which new forms of behavior can spread. There are as many different ways of being responsive as there are different gifts we possess. For some of us it can be through study or conversation, for others theater or public office, for still others civil disobedience and imprisonment. But the diversities of our gifts interweave richly when we **recognize the larger web** within which we act. We begin in this web and, at the same time, journey toward it. We are making it conscious."~ Joanna Macy, from the article Working Through Environmental Despair, http://tinyurl.com/myfdfms*

Become aware of the ways of Nature and seek to connect to them wholly ...

We can increasingly **understand the universe** by observing what is around us: the wonder, beauty, and mystery of radiant Nature …

The Rapture and Wisdom of Nature

Nature has been my solace since I was a young girl. My parents used to take us camping and backpacking. I learned to love and appreciate the vastness and stillness and the inscrutable beauty and wisdom of nature and its quiet brooks and breathtaking vistas.

What I could not put into words, I let nature absorb and dissolve. I allowed my fears and anxieties to melt into green vistas and cumulus clouds and my rapture to be the ecstasy of rain and lightning storms. Nature was and has always been my place of worship. It is where I most connected to not only myself but to God and the whole of the universe.

Nature has so much to teach us, and in some ways, we are listening.

For example, we already look to nature to improve efficiency through the field of biomimicry. *Biomimicry* is an approach to innovation by scientists, inventors, and researchers, etc. who seek to solve human issues by mimicking Nature. Some examples of biomimicry would be camouflage, shark-skin swimsuits, Velcro based on plant burrs, paint that mimics lotus petals, etc.

"Study nature, love nature, stay close to nature. It will never fail you."

~ Frank Lloyd Wright

The more our world functions like the natural world, the more likely we are to endure on this home that is ours, but not ours alone.

~ Janine Benyus (1997), scientist and writer who first popularized the term biomimicry

Of course, we also rely on herbs for effective natural medicine, and mainstream medicine relies on nature as well (40% of prescription drugs are based on herbs in some capacity). Even Western medical practitioners use herbs and other natural remedies in addition to prescription drugs: My mom was advised by her traditional physician to take red yeast rice containing monacolin K daily to help lower her LDL and overall cholesterol counts. In addition, her statin prescription was re-written to a lower dose. After following this regimen for three months, her LDL and overall cholesterol levels were reduced.

Whatever your current relationship with Nature, you can choose to be open to the *experience of* what Eckhart Tolle calls a *felt sense of oneness with all living beings. There is no more incredible feeling than this one: To know you belong. It is truly freedom.*

Our task must be to free ourselves from this prison
by widening our circles of compassion to embrace all living creatures
and the whole of nature in its beauty.
~Einstein

YOGA – Body, Mind, Spirit, Universe

A thought planted in the mind and nourished by the breath,
takes root in every cell of the body. ~ Binnie Dansby

Yoga & Lifeforce Energy

Yoga is about breath: breathing in spirit and life force. You are literally strengthening vagal tone and *every time you breathe, you breathe in life.* ...

This is what you are made up of: the breath of lifeforce or the eternal, creative nature of the universe... .

~ What you are seeking is right in front of you - your own breath ~

I am not a master of yoga, but I do know this about yoga and life:

Yoga is all about union of mind, body and soul, and, to me, most importantly: breath. It is literally breathing in spirit & life force ... Every time you breathe, you breathe in life, you breathe in *energy/spirit.* Yoga is also a *restorative* form of exercise. It heals you on *all* levels: physically, mentally, emotionally, spiritually, socially, universally...

Try it, you'll see. Don't worry about yoga being an elite or exclusive club. It is an ancient form of mind-body medicine, and it is there for you to experience. Come practice with me online or in person. You can start with meditation, breathwork, or yin or restorative yoga.

For those of us with neurally-mediated conditions, yoga is literally a godsend. *It can greatly assist the health and well-being of your nervous system. Ujjayi breathing (create a slight constriction in the back of your throat while you breathe)* activates your vagus nerve. This can strengthen vagal tone.

Do I say literally too much? Try living literally ... and you'll be saying it too! I use a lot of clip art also, but it sure is fun, and it makes me feel good, like yoga! ☺

So much of your life is what your brain is used to doing. Sounds weird, eh? But it is nonetheless true. That's why it's so hard when you're growing up because everything is "new." But, that's also why it's so thrilling and naturally blissful. The human brain loves consistency *and* novelty. In addition to building neuroplasticity, these are two ways your brain, and therefore your body, can thrive.

Neuroplasticity may be implicated in how or why the brain, i.e., the *nervous system,* changes over time due to environmental, behavioral, and/or experiential changes, etc. - and why symptoms of fatigue and/or pain may be *diminished or heightened* over time as a result.

*[Yoga may affect] an **improvement in nervous system function**, allowing messages to be carried more efficiently to and from the brain. *www.hotyogaforlife.com*

It takes about six months for remodeling in the brain to change behavior and make it second nature, ~Bruce S. Rabin, MD, PhD, medical director of the University of Pittsburgh Medical Center Healthy Lifestyle Program

My Blog Entry – April 2012 MindBodyGreen.com Article

Brain Remodeling & Brain Plasticity
Superflex vs. Rock Brain on MindBodyGreen
By Edie Summers

I was taking care of my brother's girlfriend's son, and he had this homework assignment that was all about whether you could go with the flow – Superflex – or whether you were stuck in the muck, i.e. Rock Brain. Of course, this was a homework assignment for fourth graders on skill-building, but you get the point.

According to Stephanie Madrigal, one of the creators of Superflex and The Unthinkables, "Superflex is a superhero that hangs out in our brain and helps us to think about thinking about others, being flexible, and making good choices."

It has been used to help kids with high-functioning/broad-spectrum autism, ADHD, or other social learning challenges.

All of this reminded me of brain plasticity, which may be related to being a Superflex. Brain plasticity means your brain has, among other things, the capacity to change overtime.

*Note: I do not condone "hot" yoga over 90/95 degrees, and I feel it is generally too hot for people with health challenges.

Brain plasticity or neuroplasticity is implicated in perhaps how or why the brain – read nervous system – changes over time due to environmental, behavioral, and/or experiential changes, etc. One of the implications of having a physically "flexible, plastic mind," is that neurally-mediated conditions such as chronic fatigue syndrome (CFS) or fibromyalgia could be positively impacted, diminished, or even fade away altogether over time.

Likewise, being a Superflex in the way you approach life – being open to change and going with the flow – serves you much better than being a Rock Brain, stuck in your ways. Silly? Perhaps. But being flexible in how you approach the areas of your life where you feel "stuck" can afford you multiple opportunities to move out of stagnation into greatness. It's being open to choice and change that matters.

I have what I call [positive] recovery from what has been labeled CFS. Chronic fatigue syndrome is now better understood as possibly being related, at least in part, to a dysregulation of the hypothalamus, also known as hypocortisolism.

For whatever reason, in some people – severe, on-going stress has been implicated – the hypothalamus (part of the nervous system) seems to downregulate, and stay there, causing symptoms such as unrelenting fatigue. I have managed my symptoms, which are either gone, mostly gone, by lifestyle choices such as high-quality nutrition, regular exercise, stress management, and consistent sleep habits.

My latest way to treat and manage any lingering symptoms? The superpower of yoga. I used to think people who did yoga were part of some super cool, exclusive club I had never been invited to. But, much like life, yoga isn't a club. It's just there, waiting for you, until you can no longer wait for yourself to show up...for yourself and for your life.

I have always been curious about yoga, and have practiced certain stretching techniques for years after my workouts. But it wasn't until I tried a heated vinyasa yoga class that my whole world opened up and my body began to heal on [a deeper] level. It really helps my organic authentic energy levels as well. Yoga simultaneously cleanses and restores your whole body and being.

I always thought I couldn't do yoga because of neck and knee issues due to sports injuries. But heat makes it possible to move more easily, and to sweat. Sweating out toxins, emotions, and thoughts is such an amazing feeling. You can literally sweat, move, and breathe your way through any situation.

But, also, I have felt yoga starting to heal and change my brain as well as tone, strengthen, and lengthen my body. My brain and nervous system feel more "flexible," along with my body. Let your spirit and the universe take care of the details...and leave Rock Brain in the backyard where he belongs.

Can yoga remodel my brain and heal my nervous system, as well as any lingering symptoms I sometimes still experience? Can I leave Rock Brain behind and become a superflex Yoga Brain?

It's hard to describe what yoga does to your "head" unless you experience it first hand. I've already experienced a clearer sense of myself and the world at large. Perhaps sustainable symptom-free health is to follow. Time and practice will tell. So far, so good. Stay tuned.

Has yoga helped me? Absolutely, yes. I am literally more flexible in my ability to adapt to stress. ***Here's the thing:*** yoga is a way of being and it is a practice. Do you have to practice yoga? No, you can practice meditation, or anything on a regular basis that puts your body into the relaxation response. This is the research that has shown to be effective (Bhasin, et. al., 2013). Aim for 20 minutes daily or on a regular basis of any of these practices: yoga, prayer, meditation, Tai Chi, QiGong, or even biofeedback, etc. Brain plasticity is very real, and I am proof of it. You can literally build and strengthen neural pathways that change your well-being and even your health, including genetic expression.

Riding the Wave of the Mind-Body-Spirit Connection: I AM…

First of all, what does I AM mean? Perhaps it's God consciousness. It could also have a more down-to-earth meaning: *I am aware.*

When you become *aware*, you can change your *energy*. And when you change your energy, you move into a state of increased awareness.

This is a natural, restorative, coherent, synergistic process that can lead to a new level of well-being. *It is a bi-directional effect: energy = awareness*

You can connect or re-connect to the circle of energy, the circle of life. You become *aware of* the ways and connect back to the natural order of things and the *ways of nature*…the natural ways, rhythms, and patterns of nature…

~ I AM…riding the natural wave of the mind, body, spirit connection ~

This may be how you heal: through *synergy and coherence* … because the *whole is greater than the sum of its parts.* The three parts of you - mind, body, and spirit - operate synergistically together. Indeed, you are one complete, coherent mind, body, and spirit, *and* you are already whole.

We are beginning to come full circle. This is the beauty of holistic well-being as well as integrative thought and medicine. All is connected ...

As a brief reminder: the mind-body connection, brought into popular consciousness by Candace Pert's book Molecules of Emotion *(1999), is the understanding and experience that your mind is found everywhere in your body. An example of this would be neurotransmitters, or the small molecules that send signals from one nerve cell (neuron) to another. One such transmitter, serotonin - associated with feeling happy, playing a role in the onset of migraines, helping regulate heartbeat, etc. - is produced predominantly in your digestive tract. On top of that, your gut is called your second brain. It looks similar to your brain, not to mention the fact that chemical messengers like serotonin are found there.*

Riding the Wave of Health/Well-Being

According to mind-body theory, your mind and body are the same entity. There is no delineation between where mind ends and body begins. They are, instead, both part of the same **system.** And **systems** are how Nature seems to work and operate the most efficiently.

Another way of looking at the concept of systems would be to look at the nature of **patterns.** Nature loves patterns. In fact, it's how she not only seems to survive, but to thrive and evolve.

In Nature, there are two main principles: *chi and li.* We've talked about *chi* as being your energy and lifeforce. You also know that *li organizes chi.* Li is consciousness. According to Joeseph Needham: *Li is [the] organizing principle...or the great pattern.* In fact, *li and chi* work together to create a healthy, sustainable pattern and system of living system that is Nature. In your body, this system is created by the merging of your mind, or *li,* and your body, which is *chi* or your manifested energy.

Nature operates in systems, patterns, and rhythms. Some examples would be *sound waves, heartbeats, tidal waves, fractal geometry, ecosystems*, etc. How does this play out in understanding and living the mind-body connection? First, let's look at how we create our own *chi and li:*

Chi is created by:	*Li* is created by:
Type of air you breathe & frequency	Your thoughts: *"positive/negative"*
Energy from food choices	People you hang out with
Energy from exercise patterns	Who you allow yourself to be

The food you eat, the air you draw in, the people you surround yourself with, and the thoughts you think, and who you allow yourself to be, all **create YOU.**

*In other words, the energy you take in or create, whether from food or through exercise, create your chi and create **YOU** at any given point in time.*

The thoughts you think, who you hang around, and who you allow yourself to naturally be, is the li that organizes you at any given point in time and creates a mind-body system - an ecosystem of a living being.

The goal is to allow your ecosystem to thrive by riding the wave of well-being. This way of being can affect your genomic expression too, as well as build neuroplasticity.

~ Ride the wave of well-being and synch up with the rhythm and patterns of nature ~

It's what you focus on that matters, much like a surfer who rides the waves. He must focus and stay present in order to catch and ride the waves. And when he does? Oh what an effortless and thrilling ride.

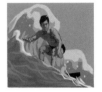

The Wave Theory and Memory

Here is one way to understand the mind-body connection and how it can help you to get into a balanced state of being.

Nature loves rhythm and balance. It's how she maintains herself, and also grows, literally. According to Irving Dardik, M.D., all of Nature is waves within waves, and the way Nature operates is part of a wave function called the **_SuperWave Principle_** (Dardik, 1983; Dardik & Waitley, 2015; Lewin, 2005).

The SuperWave Principle states that Nature operates within rhythms and what Dardik called **_wave energy._** Wave energy is how Dardik referred to the organizing principle, very similar to *li* in Chinese philosophy. The wave itself may be pure energy, but *it's the motion of the wave that is the li,* the organizing principle. It may seem overly simple, but it *does* make sense that Nature would be organized in such a way to self-propagate and also maintain herself the most efficiently.

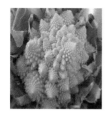 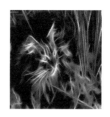 One only has to study the field of fractal geometry - which is also **considered to be a system of waves within waves** - to realize that Nature grows, thrives, and repeats herself based on patterns.

Let's look for fractals both in a forest and in your body: On one tree in the forest, the branches are duplicates of each other. In an entire forest, trees can be a duplicate of one particular type of tree. Not an exact duplicate, because this is Nature - *not perfection* - but in each tree of that forest there are patterns that are recognizable and traceable by scientific method. In the body we see fractals in our nerves and blood vessels. *Fractals seem to be everywhere. Why is this? Is this due to efficiency? What other clear patterns are relevant? Waves are clear patterns. Why is this?*

How does all of this relate to healing? In some healing traditions, such as *homeopathy*, there has been **pattern** noticed in which what may cause symptoms in the body in large doses seems to stimulate healing in the body in small doses. *Researchers postulate is that **homeopathy is based on the principle of similars**: like treats like. Yet, we are not sure exactly how it works.* Of course, much of mainstream medicine claims that homeopathy does not work. *I firmly challenge their reasoning. Homeopathy is recognized and regulated by the FDA as a branch of medicine.* Homeopathy has helped my health and well-being tremendously and consistently. **There is some principle at work here.** What is it?

*Nature operates in wave cycles – big wave, small wave, just like the tidal waves– and this represents balance in nature. Perhaps this is the **cycle that regulates** balance in the body. Is this how homeopathy works via **dispersion**? Perhaps the **small waves disperse small doses of medicine** throughout the body, stimulating it to heal. Or does homeopathy work on the principle of "like treats like" or how about via nanopharmacology, the same principle as nanotechnology?*

*Perhaps homeopathy works when **a substance of a certain vibration fits like a lock into a key** where needed in the body to regain balance. In homeopathy, substances that **produce symptoms in regular doses** in people are administered in **micro doses** over extended periods of time to **stimulate innate healing responses in the body**. This is known as "like treats like." Homeopathic substances are prepared by **shaking and/or stirring**. These **actions are necessary** to activate the micro-doses, and to create the final, **active potency**.*

Read this for research on homeopathy as nanotechnology: http://goo.gl/Mw6TjP

What is happening when the homeopathist stirs and shakes the substance? Is the liquid holding space, allowing for the transference of resonance between homeopathic substances and the cells of the body? *Does liquid hold memory?* Can liquid transfer information via wave energy or dispersion? Is this how life exists and/or propagates itself, through wave and/or fractal energy?

Memory and Morphic Resonance

The concept of *morphic resonance* may be another explanation, in addition to wave theory, of how the medical discipline of homeopathy, and other disciplines which rely on *small dose* applications, may function to encourage healing. Morphic resonance is based on *similarity of vibratory patterns.* In some regards it is like *homeopathy's principle of similars.*

Morphic resonance is the influence of like upon like through or across space and time. Similar things resonate with subsequent similar things on the basis of similarity of pattern and, particularly, of vibratory patterns of activity. A chemical of a given kind resonates with previous chemicals of that kind and is influenced by it. ~ Rupert Sheldrake (1987 and 1988).

Will we circle back to morphic resonance here. Regarding the discipline of homeopathy, *it fits into the realm of credible holistic science.* It has a track record having been founded in 1810 and actively practiced today, and, again, is *regulated by the FDA as a branch of medicine.* Practitioners and patients engage in **double-blind studies to test substances.** *It helps me, and it helped my mother heal when she was young with auto-immune issues.*

Regarding Dardik's theory of wave energy, time will tell if he's right. Dardik (2015) developed an exercise program to help people re-synch with their environments and natural rhythms to mitigate the effects of chronic stress and persistent, long-standing conditions.

*In a similar fashion, I believe this may be how some of our future integrative and holistic medicines as well as lifestyle medicines may work: by riding the waves of nature's healing pattern of self-propagation and regeneration, and tapping into and harnessing our natural biorhythms. **In time, the body finds balance in a seemingly choppy world, much like the surfer who, learns to fluidly ride the up and down cycles of the ocean's waves.** Recall, as we have discussed before, that small doses of stress encourage growth and healing. Stress can equal change and growth. It is the way we respond to stress that matters: rising to the challenge as well as allowing for rest and recovery keeps us in fluid and ever-present, dynamic balance.*

According to *Dardik (1983)*:

Smaller rhythms are imbedded within larger rhythms, and those within larger still. The short biochemical cycles of cells of the **human heart waves** *are embedded within the circadian rhythm of the whole body, and they are all embedded within the larger waves of weeks, months and years.*

Almost every cell in your body has a circadian clock in it that resets itself every 24 hours. Your body is synched up, or should be, ideally. The fact that the clock knows to reset itself indicates that these rhythms - these waves - have a *memory*. What is this memory? Is it *li*? Is it God? Is it love? Is it *I AM awareness*? Is it the Higgs boson particle, pure consciousness or organizing information?*

Waves repeat themselves as an inherent continuum of nested waves. ~ unknown

Consider this:

> *~ Fractal waves may have a memory*
> *and our bodies seem to mimic fractal designs. ~*

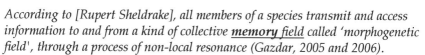

Does our body remember how to be well, based on ancient, primordial, energetic patterns?

Can we access these patterns, this field of energy and awareness at any time? Is it a connection to a collective field or higher source that makes or keeps us well? I believe intention on the physical plane is our Li.

According to [Rupert Sheldrake], all members of a species transmit and access information to and from a kind of collective **memory field** *called 'morphogenetic field', through a process of non-local resonance (Gazdar, 2005 and 2006).*

If all of this conjecture is true, then when we become ill, or out of synch, how do we enable these patterns to work correctly again?

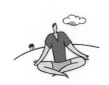

Gazdar (2005) points out that *prayer* may connect us, as humans, to our own collective memory field. I suspect *meditation is* another way, along with *mind-body fitness*, and perhaps anything that puts us into *flow*.

~ Become aware of and connect back to the ways of Nature ~

*Is the Higgs boson or Higgs field the organizing principle, or is it something beyond this we have yet to discover? The Higgs boson field and particle explained: http://goo.gl/kMgJBV
More detailed information: http://physics.info/standard/
http://www.ncbi.nlm.nih.gov/pmc/articles/PMC4247395/

A Memory of Health

From the way Dardik (1983) described the nature of waves, it appears they can and do repeat themselves, even without new stimuli. Waves* appear to have *memory*.

Where does this memory come from? Is it the driving force of the organizing principle itself? What does this kind of memory have to do with coherence or harmonic resonance (http://goo.gl/M1N37R)? And, most critically, what does it mean for you and for your health, where your health is understood as holistic well-being? (Matter as waves: http://goo.gl/BzNaRo)

Waves transmit energy and information. Is *wave energy* awareness, or *some type of duplicated memory?* Our memory of health may be *awareness* (read also: mindfulness) - the organizing principle - *coupled with energy.*

Together, *awareness and energy* may comprise *The Mind-Body Field*, and this field may not only be within you, but it extends outside of you, beyond your person. Why a *field?* Again, because everything works by connection and feedback loops.

Think of the ***mind-body connection* as a web:** touch one part of the web and the whole web reverberates and is affected by your touch.

The *mind-body field* within us seems to be a field of both *energy and awareness:* **It is the flow and nature of nature …**

Nature is a patterned flow: it's a patterned energy flow (li & chi, yin & yang)

*Organisms are resilient **patterns in a turbulent flow, that is, patterns in an energy flow**...* ~ *Molecular Biologist and Biophysicist, Carl Woese (2004).*

Note: Please read about Dr.Woese. He was an innovative thinker, explorer of the universe, and beloved professor whose former graduate student, Freeman Dyson, said:

This picture of living creatures, as patterns of organization rather than collections of molecules, applies not only to bees and bacteria, butterflies and rain forests, but also to sand dunes and snowflakes, hurricanes and thunderstorms. The nonliving universe is as diverse and dynamic as the living universe, and is also dominated by patterns of organization that are not yet understood. ~Freeman Dyson (2007).

*Matter is condensed energy & perhaps just a hierarchy of standing waves. Energy is either kinetic or potential (i.e., it organizes), and our universe may be a "feedback of information" http://goo.gl/hKzLpR.

Dr. Woese spoke of a *turbulent energy flow* operating in the scientific worlds of biology, physics, chemistry, etc. Let's look at *flow* as it operates in our bodies, minds, and spirits. When I teach yoga and mind-body fitness classes, *flow* is a natural part of my terminology: yoga flow, vinyasa flow...we have mentioned "flow" frequently in this book. *What exactly is the formal definition of flow?*

Mihaly Csikszentmihalyi - and his book *Flow: The Psychology of Optimal Experience* (1990) - is known as the architect of modern *flow psychology*. In fact, he's one of the main leaders of the *positive psychology movement*, along with Martin Seligman. *Flow* is where one can find a *conscious place* of ease and challenge, *right at and within the edge of one's growth curve.* It's a combination of one's *strengths, skillsets, passions, and intrinsic motivation* matched to the challenge at hand. When we successfully match our internal resources with the impending task or issue, things *flow* along.

Much like the concept of the organizing principle of *li*, we can *create* our own optimal state of well-being and happiness by organizing and *interpreting/experiencing* data and information we receive as *for our growth.*

We can organize and *create* our own flow, our own zone, our own optimal experience of life and well-being. Flow is about *deep enjoyment, even exhilaration,* as well as *stretching oneself* to one's limits or growth edge. It gives us a new way of looking at what we formerly perceived as stressful in our lives.

Flow is **immersion** into activities you love and which make use of your skills and strengths, despite challenges. In fact, challenges are part of creating flow. Challenges demand we use the best of ourselves, strengths, and skills. *We can become our best selves in the midst of challenge. How cool is that? This also may be a viable tool to heal the nervous system.*

Allow yourself time to enjoy activities that challenge you and/put you in the *flow and in the zone.* You have so many options: learning a new language, playing sports, mind-body fitness practices like yoga, sex, writing, dance, exercising your memory, math, meditation, solitude, music, composing, creative projects, connection with others, etc.

Flow is about *creating order* in your life and mind. From order springs integration, harmony, coherence, and a deep sense of feeling truly *alive.*

I believe the state of well-being is not only when we achieve *flow* in our lives, but also when we connect to a greater source than ourselves. This source is creative and coherent consciousness. It is omnipresent. It is whole.

Be really whole and all things will come to you. ~ Lao Tzu

Consciousness/Presence is exquisitely *aware*. Instead of running from it, sink into it. It's where *well-being lives*, and where your *peace* and *freedom* live. In fact, it is *wholly you….*you in wholeness, where your life flows

~ Awareness is you and it is your body's memory of health. ~

Awareness is *li* - the organizing principle. When you *allow yourself to follow the signals of your body* – the natural ways of Nature - your energy, your *chi* realigns and you find your way back into *active balance.*

Energy, and therefore healing, are based on the principles of

focus *and* expansion

Your job, as you walk on your chosen pathway toward increased well-being, is to *focus* on your goal. Attract that positive healing energy, then *expand* the energy you receive. *Let it light you and radiate out from you…*

Here's how you can expand healing energy: Picture it as *wave upon wave* of healing energy. Keep in mind, always, that in your body *everything may be waves within waves, and these waves may have a memory.* They know instinctively your ideal state of well-being. *Picture synchronous waves of health - healing energy - flowing throughout your body just like music flows (sound waves) throughout your body.*

focus expand focus
expand focus expand

Don't be surprised if you feel a little disorder in your wave, or in your progress, now and then. This is normal. This is life

Even though there seems to be order in the universe, *superwaves*, which is the way *Dardik* referred to them, *are both yin and yang, order and chaos.*

It turns out that an eerie type of chaos can lurk just behind a façade of order – and yet, deep inside the chaos lurks an even eerier type of order. ~Douglas Hostadter

The Tao of Health and Well-Being

The yin and yang principles act on one another,
affect one another and keep one another in place.
~ Chuang Tzu, ancient Taoist

Life is naturally about *ebb and flow, yin and yang.* Ebb and flow are opposites. Yin and yang are opposites. Life is about finding balance between opposites. Achieving balance between opposites is the key to living in a state of well-being ... body, mind, and spirit all together.

When you adopt, or even fall into, a pattern of sustainable, healthy living that works for you, then you will effortlessly find your authentic natural health and happiness. It's that simple and yet ... profound.

This is why yoga or any mind-body fitness routine, or anything that truly helps you engage in life, works. It is because engaging in life puts you into the frame of mind and framework of the natural *ebb and flow, the yin and yang* Nature of life. Within this framework, the brain can create new neural pathways and find *holistic, dynamic* balance again.

Well-being exists within patterns of energy flow, I believe. What pattern do you wish to be yours? What is your ideal pattern of living? What is an optimal pattern of well-being for you? On what frequency does your health and well-being vibrate? What is your vibration of well-being? Remember your intrinsic, and essential whole Nature....

When you are in vibrational harmony, your body produces whatever it needs to remain in perfect balance. ~Abraham

More on Memory and Morphic Resonance

How do monarch butterflies, from Canada and North America, know the exact town to fly home to in Mexico - all at the same time, no less? Why do geese and other birds fly together (hint: it may have to do with speed and efficiency). How does a lone bird find its flock again?

For that matter, how does DNA know to become a leg vs. a hand? Your DNA starts out as potential, as a blueprint of life. But the DNA that makes your legs is not distinguished from the DNA that makes your hands or hair. *Is this blueprint connected to our light body's blueprint?* What informs our DNA? A mind-body field? Consciousness?

What teaches us and shapes nature? Is there an electromagnetic field we tap into that informs our actions? Does this field shape our genetic raw material across generations? Does this field inform our development as well? Is Jung's collective unconscious an example of morphic resonance? What about archetypes? Is the sum truly greater than the whole of its parts as Nature suggests and provides examples for in the synergistic effects of food and herbs? What is consciousness? Is it more than a developed pre-frontal cortex?

These questions relate to a concept we mentioned earlier called morphic resonance, which is the theory of like influencing like. Such impact, or resonance, among similar things operates over time, within patterns and especially vibratory patterns of activity, and may imply the existence of held memory. Here is a quote from Robert Sheldrake to help us understand the possible universal presence of morphic resonance.

*Obviously, if there are habits in Nature, then there must be a **memory** in Nature. Our own habits depend on memory, largely unconscious memory. There is no need to assume the habits of Nature are any more conscious than our own. So what I suggest is an **inherent memory process in Nature**. The basis of it is [what] I call morphic resonance.*

***The morphic field is the organizing field of a system.** Each crystal has its own kind of morphic field; each species has its own kind of morphic field. Then, say, within the body, each organ has a morphic field, each tissue, each cell, each kind of organelle, each molecule. There are nested hierarchies of fields within fields. **The whole of Nature is built up of systems within systems**: solar systems within galaxies, the Earth within the solar system, ecosystems within the Earth, and so on. Each of these, I suggest, has a morphic field which organizes it in accordance with habit, in accordance with the habits of that kind of thing. ~ Rupert Sheldrake (1987)*

As we understand more about the tools available to us for healing and improved well-being, we realize *our part in the equation* is awareness itself: to receive and act, to focus and expand, to be mindful as much as possible.

The universe is a self-organizing system, always designing new patterns of possibility and perfection, and lifting all living things to their highest manifestation. Your job is to receive that power (through prayer, forgiveness and meditation) so that it can redeem your own life and then extend through you to redeem others. To... do so is the only thing that provides the joy we all long for.
~ Marianne Williamson

I believe we seek joy, and one great joy may be realizing our deeply intimate, inevitable connection with others, nature, and the universe. It's maybe even more of a connection than we can possibly imagine, no doubt. *Is "relationship" our connection to Source, a direct experience of God?*

He who lives in harmony with his own self ... lives in harmony with the universe; for both the universal order and the personal order are nothing but different expressions and manifestations of a common underlying principle. ~ unknown

Any way you look at it, what our body and mind seek and yearn for is an active, dynamic balance, where you can *Flow* and be with Life ...

Balance - How To Find and Keep It

*Energy seeks balance, harmony, wholeness, [and] peace. **Energy** does not like to be out of balance. ~ Joe Nunziata*

It is not your role to make others happy; it is your role to keep yourself in balance. When you pay attention to how you feel and practice self-empowering thoughts that align with who-you-really-are, you will offer an example of thriving that will be of tremendous value to those who have the benefit of observing you. ~ Abraham

This is ideally how your mind, body, and spirit operate: in harmonious balance with one another - self-awareness in *mind*, wholeness in *body*, and peace in spirit. With a little effort, we can ease into *Flow...*

Balance is effortless effort. When you draw from your center, that is your internal power, balance is natural and spontaneous. This is how the practice of Qi Gong works. With slow, gentle, precise movement, often with eyes closed, energy is freed to flow throughout the being to bring balance and coherence between and among mind, body, and spirit. With practice, finding your dynamic balance becomes effortless.

At the same time: extremes are easy. It's easy to be angry. It's easy to give up. It's being in the middle and holding your balance at first that's the challenge. It's being in the middle of a yoga pose (asana), or a tough assignment at work, or a problem with your kids, and holding your balance, waiting for results, adjusting to loss or grief or pain or fatigue - these are the real challenges that test your strength and resolve. *The challenge is to find the sweet spot between effort and surrender.*

Again, achieving dynamic balance in body, mind, and spirit is an effortless effort. At first, it takes practice. But, then you will reach cruising altitude, and it can get really fun to see results. Stay focused on the *positive*, observe what *is* going right and what *can* go right in your life. These behaviors can signify resiliency. They exhibit your harnessed *chi* and life-force. *Find your positive growth/healing edge and Flow*

In flow, what used to be challenging is now exhilarating. The following ten sub-sections are *ten tips for balanced living*. Beyond the habits of *self-care and positive mindset*, here are suggestions to *boost joy, love, and flow* in your life, all of which may help you to achieve and maintain balance.

✦ First Tip for Balanced Living
Understand That Energy Is Alive! It Flows In and Out of You

Energy and wellbeing are balanced, yes, but with a growth edge. Balanced energy and wellbeing are in a state of flow. **Your energy is evolving and dynamic.**

Just because something is balanced, doesn't mean it's static. Balance is not homeostasis. So, when you're in a state of wellbeing, you are *constantly growing and utilizing all of your skills and strengths.* You're also recalibrating responses to the feedback loops of information and communication in your body. Balanced energy is about the continual flow of both the *input and output* of energy. It's an ever-evolving, ever-adjusting, ever-expanding *healthy system.* Thus, to have good energy and health, there has to be an equal, dynamic exchange of energy *coming in and going out.*

Again, these ideas about energy balance and flow are based on the concepts of cybernetics (Wiener, 1965) and living systems theory (James Grier Miller, 1978 and 1995).

✦ Second Tip for Balanced Living
Love Yourself and Exchange Positive Energy with Others

Find the energy that animates your heart and gives you peace in living as yourself, who you are. You are that perfect you. You can spark an awareness - a consciousness - everywhere. ~ misty tripoli

Balanced energy is also about loving yourself deeply, unconditionally, and with a true sense of celebration. When you love yourself and feel energetically balanced, you will confidently invest some of your energy in an exchange of energy with others. All relationships - both personal and professional - include the concept of *energy exchange.*

~ Relationships are about the exchange of energy and love ~

I've had snags in energy exchange between others and myself. In my marriage, ultimately, we both used each other in some capacity, unconsciously, whether or not we admitted it. I've also had difficulty with energy exchange within myself - in my own feedback loops of communication. Both issues may have contributed to my chronic health condition. Recovery depended on my power to engender a loving, unconditional, respectful relationship with myself, which led to my ability to engage in healthy relationships with others. You come from a deep well of love. *Remember and reconnect with your essential nature.*

My advice? Get to know and love yourself. Appreciate and honor your own needs, wishes, dreams, and desires, and then act on them. Practice self-care, practice moving around in your own energy. Get grounded in your authentic self and voice. Be 1000% yourself.

↓ Third Tip For Balanced Living
Focus on Expansion of Energy, Avoid Contraction-Type Behaviors

When we're exhausted, there's a tendency and temptation to contract and literally shut down. While one should rest if truly burned out, shutting down is really a *lock-down of life-force*, or a drawing-in, much like a turtle or snail. Rest, of course, but when you awaken, be sure to at least *keep your mind expanded in hope, faith, and possibility*. Remember to seek and accept authentic connection and love from others as well.

There's also a difference between contracting and surrendering. *Surrendering* is allowing life and your body to flow and be as it is. *Contracting* is putting the lid on energy ... the last thing you want to do. Try applying the opposite energy to your situation. In other words, when you feel tired, expand your energy to create more ... try gentle movement practices such as yin/restorative yoga, Tai Chi or Qi Gong, which can be enjoyed by any age and persons in almost any condition.

↓ Fourth Tip For Balanced Living
Support vs. Stimulate & Build Energy Reserves

What our bodies need to thrive, more than anything, is the support of vital breath, love, chi, inspiration, and nutrition to harness the energy and vitality of the day. Take deep, long breaths to activate your vagus nerve to help you relax. Even if you don't have time for a formal yoga or meditation class any day, just take slow, deep breaths to reconnect to your core. Out of this space, notice any fearful/contracting thoughts that come up, and transform them into positive energy and excitement and anticipation for your day and life!

Build your energy reserves so you aren't running on empty, which is when you reach for the caffeine and sugar fix. Build energy reserves by supporting your body as much as possible and giving yourself what you need: rest, food, nutrition, touch, love, inspiration, exercise, downtime, playtime, faith, fun, etc. Stay in a healthy range of cortisol levels. Focus on building your chi through breath & awareness of where your bodymind is in time and space. Slow down to reboot...take breaks when you need them...and give yourself permission to do so. Of course, energy can be affected by physical circumstances, but try changing your thoughts to change your energy. Even a subtle shift from fear to knowing everything is not only going to be okay, but IS okay exactly as it is NOW is liberating.

My hope for you is that you realize you have more than enough energy to live your authentic life. My hope for you is that you realize you only have energy to be your Self.

⚜ **Fifth Tip For Balanced Living**
Music - Remember Where You Came From

"The earth has music for those who listen." ~William Shakespeare

Music gives a soul to the universe, wings to the mind, flight to the imagination and life to everything. ~ Plato ☼ ´℘ *•.,, ✿☆

If you truly want to see and understand how all meaning emerges out of the flesh, blood, and bone of embodied experience, philosopher Mark Johnson suggests that you start with music. ~Carla Scaletti - The Meaning of the Body: Aesthetics and Human Understanding by Mark Johnson

Why music? How can music help you achieve balance in your life?

I like to think *that music feeds our bodies and souls.*   Perhaps our bodies are instruments that the universe plays through. I believe your nerves are similar to strings on a violin or harp. Your nervous system heals and responds to different tones, different *vibrational energies*. At the very least, sound waves are incredibly healing and music is inspirational.

*In the span of a single second, our lives can change immeasurably because energy moves at a pace more rapid than anything we can consciously fathom. Though we may not at first be sensitive to the **vibrational shifts** taking place, our choices are ultimately at the heart of these transformations. ~Daily OM ~Much gratitude to The Daily Om for this quote: http://www.dailyom.com/*

Music is sheer therapy for your body, mind, and soul. Music also *engages both sides of your brain* - just like writing (on paper as well, to access your subconscious mind) and metaphorical thinking - whether you play it, dance to it, sing it, or *listen.*

Music is one of the few activities that activates, stimulates, and uses the entire brain. ~ unknown

We sing when we're joyful *and* when we're sad, too. We create music and our bodies and souls respond to it because that may be what we're made of. Instrumental music and song are some of the deepest expressions of ourselves and our souls. Perhaps we are song itself:

Now…we can let the song sing through us. ~ Joanna Macy

My firm belief is that…the majority of us do not live out the song of our soul … the vibrations of our voice echo the vibrations of our body, which, when tuned, echo the vibrations of nature and the Cosmos. ~ Stewart Pearce

,~Thanks to musician Natalie Whitfield for graphics ~

Yes, the Cosmos. Indeed, we may be born of ancient sound, song, or word. Was it the silent collision of dimensions and then awareness breathing life into existence with OM, I AM? The sound of the earth itself may be OM or AUM (different aspects of infinite consciousness or God). Recall, the Chinese character for medicine means music. Regardless, when we are well, we are in harmony with all that is…

What is first-created or primordial sound?   Perhaps it is composed of the most elemental sounds of nature and of the universe. It is ocean waves, whale song, a chorus of frogs, a symphony of crickets, and birds, *the ancestors of long-ago dinosaurs, singing joyously in the trees.* It may be the motion of the planets, and *Tibetan and crystal bowls used in healing.*

In English classes at school, we pondered the *word of God* and *the music of the spheres.* For me, at that time, these were mysterious concepts, a wondering of *what this word of God and music of the spheres?* What were these elemental, lofty, yet strangely familiar concepts? Today, planets - along with their moons and rings - can made to sound like whale song, dolphins, even Tibetan bowls. *Some say these sounds of space are re-created to represent sounds we can recognize vs. real sound of planets, etc. Either way, real or created, they seem alien and yet hauntingly familiar all at the same time.*

Space is a vacuum, but, again, electromagnetic waves and charged particles have been interpreted by NASA as similar to whale song and other seemingly familiar sounds. Was NASA correct to interpret space sounds this way? Whether you answer *yes* or *no*, it is fascinating to consider. We are a hopeful, imaginative race. To hear sounds from earth's high atmosphere, click on this link: Music\Chorus of Radio Waves within Earth's Atmosphere.mp3 You can hear other sounds from outerspace by going to www.nasa.gov/connect/sounds/index.html

What is your relationship to sound and song? Perhaps primordial sound may even affect you on deep, physical levels – *perhaps even allowing your body to relax and reboot and recall its inherent wholeness -* reminding you of where you came from, and, most importantly, *your inherent worth,* just by being here. *You are a valuable, inherent, one-of-a-kind part of the whole picture. What song is in you? What song is unsung in you still to be expressed? How can you live at the level of joy and rapture expressed in song?*
http://www.chopra.com/ccl/what-is-oneness

Primordial sound is everywhere if you listen and absorb. It is used in meditation as well to reconnect you with your energy currency. Listen deeply to the earth: the wind, the rain, the singing of crickets, the waves on the ocean, the hum of the earth. Use it to reconnect with your energy currency and to find balance again. If you use the mantra *Om*, contemplate it. Does Om mean I Am? Consciousness? Or, is it the sound of the earth? It is a unified sound, and its implications can be profound. There are different ways to describe the meaning of the word or sound of OM or AUM. One interpretation is that OM itself is the source of all existence, and that this sound of OM – or AUM - comes from vibration. Is it the vibration of sound that makes us whole again or resonates with us? Some would say that OM as AUM is infinite consciousness, *the unity of all levels of consciousness.*

Sounds have such power to heal us at the deepest level, I believe. The Chopra Center for Wellbeing, in Carlsbad California, specializes in primordial sound applications. Deepak Chopra, in his book *Quantum Healing* (1989), mentions it as being one way to heal fully. If you haven't read Chopra's classic book, take time to check it out.

Edgar Cayce suggested that sound would be the medicine of the future. Along those lines, one of my musician friends believes that *the harmony of sound through resonance* can contribute to the healing of the body, mind, spirit, and emotional states of being and *bring us back into balance.* He also says we each have a *signature note* that is powerfully helpful to us. *Signature notes* correspond with the *chakras.* My signature note is *C* and matches with the root chakra. I found my note by going to a bookstore and playing different Tibetan bowls, fake ones, until I found the tone that resonated with me. Probably the easiest way to you're your note is to play keys on a piano or any instrument. However, keep in mind there are more tones than what we hear, i.e., tones in between tones. Your note could be in the spaces between audible tones. Don't worry if you can't find your note; just rest assured you have one.

One of the coolest things I've found is musical acupuncture. The music feels amazing and healing to my body. You can google it to check it out. Sound is healing and music is mysterious and alchemical.

At any rate, how can music help you return to a balanced state of being? The following are suggestions to consider in regards to music:

Listen to music again: at home, in your car, at concerts, dance classes, drum circles … what music resonates with you? Just like food, find the music that feeds your body, heart, and soul. *Feel the joy and sheer rapture of music…*

Find your signature note: Go on a treasure hunt. Identify which note grounds you, resonates with you. Use it in your meditations. I bought a fake Tibetan bowl and love it and play it. Let your signature note remind you of *the joy and authenticity of being you.*

✦ Sixth Tip For Balanced Living
Joy - Remember Who You Are and Live Your Truth

> *What I know for sure is that you feel real **joy** in direct proportion to how connected you are to living your truth. ~ Oprah Winfrey*

I've touched a little in this book on what it means to have *authentic health.* But what you need to know - in order to enter into balanced living - is that following your *truth*, your *joy*, your *bliss* and your *body* has so much to do with getting into better balance. The path of healing leads you to yourself. It comes full circle. *What a journey and what a joy.*

✦ Seventh Tip For Balanced Living
Follow Your Bliss to Improved Well-Being and Never Give Up

Effortless bliss is a sensation of floating, of feeling transcendent of not only your body but of your immediate problems which seem to disintegrate, if not disappear entirely. You feel as if you are breathing cosmic oxygen not of this earth that is recharging you all the way down to the atoms in your cell tissue. ~ unknown

Bliss is the key to vibrant well-being! Do as Joseph Campbell said and follow your bliss. Focus on what makes you feel good. Eat what makes you feel good, but not just *temporarily good* like sugar, which may lead to a crash and steal your vitality, or *chi*. If you're sick you'll need to do more than follow your bliss. Take your supplements/medicine, eat extra well, get acupuncture, etc. But if, at the same time, you're living in a *blissful state*, the *difference between not feeling well* and *feeling truly well in your body and mind* could literally be days or months as opposed to years.

Bliss and positive thinking lead you to make decisions that change the nature of your life, including your well-being of mind, body and soul, which are the roadmaps of your life.

The body has its own innate healing response. In many cases it will heal itself if you allow it. No matter what healing system you follow, above all else, believe that you can heal and regain balance in life. That is your greatest role as a patient. Even more important, is to believe in yourself, even if you're the only person that currently does. Don't ever doubt for a second that what you're experiencing isn't real. Yet, you must be your own cheerleader because your happiness and life depend on it. *Fight for your life and your well-being. You're worth it. Don't ever give up.*

Also, surround yourself with people who make you feel good. People who have negative energy may suck the life force out of you. Even then, you have control over how you respond. Stay in bliss, and keep your intention on regaining balance. This is the key. You have the power to change your life. And remember that you have a beautiful soul that is yours forever and no matter what. You are already whole.

Give yourself abundant pleasure and you will have abundant pleasure to give to others. You are what you experience. You experience what you express. You express what you have to express. You have what you grant yourself.
~ Neale Donald Walsch

*Now, and for the rest of my life, I will enjoy myself as much as possible and try to create a good situation around me by giving to others the best part of my divine qualities and **blissful energy**. May this joyful present lead to unsurpassed joyful realizations in the future. ~ The Bliss of Inner Fire*

Energy *is the word we use for **grace**. You are never outside the field of **working** **grace**. It's impossible, just as it's impossible to exist outside the field of energy.*
~ Carolyn Myss

✢ Eighth Tip For Balanced Living
Consider the Relationship of Spirituality and Health

Sometimes the only available transportation is a leap of faith. ~Margaret Sheperd

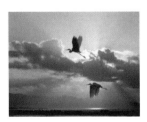
Faith is the strength by which a shattered world shall emerge into the light.
~ Helen Keller

There is only one temple in the world and that is the human body. Nothing is more sacred than that human form. ~ Novalis

You are the creative force from which all things flow. ~ Wallace Wattles

You don't ask God for too much, you ask for too little. ~ A Course In Miracles

Remember Einstein's equation, $E = MC^2$? Energy equals matter times the speed of light, squared. That's a lot of light, isn't it? Do you ever wonder what that light exactly is? Doesn't this concept of so much light fill you with wonder and mystery?

What about the energy and matter part of the equation? Einstein deduced that matter could be turned into energy and energy into matter. Remember our discussion of wave energy? Is wave energy God consciousness? Perhaps it is, at least, the organizing principle, whatever that may be, or even awareness or consciousness itself.

Here's the way I think about spirituality: love is energy. Light is energy too, and perhaps awareness and consciousness. You, as light, are an inherent part of this universe. Stay connected to that energy.

Body is the vehicle we are in, the alchemical mystery that we drive. With this instrument we can choose to make love or destroy cities. Our physical Be-ing demonstrates who we appear to be, who we want to be, and betrays quite often who we really are inside. Soul is the spark of God, the flame within that is Eternal and cannot be destroyed by man. This is the real You, the You that you hide from the world and wonder in sorrow whether anyone truly sees You.
~ William Patrick Corgan

"The sun never says to the earth, "You owe me." Look what happens with a love like that, it lights up the whole sky."~Hafiz

Remember the play *Waiting for Godot*? It's about two men who wait - and keep waiting - for this man, Godot, to show up. He never does. I think it was meant to be a commentary on the existence of God, or in this case, perhaps, the concept of *no existence.*

I can't tell you whether or not to believe in God. That's your path. I've had mystical experiences - even forgotten in detail - *that leave me only with faith.* I may not remember all of the occurrences, but I *remember* the *feeling of grace* or divine or unconditional love touching my soul and life. And out of these encounters, I have developed faith. Faith is trust in the unknown, the inscrutable mystery of existence …

In my experience, you don't wait for God or your Life …

You just open your heart and let the light in … Turn toward the Sun

Relationship is synonymous with *life*. Our relationships help us heal. I've chosen to engage on a transpersonal level. I let the fluid nature of life itself carry my burdens. My job is to show up, which I do every day, through yoga, QiGong, and other meditative practices.

Whatever your beliefs of the infinite are, remember you are whole and know you are loved. Here are some mantras/meditations to increase your positive energy, improve your well-being, and reset your balance.

Breathe in light and wholeness, exhale fear and suffering
Breathe in Light & Love, exhale darkness and suffering
I AM: I am whole and filled with light
Let each exhale dissolve suffering and darkness.
Your body is a hologram, a light body, and it's already whole. The root of *hologram* and *holistic* is the Greek word *holos* meaning *whole, healing, and holy*. When you breathe in the sacred spirit of life, light, love and energy, you know already you are whole on one plane of being…

Breathe in courage, exhale fear.
Breathe in the Spirit of Light & Love, exhale lack, fear, separation
I AM: I have courage, I am love and I am loved – I AM Free
Exhale fear and dissolve all thoughts/experience of separation

✛ Ninth Tip For Balanced Living
Accept the Invitation to Inhabit the Love Field:
Love Yourself, Love Others

Life is only ever offering its invitation to fall heart-first into an immense field of not-knowing … and no matter what the details, love has somehow configured itself as your unique life, and has offered itself as a gift … only forever waiting for you to receive it, as it is. ~ Matt Licata

Let's start at the beginning. You've been given the gift of love. Being *alive* means you exist out of love. Let the gift of *love* live inside of you. *Let all else fall away. There is a **well of infinite love** inside of you.*

To inhabit the mind-body field of love, you must first *love yourself.*

*Loving yourself is not only accepting but embracing and celebrating all of you and your uniqueness … ! No one can do this for you. It's an individual choice and the potential for unlimited **love, peace and acceptance** are possibilities that exist within you. A vibrant body is only possible when [you've accepted who you are.]*
~ misty tripoli

Loving yourself means *seeing yourself clearly. Your essence is whole and perfect and magical. Your essence is already whole. Use your spirit/light body to inform your physical body. Use this wholeness to create wholeness.* What is the deepest expression of your loving self? *See, know, be, and feel* who you truly are.

Love is energy, and may be the most powerful energy in the universe. When you inhabit and radiate the energy of love, your heart rate slows, you exude a peaceful energy, and you vibrate at a very high frequency.

If you only remember one thing from this book, please remember this: *Stay in the vibration of **love***. When you carry out your life from a place of love, instead of fear, the whole world changes.

Loving yourself is loving everything.
Love integrates. Kindness lubricates.
Lovingkindness is love in kindness.
Listening to the body is wisdom.
When barriers go, energy flows.
The more energy you spend, the more you have.
The two constituents of life are energy and love.
There is no social status, only energy-flows or blockages.
Transcending the self is becoming immanent in the universe.
~Jeremy R. Lent

Jeremy Lent uses the word *immanent* in his final line. *When referring to God it means present in the universe.* It's used by philosophers and theologians, most commonly. Immanent means inherent. *Perhaps we can go beyond ourselves, reach out to others, and acknowledge the space we inhabit, and realize we are not only an inherent part of the universe, but unfolding into and as the universe as infinite, creative energy. We can ground ourselves in love, and then extend out beyond ourselves to join in the mind-body field of love and service.*

Find the courage to love and believe in yourself, and to reach beyond yourself to develop healthy, loving, wholly sustainable, relationships:

What if your preoccupation was with love? What would change? My experience is ... everything changes. Your relationships change. Your physical body changes. Your business changes. Your bank account changes. You change. ~Melani Ward, Finding Your Mojo

Finally, with your loved ones, show your love, always and in all ways:

Tender words we spoke to one another are sealed in the secret vaults of heaven. One day like rain, they will fall to earth and grow green all over the world. ~Rumi

⤋ **Tenth Tip For Balanced Living**
Cultivate the Energy of Peace, Presence, Love and Creativity
to Gain Union of Mind, Body, and Spirit

When stress is removed from the system of energy that you are, your true nature expresses itself as presence, peace, love, and creativity. ~ Joan Borysenko

The energy that Dr. Borysenko describes is the energy you continuously cultivate. We've discussed the components of that energy extensively in this book. *Allow yourself to relax into well-being:*

➢ Relax into *peace* within your *spirit*.
➢ Let your *mind* dwell on the *present*.
➢ Express *love* for yourself and for others.
➢ *Create* stimulating experiences to keep your *mind, body, and spirit* united in the flow of life.

When I worked at The Beaverton Healing Center, our motto was that *well-being is mind, body, and spirit*. All three work together *in harmony* to create well-being. If one of the trio is out of balance, it affects the rest of the system. Let's look a little deeper into each one and how they work synergistically to produce the effect of well-being in your body.

Mind - Mindfulness is about being aware of what's going on *right now* in your body and in your life. Mindfulness is about being present, curious, and accepting of yourself exactly where you are right now. When you witness your pain, your fears, your fatigue, your eating habits, or anything else - the non-judgmental presence you create can diminish the burdens you carry. *That which you shine a light on is illuminated and becomes clear.* The more you choose to be aware and mindful, the more *your body* responds with the presence of well-being. Accepting yourself just as you are dissolves all fear and suffering...

Body - Your body is filled with consciousness, breath, joy, and love. It's perfectly suited for you. It's your vehicle to experience this amazing world. Make friends with your body, and make peace with it. Listen to it deeply, as well. Your body talks to you and it wants you to hear it. Give it what it needs. It's on your side. It uses the language of feelings and symptoms, which are your keys to authentic health. Listen to your body and *honor* what it says. Taking care of your body's simple needs will result in a profound feeling, in both *body and mind*, of well-being. Also, when you take care of your body, you honor yourself at the highest level: you honor yourself as eternal (spiritual) energy

Spirit - Tending to your spirit can help keep you well. You tend to your spirit by being aware of what your spirit craves. *Your spirit craves union.* Union can be thought of as the *awareness and feeling* of a unified mind-body-spirit connection. Mindfulness could be thought of as being conscious that your mind and body are one living field of energy that responds to your light-bulb of awareness.

In return, your spirit gives you the gifts of courage, faith, hope, and the experience of unconditional love. As you seek improved well-being, you must be infinitely, indefinitely brave, never lose faith or hope in possible outcomes, nor in loving yourself. Your spirit is your connection to infinite source. It's your connection to your spirit that allows eternal energy to flow through you to create vital well-being.

The Memory of Health

What is my memory of health? My memory of health is the memory of the *joy of being alive and that I'm not alone* ... that I'm connected to all living beings. *I can live in a lucid state of being at all times, if I choose.* I can allow this *awareness, mindfulness, and energy* to flow effortlessly both in my body and in the universe all at once. *This is my eternal peace ...*

I will not allow anyone or any experience to take this peace from me again: not abuse, not trauma, not chronic illness ... not anyone else's agenda or judgment about me or my value or inherent worth.

I can match up my energy with the subtle, ecstatic energy of the earth and vibrate at this frequency. This not only grounds me, it instantly fills me with *joy.* No matter what, I AM at peace with All that is...

This is what the Buddha knows and taught ...

They say water holds memory. I say our cells and our souls hold the memory of our authentic blueprint of *love and well-being.* All we have to do is *trust* ourselves to *be it and feel it* authentically.

Trust your body. Every cell is on your side, which means you have hundreds of billions of allies. ~Deepak Chopra

You know I love quotes. But Emerson didn't:

> *I hate quotations. Tell me what you know. ~ Ralph Waldo Emerson*

I know this: I was out of balance, so I lost my balance. Now I'm in a new dance with my body. My body is different now. I'm stronger and more awake than I've ever been in my ever-changing body. I have a new story I'm telling. I've let the old storyline go. Where did it go? I let it burn away, like once it burned me away, a long time ago.

What about you? Tell your story, acknowledge it, and then let it burn away. Or, step outside of your story, if you can, and release it. And if you can't let it go? Then make sure it's a story you wish for the world to know about you.

I'm a dancer, and one of the first things they teach you is how to maintain your balance, how to hold your center so you don't fall. And if you do fall, you should try to make it look like it was intentional, or part of the choreography. Then get back up. Always get up. You have a dance to finish. You have a life to live. And who knows what chapters you have left to write. Who knows what the rest of your story or journey will be. This book contains my story thus far. What's yours?

One does not discover new lands without consenting to lose sight of the shore for a very long time. ~ Andre Gide

As a yoga instructor, I help people to get stronger and more flexible in both mind and body, by helping them move through both flow *and* challenge in vinyasa yoga. What you finally realize is that when you engage right at the edge of your comfort zone, yet still stay in flow and accept yourself as you are, that's when the deepest *transformation* occurs.

Here's one yoga asana for your *life*:

Inhale into Life.
Plant your feet firmly on the ground.
Press your palms together at your heart center.
Open your heart and send the crown of your head toward the sky.
Gaze forward, or close your eyes and look inward.
See in your mind's eye a positive, fulfilled, blissful present.
Remember to keep breathing. Inhale, exhale, inhale, exhale ...

Whatever your circumstances, choose a positive, heart-centered stance.

Remember to be well in mind. You can do this ...

This Is My Home

This is my home…
Despite all my difficult paths, I realize that
I am deep in beauty here.
The woods outside my window hold serenity of soul,
and an auric certainty that maybe the only very wise know.
The moon hangs back in the dark blue sky
Like a small light on a wristwatch, and patiently glows.
I notice it out of the corner of my eye, and wonder about it all.

This is my time…
It's complex, it's organic, and it
really is all mine.
I see the rim of foreign beauty as I
drive by the Ponderosa,
and the image of eternity move*
as the wind blows through the pines,
and I behold the silent darkness in
the corner of my mind.

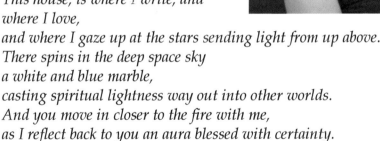

This is my life…
This house, is where I write, and
where I love,
and where I gaze up at the stars sending light from up above.
There spins in the deep space sky
a white and blue marble,
casting spiritual lightness way out into other worlds.
And you move in closer to the fire with me,
as I reflect back to you an aura blessed with certainty.

*Plato

From Frozen Light A Collection of Poems
by Edie Summers

Resources

The Holistic Coach

Wellness for Life

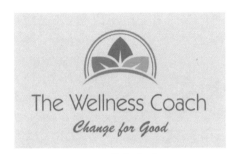

The Wellness Coach
Change for Good

Self and Group Coaching, Free Yoga Videos, SEID Support:
http://www.ConnektWell.com

http://www.PortlandWellnessCoach.com

https://www.facebook.com/ChronicFatigueSupport?ref=hl

Allergies
Asthma & Allergy Foundation of America
http://www.aafa.org/display.cfm?id=9&sub=30 Facts & Figures

Animals
http://www.asknature.org/
http://www.biomimicry.net/
http://www.TheHumaneSociety.org
http://www.wspa-international.org/ World animal protection

Anti-Aging
Aging and Smoking
http://www.freeclear.com/quit-for-life/ American Cancer Society Smoking Cessation Program: Tobacco use is the **#1 cause of preventable death and disease in the U.S.**
Aging and Telomeres
http://www.wellnessresources.com/health/articles/how_nutrition_makes_a nti-aging_possible_secrets_of_your_telomeres/
http://www.naturalnews.com/034513_telomeres_longevity_nutrition.html#ix zz3c8WFbl5d

Auto-Immunity
http://www.cortjohnson.org/blog/2013/12/10/study-suggests-specific-gut-bacteria-may-able-provoke-autoimmune-disorder/

Autism
http://medicalxpress.com/news/2014-02-causal-link-vitamin-d-serotonin.html

Any Treatment – *The Best Treatments for Your Condition*
https://www.anytreatment.com/

Body Care/Cosmetics/Sunscreen
http://www.ewg.org/skindeep/ cosmetics database; safety information
http://www.fda.gov/cosmetics/productandingredientsafety/selectedcosmeticingredi
ents/ucm128042.htm
http://www.wholefoodsmarket.com/about-our-products/premium-body-care-
standards
http://www.wholefoodsmarket.com/sites/default/files/media/Global/Company%20
Info/PDFs/Whole_Body_Supplier_Guidelines.pdf
http://www.wholefoodsmarket.com/sites/default/files/media/Global/Departments/
Department%20Article/WFM-Premium-Unacceptable-List-Dec5-2013_0.pdf
Update on Lead in Lipsticks:
http://www.motherjones.com/environment/2013/05/study-lead-metals-lipstick-top-
20
Sunscreens
Are they beneficial for health? An overview of endocrine disrupting properties of
UV-filters. **International J of Andrology, 35: 424–436** http://goo.gl/AH9XR4

Bumblebees
http://www.livescience.com/51502-bumblebee-range-shrinking.html?

Cell Food
http://www.oxywave.com/landing/cellfood/dyer-cellfood-book.pdf
http://manifestliving.com/bio/

Children
http://futureofchildren.org/futureofchildren/index.xml
www.generationrescue.org Jenny McCarthy's Autism Organization
http://earthweareone.com/mit-researchers-new-warning-at-todays-rate-half-
of-all-u-s-children-will-be-autistic-by-2025/
http://www.imdb.com/title/tt0104756/ Lorenzo's Oil, an American film (PG-13
| 129 min | Drama | 15 January 1993 A boy develops a nerve disease so rare that
nobody is working on a cure, so his father tackles the problem himself. Stars: Nick
Nolte, Susan Sarandon, Peter Ustinov.

Chronic Fatigue, ME/CFS/SEID, MCS, Fibromyalgia, Environmental Illness, etc.
http://www.prohealth.com Dedicated to patients with CFS, ME, and FM.
Founder, Rich Carlson, was diagnosed with CFS in 1981; a top US fundraiser for
research; represented the CDC in their $4 million CFS awareness campaign. In
1997, he launched the *Campaign for a Fair Name*, which succeeded in changing CFS
to ME/CFS. Posts news, information, and resources, etc.

http://www.womenshealth.gov/faq/chronic-fatigue-syndrome.cfm
http://www.healandintegrate.com/?pageClass=CPFR3
http://www.fallonpharmacy.com/Chronic-Fatigue-Syndrome-and-
Fibromyalgia-c16.html
http://arthritisconsult.com/what-causes-fibromyalgia/

Multiple chemical sensitivity: a 1999 consensus. Arch Environ Health 1999;
54:147-49 [Note: This was a seminal report.] http://goo.gl/jwJDrT

Cover Design by Richard Crookes
http://richardcrookes.co.uk/

Detoxification
http://www.carahealth.com/health-conditions-a-to-z/digestive
system/detox/365-phase-1-and-2-liver-detoxification-pathways60.html

Epstein-Barr Virus and other theories (EBV, vagus nerve)
http://goop.com/the-medical-medium-and-whats-potentially-at-the-root-of-
medical-mysteries/
http://www.nytimes.com/health/guides/disease/chronic-fatigue-
syndrome/print.html

http://thelowhistaminechef.com/harvard-neuroscientist-dr-michael-van-elzakker-
chronic-fatigue-vagus-nerve-link/

Feelings
http://www.binnieadansby.com/ecstatic-life/Feelings
http://drdansiegel.com/about/mindsight/ Name and
tame emotions

Freedom to Move
http://www.freedom2move.org/ Customized exercise
videos for any level!
M. Csikszentmihalyi

Happiness & Joy
http://www.pursuit-of-happiness.org/history-of-happiness/mihaly-
csikszentmihalyi/ Mihaly Csikszentmihalyi discovered genuine satisfaction is a state
of consciousness called Flow
Mihaly Csikszentmihalyi talks about Flow (TED Talks)
A Life Worth Living: Contributions to Positive Psychology (Series in Positive
Psychology). Oxford University Press [edited by M. Csikszentmihalyi & I. S.
Csikszentmihalyi

Health Care Providers
Physicians Committee for Responsible Medicine
http://www.pcrm.org/

High Fructose Corn Syrup (implicated in NAFL)*
http://goo.gl/Gr7EL9 / *http://aje.oxfordjournals.org/content/178/1/38*

Highly Sensitive People
http://www.hsperson.com/index.html
http://www.ei-resource.org/

*Non-alcoholic fatty liver. About 1/3 of the population has a fatty liver. Fructose, HFCS, and inability to
metabolize polyunsaturated fats properly are implicated in the cause; can lead to cirrhosis of the liver.

Information and Social Networking

http://www.ei-resource.org/ Environmental Illness Resource
http://www.anhinternational.org/ Alliance for Natural Health

Community

http://www.ConnektWell.com/ Free Yoga Videos, Group Wellness Coaching
https://www.smashon.com/ Your local health & fitness community
https://www.anytreatment.com/
A website to help patients find what works for others who have symptoms similar to yours: MS, ME/CFS/SEID, RA, etc.

https://www.facebook.com/ChronicFatigueSupport?ref=hl

Li & Chi - Enlightenment

http://liology.com/tag/enlightenment/

Magnesium

http://www.collective-evolution.com/2015/02/13/why-a-magnesium-deficiency-is-invisible-how-its-affecting-your-health-right-now/

Medical Errors Fact Sheet

http://go.nationalpartnership.org/site/DocServer/Fact_Sheet_Medical_Errors_Not_Just_a_Headline.pdf?docID=5482

Methylation

http://www.drmyhill.co.uk/wiki/CFS_-_The_Methylation_Cycle

Microbiome

http://www.theatlantic.com/health/archive/2015/01/joint-pain-from-the-gut/383772/

Mind/Body Health

http://www.lifepositive.com/Spirit/Faith_Healing/Healing_the_World122005.asp
http://newhope360.com/supplements/profile-todays-core-supplement-user?page=1

How Cells Communicate

http://learn.genetics.utah.edu/content/cells/fight_flight/

MS

http://multiplesclerosisradio.com/
http://kineticchainspecialist.com/142/neurological-laws-part-1-the-law-of-facilitation-and-the-magic-of-myelin/

Prescription Drugs
http://pubs.acs.org/doi/full/10.1021/cn3000923
http://www.drugfreeworld.org/drugfacts/drugs/prescription-drugs.html
http://www.forbes.com/2009/08/17/most-medicated-states-lifestyle-health-prescription-drugs.html

Psychoneuroimmunology
http://www.dana.org/Publications/Brainwork/Details.aspx?id=43669#sthash.r5ZFABT9.dpuf

PTSD
National Center for PTSD. Treatment of PTSD.
http://www.ptsd.va.gov/public/pages/treatment-ptsd.asp

RA, Auto-Immunity, and the Microbiome
http://www.cortjohnson.org/blog/2013/12/10/study-suggests-specific-gut-bacteria-may-able-provoke-autoimmune-disorder/

Relaxation Response
http://www.psychologytoday.com/basics/oxytocin

Sugar Controversy
http://cip.cornell.edu/DPubS/Repository/1.0/Disseminate?view=body&id=pdf_1&handle=dns.gfs/1200428197
http://www.youtube.com/watch?v=dBnniua6-oM Sugar: The Bitter Truth. Research on sugar, including its effect on health & food policy issues surrounding it.
Marty Taylor, Clker.com

Toxic Substances
Agency for Toxic Substances
http://www.atsdr.cdc.gov/
http://www.atsdr.cdc.gov/toxfaqs/index.asp#
Agent Orange
www.veteranstoday.com
http://www.publichealth.va.gov/PUBLICHEALTH/exposures/agentorange/conditions/index.asp
http://www.ewg.org/Chemicals_Law_Overhaul_Proposed_In_House
http://www.diabetes.org/living-with-diabetes/complications/related-conditions/agent-orange.html
http://www.cancer.org/cancer/cancercauses/othercarcinogens/intheworkplace/agent-orange-and-cancer
American Convention on Human Rights
http://www.oas.org/dil/treaties_B-32_American_Convention_on_Human_Rights.htm

Toxic Substances (continued)

BPA Chemical
http://www.ewg.org/Europe-Steps-Up-to-Protect-Babies-from-BPA
http://www.ei-resource.org/myblog/bisphenol-a-bpa-sources-and-health-effects.html

Endocrine Disruption
http://endocrinedisruption.org/
http://www.issues.org/16.3/br_stegeman.htm

Environmental Chemicals (from Food, Air, Water) and Body Burden
http://www.cdc.gov/exposurereport/
http://www.ewg.org/
http://www.chemicalbodyburden.org/rr_cheminus.htm
http://www.trwnews.net/Documents/Dioxin/BBreport_final.pdf
http://www.chemicalbodyburden.org/whatisbb.htm
http://www.envirohealthaction.org/bearingtheburden
www.foodincmovie.com
www.gaslandthemovie.com

R.E.A.C.H. European Union Community Regulation on Chemicals:
http://ec.europa.eu/environment/chemicals/reach/reach_intro.htm

Triclosan /Dioxins
http://www.who.int/mediacentre/factsheets/fs225/en/
http://www.epa.gov/oppsrrd1/REDs/factsheets/triclosan_fs.htm
http://www.bostonparentspaper.com/article/antibacterial-soap-vs-regular-soap.html
http://www2.conchovalleyhomepage.com/webmd/beauty/bodycare/story/FAQ-Triclosan-and-Your-Health/6-SZFj0Vpkmn8fCtpSKBBw.cspx

Veterans: to file a claim, click here:
http://www.benefits.va.gov/compensation/claims-postservice-questionnaire-claimherbicide.asp

VOCs and Plants
http://www.ncbi.nlm.nih.gov/pmc/articles/PMC3230460/
http://phys.org/news/2013-07-air-hidden-indoor.html
http://phys.org/news176571050.html#nRlv
http://www.euro.who.int/__data/assets/pdf_file/0009/128169/e94535.pdf
http://www.greenguard.org/en/index.aspx Indoor air quality: products, reviews, contractors, certifications.

World Trade Center Cough
http://www.nejm.org/doi/full/10.1056/NEJMoa021300#t=articleResults
http://www.nejm.org/doi/full/10.1056/NEJMoa021300#t=references

The Acid Sea
http://ngm.nationalgeographic.com/2011/04/ocean-acidification/kolbert-text

Detoxifying Estrogens
http://www.afmcp-sa.com/ansr/MET451%20Endocrine%20ANSR.pdf

Read the Labels. Setting Standard for Supplements:

USP
http://www.usp.org/

REFERENCES

Acute exposure guideline levels for selected airborne chemicals. (April 27, 2012). Committee on Acute Exposure Guideline Levels; Committee on Toxicology; Board on Environmental Studies and Toxicology; Division on Earth and Life Studies; National Research Council (NRC). Washington (DC): National Academies Press. Retrieved from:
http://www.ncbi.nlm.nih.gov/books/NBK201461/

Agency for Toxic Substances and Disease Registry (ATSDR) Division of Toxicology and Human Health Sciences (June 24, 2014) [data file containing profiles of toxic substances]. *ToxFAQs Toxic Substances Portal and Index*. Retrieved from: http://www.atsdr.cdc.gov/toxfaqs/index.asp

Alford, J. (September 3, 2014). Current extinction rate 10 times worse than previously thought. Retrieved from: http://www.iflscience.com/plants-and-animals/current-extinction-rate-10-times-worse-previously-thought

Allergy facts and figures. (2016). Asthma and Allergy Foundation of America Asthma & Allergy Foundation of America. Retrieved from: http://www.aafa.org/display.cfm?id=9&sub=30

American Cancer Society. (February 18, 2014). DES exposure: questions and answers. Retrieved from: http://www.cancer.org/cancer/cancercauses/othercarcinogens/medicaltreatments/des-exposure

Americans gulping down 80 percent of world's opiates. (2012). Retrieved from: http://www.drugrehab.us/news/americans-gulping-down-80-percent-of-worlds-opiates/

Applied Nutritional Science Reports. (2001). Nutritional influences on estrogen metabolism. Met451. 1/01 Retrieved from: http://www.afmcp-sa.com/ansr/MET451%20Endocrine%20ANSR.pdf

Aron, E N. (1996). *The highly sensitive person*. New York, NY: Broadway Books.

Argueta, L. (January 31, 2014). Monarchs face new threats, losses along migration route. *National Wildlife Federation: Wildlife promise, blogs from around the federation*. Retrieved from: http://blog.nwf.org/2014/01/monarchs-face-new-threats-losses-along-migration-route/

Arora, B.P. (2008). Anti-aging medicine. *Indian Journal of Plastic Surgery*. 41(Suppl): S130–S133. Retrieved from: http://www.ncbi.nlm.nih.gov/pmc/articles/PMC2825135/

Aten, D., Kuo, A., & Questell, A. (Sept. 6, 2007). Facts about telomeres and telomerase. Retrieved from: http://www4.utsouthwestern.edu/cellbio/shay-wright/intro/facts/sw_facts.html

Azar, B. (2001). A new take on psychoneuroimmunology. [Research connecting illness, stress, mood and thought in a new way]. *American Psychological Association 32*(11), 34. Retrieved from: http://www.apa.org/monitor/dec01/anewtake.aspx

Azar, B. (2011). The psychology of cells. *American Psychological Association 42*(5), 32. Retrieved from: http://www.apa.org/monitor/2011/05/cells.aspx

Bell, G., Bloomfield, J., Byrne, R., Goldenfein, M., Harrington, P., McAvoy, J. (producers) & Heriot, D. (director). (2006). *The Secret* [Motion Picture]. Melbourne, Australia: Prime Time Productions.

Bandura, A. (1997). *Self-efficacy: The exercise of control*. New York, NY: Freeman.

Barrett, M. J. (January 3, 2014). *A woman's truth: A life truly worth living*. USA. Published by The Food of Life.

Bast, J. (March 1, 2000). Instant expert guide: Facts about chlorine and dioxins. Retrieved from: https://www.heartland.org/policy-documents/instant-expert-guide-facts-about-chlorine-and-dioxins

Best, S. (2016). Are you a highly sensitive person? Retrieved from: http://www.sarahbesthealth.com/are-you-a-highly-sensitive-person/

Bhasin, M.K., Dusek, J. A., Chang, B., Joseph, M. G., Denniger, J. W., Fricchione, G.L., Benson, H., & Libermann, T.A. (May 1, 2013). Relaxation response induces temporal transcriptome changes in energy metabolism, insulin secretion and inflammatory pathways. *PLoS ONE* 8(5): e62817. doi:10.1371/journal.pone.0062817. Retrieved from: http://journals.plos.org/plosone/article?id=10.1371/journal.pone.0062817

Bjarnson, I., Zanelli, G., Prouse, P., Williams, P., Gumpel, M.J., & Levi, A.J. (1986). Effect of non-steroidal anti-inflammatory drugs on the human small intestine. *Drugs*. 32 Suppl 1:35-41. Retrieved from: http://www.ncbi.nlm.nih.gov/pubmed/3780475

Begley, S. (January 19, 2007). The brain: How the brain rewires itself. *Time.com*. Retrieved from: http://www.time.com/time/magazine/article/0,9171,1580438,00.html

Beinecke, F. (March 20, 2014). [email campaign - paraphrased] Let monarchs fly! *NRDC, Serbian Animals Voice*. Retrieved from: http://serbiananimalsvoice.com/2014/03/20/usa-let-monarchs-fly/*

Benson, H. (1975). *The relaxation response*. HarperTorch. Benson, H. & Klipper, M.Z. Retrieved from: http://www.amazon.com/Relaxation-Response-Herbert Benson/dp/0380006766/ref=sr_1_1?s=books&ie=UTF8&qid=1434475475&sr=1-1&keywords=relaxation+response

Benson, H., & Proctor, W. (March 2, 2004). *The breakout principle: How to activate the natural trigger that maximizes creativity, athletic performance, productivity and personal well-being*. New York, NY: Scribner.

Benson, J. (2015). MIT doctor reveals link between glyphosate, GMOs and the autism epidemic. Retrieved from: http://www.naturalnews.com/049065_glyphosate_autism_GMOs.html

Benyus, J. M. (1997). [Paperback 2002]. *Biomimicry: Innovation inspired by nature*. Biomimicry Guild. New York, NY, Harper Perennial.

Benyus, J. (2007). Janine Benyus shares nature's designs. TED. http://www.ted.com/talks/janine_benyus_shares_nature_s_designs.html

Benyus, J. (2009). *Biomimicry in action*. TED. Retrieved from: http://www.ted.com/talks/janine_benyus_biomimicry_in_action.html

Bergamini, C., Moruzzi, N., Sblendido, A., Lenaz, G., & Fato, R. (2012). A water soluble CoQ10 formulation improves intracellular distribution and promotes mitochondrial respiration in cultured cells. Retrieved from: http://journals.plos.org/plosone/article?id=10.1371/journal.pone.0033712 DOI: 10.1371/journal.pone.0033712

Bernstein, J. A., Bernstein, I. L., Bucchini, L., Goldman, L. R., Hamilton, R. G., Lehrer, S.,... Sampson, H. A. (2003). Clinical and laboratory investigation of allergy to genetically modified foods. *Environmental Health Perspectives, 111*(8), 1114-1121.

Biennial report of the director; summary of research activities by disease category chronic diseases and organ systems (2009). Retrieved from: http://www.report.nih.gov/biennialreport0809/ViewSection.aspx?sid=11&cid=2

Bisphenol-a (bpa) and phthalates. (2014, July 14, updated). Retrieved from: http://health.westchestergov.com/bisphenol-a-and-phthalates

Bland, J. (January 23, 2014). Candace Pert and Tony Pawson: Honoring 2 revolutionary scientists. Retrieved from: http://www.huffingtonpost.com/jeffrey-bland/healthy-living-news_b_4159049.html

Bonanno, G. A., Papa, A., Lalande, K., Westphal, M., & Coifman, K. (2004). The importance of being flexible: The ability to both enhance and suppress emotional expression predicts long-term adjustment. *Psychological Science, 15*, 482-487. Retrieved from: http://dept.kent.edu/psychology/coifmanlab/2004_BonannoPapaLalandeWestphalCoifman.pdf

Bounous, G., & Molson, J. (1999). Competition for glutathione precursors between the immune system and the skeletal muscle: pathogenesis of chronic fatigue syndrome. *Medical Hypotheses 53*(4), 347-349. DOI: http://dx.doi.org/10.1054/mehy.1998.0780

Broderick, P.C., & Blewitt, P. (2010). *The life span: Human development for helping professionals*. Upper Saddle River, NJ: Pearson Education, Inc.

Brown, J. (March 11, 2013). How exercise affects immunity. *EXOS.com EXOS Knowledge - Wellness*. Retrieved from: http://www.coreperformance.com/knowledge/wellness/how-exercise-affects-immunity.html

*additional reference

Bruckner, T. A., Catalano, R., & Ahern, J. (May 25, 2010). Male fetal loss in the U.S. following the terrorist attacks of September 11, 2001. *BMC Public Health 10*(1), 273 PMCID: PMC2889867 doi: 10.1186/1471-2458-10-273.

Brudnak, M. (2000, June). Cancer-preventing properties of essential oil monoterpenes d-limonene and perillyl alcohol. Retrieved from: http://www.positivehealth.com/article/cancer/cancer-preventing-properties-of-essential-oil-monoterpenes-d-limonene-and-perillyl-alcohol

Bunge, M. B., Bunge, R. P., & Ris, H. (May 1, 1961). Ultrastructural study of remyelination in an experimental lesion in the adult cat spinal cord. *J Biophys Biochem Cytol. 10*(1), 67–94. doi: 10.1083/jcb.10.1.67 © 1961 Rockefeller University Press.

Calafat, A. M., Wong, L. Y., Ye. X., Reidy, J. A., & Needham, L. L. (2008). Concentrations of the sunscreen agent benzophenone-3 in residents of the United States: National Health and Nutrition Examination Survey 2003–2004. *Environ Health Perspect. 116*(7):893-7. doi: 10.1289/ehp.11269.

Carson, R. L. (1992). *Silent spring* (pg.16). New York, NY: Houghton Mifflin Company.

Campaign for Safe Cosmetics (CSC). (2007). Lead in lipstick. Retrieved from: http://www.safecosmetics.org/get-the-facts/regulations/us-laws/lead-in-lipstick/

Campbell, B. (2005). Key 4: Finding your limits. Retrieved from: http://www.cfidsselfhelp.org/library/key-4-find-your-limits

Costandi, M. (2014). White matter might matter much more than we thought. Retrieved from: http://www.theguardian.com/science/neurophilosophy/2014/apr/24/white-matter-synaptic-plasticity

CDC, Centers for Disease Control and Prevention. (August 5, 2014). Arthritis basics, definition. Retrieved from: http://www.cdc.gov/arthritis/basics.htm

CDC, Centers for Disease Control (April 7, 2015). Chronic fatigue syndrome (CFS). Retrieved from: http://www.cdc.gov/cfs/

CDC, The Center for Disease Control (October 23, 2015). Cigarette smoking among U.S. adults aged 18 years and older. Retrieved from: http://www.cdc.gov/tobacco/campaign/tips/resources/data/cigarette-smoking-in-united-states.html

CDC, Centers for Disease Control and Prevention. (2013, July 23). National biomonitoring program factsheet: Triclosan. Retieved from: http://www.cdc.gov/biomonitoring/Triclosan_FactSheet.html

Chan, D. M. (2007). Remyelination in multiple sclerosis. *Int Rev Neurobiol. 79*, 589-620. Retrieved from: http://www.ncbi.nlm.nih.gov/pubmed/17531860

Chang, J. (September 6, 2010). Endometriosis pains million of women yet remains misunderstood and misdiagnosed. San Jose Mercury. Retrieved from: http://www.mercurynews.com/ci_16006045

Chaudhuri, A., & Behan, P. O. (March 20, 2004). Fatigue in Neurological Disorders. *The Lancet,* 363(9413), 978-988, doi:10.1016/S0140-6736(04)15794-2 Elsevier Ltd Choudhari, N., Roper, S. D. (August 9, 2010).

Choudhari, N., & Roper, S. D. (August 9, 2010). The cell biology of taste. *JCB* vol. 190 no.3 285-296. doi: 10.1083/jcb.201003144. Retrieved from: http://jcb.rupress.org/content/190/3/285.full

Chhabra, S. K., Reed, C. D., Anderson, L. M., & Shiao, Y-H. (1999). Comparison of the polymorphic regions of the cytochrome P450 *CYP2E1* gene of humans and patas and cynomolgus monkeys. *Carcinogenesis, 20*(6), 1031-1034. ISSN: 0143-3334. e-ISSN: 1460-2180. DOI: http://dx.doi.org/10.1093/carcin/20.6.1031

Chiesa, A. (2013). The difficulty of defining mindfulness: Current thought and critical issues. *Mindfulness Journal, 4*(3), 255-268. Springer. DOI 10.1007/s12671-012-0123-4

Chopra, D. (1989, April 1). *Quantum Healing: Exploring the Frontiers of Mind/Body Medicine.* New York, NY, Bantam Books.

Church, D. (2009). *The Genie in Your Genes.* Santa Rosa, CA. Energy Psychology Press.

Chronic fatigue syndrome (February 2, 2012). A.D.A.M., Inc. (as cited by the New York Times, 2012). Retrieved from: http://www.nytimes.com/health/guides/disease/chronic-fatigue-syndrome/diagnosis.html

Claudio, L. (2001). Environmental aftermath. *Environ Health Perspect 109*, A528-A537. PMID:11713010 PMC1240484 Retrieved from:
http://www.ncbi.nlm.nih.gov/pmc/articles/PMC1240484/pdf/ehp0109-a00528.pdf

Claudio, L. (2011). Planting Healthier Indoor Air. *Environ Health Perspect 119* a426-a427.
http://dx.doi.org/10.1289/ehp.119-a426

Coppola, S., Singer, T., & Ombelets, J. (2014). The Hidden Impact of Trauma. *Northeastern Magazine.*
Retrieved from: http://www.northeastern.edu/magazine/the-hidden-impact-of-trauma-2/

Csikszentmihalyi, M. (1990). *Flow: The psychology of optimal experience.* New York, NY: Harper and Row.
Retrieved from http://www.pursuit-of-happiness.org/history-of-happiness/mihaly-csikszentmihalyi/

Cox, I.M., Campbell, M.J., & Dowson, D. (March 30, 1991). Red blood cell magnesium and chronic
fatigue syndrome: *Lancet.* 337(8744):757-60. Retrieved from:
http://www.ncbi.nlm.nih.gov/pubmed/1672392

Cyanotech (May 26, 2009). Key constituent in spirulina "phycocyanin" shows anti-inflammatory and anti-
hyperalgesic action. Retrieved from: http://newhope360.com/trends/key-constituent-spirulina-phycocyanin-shows-anti-inflammatory-and-anti-hyperalgesic-action

Dansby, B. A. (2015). Archetypal affirmations and how they work. Retrieved from:
http://binnieadansby.com/ecstatic-life/Archetypal-Affirmations/

Dantzer, R. (October 1, 2004). Cytokine-induced sickness behaviour: a neuroimmune response to
activation of innate immunity. *Eur J Pharmacol., 500*(1-3), 399-411. Retrieved from:
http://www.ncbi.nlm.nih.gov/pubmed/15464048

Dantzer, R. (2006). Cytokine, sickness behavior, and depression. *Neurol Clin.* 24(3), 441–460.
doi:10.1016/j.ncl.2006.03.003 PMCID: PMC2909644 NIHMSID: NIHMS214073

Dantzer, R., O'Connor, J. C., Freudn, G. G., Johnson, R. W., & Kelley, K. W. (2008). From inflammation
to sickness and depression: when the immune system subjugates the brain. *Nat Rev Neurosci.* 9(1): 46–
56. doi:10.1038/nrn2297. Retrieved from:
http://www.ncbi.nlm.nih.gov/pmc/articles/PMC2919277/pdf/nihms213147.pdf

Dantzer, R. (2009). Cytokine, sickness behavior, and depression. [republication of 2006 study, with
updates]. *Immunology and Allergy Clinics of North America. 29*(2):247-64. DOI:10.1016/j.iac.2009.02.002

Dardik, I. (December 17, 1983). *Breakthrough to excellence quantum fitness.* New York, NY, Pocket Books.

Dardik, I. & Waitley, D. (April 29, 2015). [audio narrated by Dardik & Waitley]. *Quantum breakthrough to
excellence.* Wheeling, IL, Nightingale Conant.

Delaney, L., & Smith, J. P. (2012). Childhood health: Trends and consequences over the life course. *The
Future of Children* Volume 22, Number 1, Spring 2012. 43-63 | 10.1353/foc.2012.0003.Retrieved from:
https://muse.jhu.edu/login?auth=0&type=summary&url=/journals/future_of_children/v022/22.1.
delaney.html

Deans, E. (June 12, 2011). Magnesium and the brain: The original chill pill. Retrieved from:
https://www.psychologytoday.com/blog/evolutionary-psychiatry/201106/magnesium-and-the-brain-the-original-chill-pill

Deans, E. (Feb. 4, 2012). Magnesium deficiency and fibromyalgia. Retrieved from:
http://evolutionarypsychiatry.blogspot.com/2012/02/magnesium-deficiency-and-fibromyalgia.html

De Vos, J. M., Joppa, L. N., Gittleman, J. L., Stephens, P. R. & Pimm, S. L. (April 26, 2015). Estimating
the normal background rate of species extinction. *Conservation Biology 29*(2), 452–462.
DOI:10.1111/cobi.12380

Doheny, K.(April 9, 2010). [FAQ: Triclosan and Your Health]. FDA reviewing antibacterial chemical
widely used in soaps and body washes. WebMD Health News. Retrieved from:
http://www2.conchovalleyhomepage.com/webmd/beauty/bodycare/story/FAQ-Triclosan-and-Your-Health/6_SZFj0Vpkmn8fCtpSKBBw.cspx

Duke, A. (September 23, 2009). New charges filed in investigation of Anna Nicole Smith death. *CNN -
Los Angeles.* Retrieved from:
http://www.cnn.com/2009/SHOWBIZ/09/23/anna.nicole.case/index.html?iref=nextin

Dychtwald, K. (1977). *Bodymind.* New York, NY. Pantheon Books.

Dykema, R. (2006). How your nervous system sabotages your ability to relate: An interview with Stephen
Porges about his polyvagal theory. Retrieved from:
https://nexusalive.com/articles/interviews/stephen-porges-ph-d-the-polyvagal-theory/
http://www.naturalworldhealing.com/images/polyvagal_interview_porges.pdf

Dyson, F. (July 19, 2007). Our biotech future. The New York Review of Books. Retrieved from: http://www.nybooks.com/articles/archives/2007/jul/19/our-biotech-future/

Edwards, J. (June 7, 2015). Doctors against vaccines – Hear from those who have done the research. Retrieved from: http://www.organiclifestylemagazine.com/doctors-against-vaccines-hear-from-those-who-have-done-the-research

Edwards, L. D. (April 7, 2011). *Adrenalogic.* Toronto. TUPH Canada, Inc.

Edwards, L. D. & Heyman, A. H. (2011). Hypocortisolism: An evidence-based review. *Integrative Medicine, 10*(4). Retrieved from: http://www.scribd.com/doc/79297929/Hypocortisolism-an-Evidence-Based-Review

Edwards, S. P. (2006). *The other side of cytokines.* Retrieved from: http://www.dana.org/Publications/Brainwork/Details.aspx?id=43669#sthash.r5ZFABT9.dpuf

Eisen, S. A., Kang, H. K., Murphy, F. M., Blanchard, M. S., Reda, D. J., Henderson, W. G., Toomey, R., Jackson, L.W., Alpern, R., Parks, B. J., Klimas, N., Hall, C., Pak, H.S., Hunter, J. Karlinsky, J., Battistone, M. J., Lyons, & M. J. (June 7, 2005). Gulf War veterans' health: Medical evaluation of a U.S. cohort. *Ann Intern Med.* 142(11):881-90. Retrieved from: http://www.ncbi.nlm.nih.gov/pubmed/15941694

Ellis, J. S., Greenlee, M., Stone, J. (producers) & Greenlee, M., Stone J. (directors). (2009). *The Compass* [Motion Picture]. USA: 363 Productions, Spencer Media.

Entine, J., & Wendel, J. (Oct. 14, 2013). 2000+ reasons why GMOs are safe to eat and environmentally sustainable. Forbes. Retrieved from: http://www.forbes.com/sites/jonentine/2013/10/14/2000-reasons-why-gmos-are-safe-to-eat-and-environmentally-sustainable

Environmental Justice and Health Alliance for Chemical Policy Reform (2014). Who's in danger? Race, poverty, and chemical disasters. Retrieved from: http://www.comingcleaninc.org/assets/media/images/Reports/Who's%20in%20Danger%20Report%20and%20Table%20FINAL.pdf

Environmental Working Group (July 14, 2005). A benchmark investigation of industrial chemicals, pollutants and pesticides in umbilical cord blood. Retrieved from: http://www.ewg.org/research/body-burden-pollution-newborns

Environmental Working Group (October 3, 2013). BB and CC creams: Where the FDA fails consumers. Retrieved from: http://www.ewg.org/research/bb-and-cc-creams/where-fda-fails-consumers

Environmental Working Group (2015). EWG's 2015 guide to sunscreens. Retrieved from: http://www.ewg.org/2015sunscreen/report/the-trouble-with-sunscreen-chemicals/

Erasmus, U. (1993). *Fats that heal, fats that kill, the complete guide to fats, oils, cholesterol and human health.* Summertown, TN, Alive Books.

Ewis, S. A. & Abdel-Rahman, M. S. (1995). Effect of metformin on glutathione and magnesium in normal and streptozotocin-induced diabetic rats. *J Appl Toxicol* 15(5), 387 -390. DOI:10.1002/jat.2550150508

Fernandez, E. (September 16, 2013). [Study conducted at UC San Francisco and Preventive Medicine Research Institute. Full study published on Lancet Oncology at thelancet.com]. Lifestyle changes may lengthen telomeres, a measure of cell aging. Diet, meditation, exercise can improve key elements of immune cell aging. *UCSF Scientists Report.* Retrieved from: https://www.ucsf.edu/news/2013/09/108886/lifestyle-changes-may-lengthen-telomeres-measure-cell-aging
DOI: http://dx.doi.org/10.1016/S1470-2045(13)70366-8

Fiedler, N., Udasin, I., Gochfeld, M., Buckler, G., Kelly-McNeil, K., & Kipen, H. (1999). Neuropsychological and stress evaluation of a residential mercury exposure. *Environ Health Perspect.* 107(5):343-7. Retrieved from: http://www.ncbi.nlm.nih.gov/pmc/articles/PMC1566413/

Flatow, I. [Interviewer] & Kipnis, J. [Interviewee]. (2015). Retrieved from: http://www.pri.org/stories/2015-07-04/scientists-have-discovered-missing-link-between-brain-and-immune-system

Forsgren, S., Nathan, N. & Anderson, W. (2014). Mold and mycotoxins: Often overlooked factors in chronic lyme disease. *Townsend Letter.* Retrieved from: http://www.townsendletter.com/July2014/mold0714.html or http://www.gordonmedical.com/unravelling-complex-chronic-illness/mold-and-mycotoxins-often-overlooked-factors-in-chronic-lyme-disease/

Fox, J. (writer & director). (2010). *Gasland* [Motion Picture]. Winger, D., Gray, H., Adlesic, T., Fox, J., Gandour, M., & Roma, D. (producers). USA. New Video Group/HBO/International WOW Company (distributors). Retrieved from: https://www.youtube.com/watch?v=6mp4ELXKv-w

Fox, J. (writer & director). (2013). *Gasland Part II* [Motion Picture]. Fox, J., Adlesic, T., Sanchez, M., Wallace, D., & Ziesche, L. (producers). USA. International WOW Company. Retrieved from http://www.gaslandthemovie.com/whats-fracking

Friedrich, B. (writer & director). Akin, C. People for the Ethical Treatment of Animals [PETA] (2002). *Meet your meat*. [Video File]. Friedrich, B. (producer) & Akin, C. (co-producer). USA. PETA. Retrieved from: https://www.youtube.com/watch?v=32IDVdgmzKA

Garber, A. K. & Lustig, R. H. (September 4, 2011). Is fast food addictive? *Curr Drug Abuse Rev.*, *4*(3), 146-162. PMID: 21999689. Retrieved from: http://www.ncbi.nlm.nih.gov/pubmed/21999689

Gates, D., & Schatz, L. (2011). *The body ecology diet: Recovering your health and rebuilding your immunity*. Carlsbad, California. Hay House, Inc.

Gazdar, R. (2005). Healing the world. Life Positive Magazine. Retrieved from: Lifepositive.com/healing-the-world/

Gazdar, R. (2006). In resonance. Life Positive Magazine. Retrieved from: Lifepositive.com/in-resonance/

General Mills accelerates plan to double organic acreage for sourcing natural foods. (March 10, 2016). [PR carried by NewHope.com]. Retrieved from: http://newhope.com/organic/general-mills-accelerates-plan-double-organic-acreage-sourcing-natural-foods?NL=NP-01&Issue=NP-01_20160311_NP-01_294&sfvc4enews=42&cl=article_1&utm_rid=CNHNM000000256146&utm_campaign=15636&utm_medium=email

Gerrard, P., & Malcolm, R. (2007). Mechanisms of modafinil. *Neuropsychiatric Disease and Treatment*, *3*(3), 349–364. Retrieved from: http://www.ncbi.nlm.nih.gov/pmc/articles/PMC2654794/

Gratix, N. (May 17, 2014). Limbic kindling: Hardwiring the brain for hypersensitivity and chronic fatigue syndrome. Retrieved from: http://www.cortjohnson.org/blog/2014/05/17/limbic-kindling-hard-wiring-brain-hypersensitives-chronic-fatigue-syndrome/

Goldenfeld, N. & Woese, C. (January 25, 2007). Biology's next revolution. *Nature, 445*, 369-369. doi:10.1038/445369a [PDF]

Goode, E. (September 2, 2003). Power of positive thinking may have a health benefit, study says. [paragraphs 6, 13 & 14 are about Dr. Richard J. Davidson]. Retrieved from: http://www.nytimes.com/2003/09/02/health/power-of-positive-thinking-may-have-a-health-benefit-study-says.html

Gottfried, S. (2014). *Origins* [Motion Picture], Section 43:11-45:23; Shojai, P. (Producer), & Shojai P. (director). USA. Retrieved from: http://origins.well.org/movie/

Gottfried, S. (March 11, 2014). *The hormone cure: Reclaim balance, sleep and sex drive; lose weight; feel focused, vital, and energized naturally with the Gottfried protocol*. New York, NY. Scribner.

Grey, C. (June 8, 2011). Vitamin B12 and intrinsic factor. Retrieved from: http://www.livestrong.com/article/466841-vitamin-b12-and-intrinsic-factor/

Guerry, J. D. & Hastings, P. D. (2011). In search of hpa axis dysregulation in child and adolescent depression. *Clinical Child and Family Psychology Review, 14*(2), 135-160. DOI; 10.1007/s10567-011-0084-5

Guide to safe cosmetics: 9 facts about the personal care industry. (2015, May 19). Retrieved from: http://www.honeycolony.com/article/myths-on-cosmetics-safety/

Guilliams, T. G. & Edwards, L. D. (2012). Chronic stress and the hpa axis: Clinical assessment and therapeutic considerations. *The Standard, 9*(2). Retrieved from: http://www.pointinstitute.org/wp-content/uploads/2012/10/standard_v_9.2_hpa_axis.pdf

Gulf war syndrome. (January 27, 2015). Environmental Illness Resource. Retrieved from: http://www.ei-resource.org/illness-information/environmental-illnesses/gulf-war-syndrome/

Gulf war veterans' medically unexplained illnesses (n.d.). US Department of Veterans Affairs. Retrieved from: http://www.publichealth.va.gov/exposures/gulfwar/medically-unexplained-illness.asp

Gratrix, N. [interviewer], Gupta, A. [interviewee] (2015). Amygdala retraining: Rewire your brain for optimum energy. Retrieved from: http://abundantenergysummit.com/

Gupta, S. (writer), & Selig, R. (director). (June 2, 2010). Toxic towns: USA. Part one of a two night CNN special investigation television broadcast. Martin, D. S., & Hellerman, C. (producers), Martin, S., Young, S., Bonifield, J., Hellerman, C., & Gupta, S., (researchers). Retrieved from: http://www.cnn.com/2010/HEALTH/02/26/toxic.town.mossville.epa/

Gupta, S. (July 31, 2012). More treatment, more mistakes. NY Times. Retrieved from: http://www.nytimes.com/2012/08/01/opinion/more-treatment-more-mistakes.html

Gurule, K. (June 5, 2013). What is the halliburton loophole? Frackwire.com, What is Fracking? Our Position. Retrieved from: http://frackwire.com/halliburton-loophole/

Hamilton, D. R. (June 26, 2008). *It's the thought that counts: The power of thought, feeling, and faith.* UK: Hay House.

Haynes, T. (writer & director). (1995). *Safe.* [motion picture]. Christine Vachon (producer). USA/Britain. Sony Pictures Classics.

Heathers, J. (2011). A basic introduction to vagal tone. Retrieved from: http://www.psych.usyd.edu.au/staff/jamesh/

The highly sensitive person (HSP) explained. (February 8, 2015). Retrieved from: https://bookofresearch.wordpress.com/2015/02/28/the-highly-sensitive-person-hsp/

Hillenbrand, L. (July 7, 2003). A sudden illness. Retrieved from: http://www.newyorker.com/magazine/2003/07/07/a-sudden-illness

Hillenbrand, L. (2002) *Seabiscuit: An American legend.* USA. Ballentine Books, Random House Publishing Group.

Hillenbrand, L. (2014) *Unbroken: A World War II story of survival, resilience, and redemption.* USA. Random House LLC.

Hoffman, J. W., Benson, H., Arns, P. A., Stainbrook, G. L., Landsberg, G. L., Young, J. B., & Gill, A. (January 8, 1982). Reduced sympathetic nervous system responsivity associated with the relaxation response. *Science, 215*(4529), 190 -192. *DOI:* 10.1126/science.7031901 Retrieved from: http://www.gpo.gov/fdsys/pkg/CHRG-105shrg54619/pdf/CHRG-105shrg54619.pdf

Hölzel, B. K., Lazar, S. W., Gard, T., Schuman-Olivier, Z., Vago, D. R., & Ott, U. (2011). How does mindfulness meditation work? *Perspectives on Psychological Science, 6*(6), 537-559. doi: 10.1177/1745691611419671

Houlihan, J., Wiles, R., Thayer, K., & Gray, S. (2003). Body burden: The pollution in people. Environmental Working Group. Retrieved from: http://www.trwnews.net/Documents/Dioxin/BBreport_final.pdf

Hudson, K. (February 13, 2013). What are your dishes made of? Why avoid melamine dishes. Retrieved from: http://www.organicauthority.com/sanctuary/why-avoid-melamine-dishes.html

Hurley, D. (June 25, 2015). Grandma's experiences leave a mark on your genes. Retrieved from: http://discovermagazine.com/2013/may/13-grandmas-experiences-leave-epigenetic-mark-on-your-genes

Hyman, M. (Nov 17, 2011). Glutathione: The mother of all antioxidants. Retrieved from: http://www.huffingtonpost.com/dr-mark-hyman/glutathione-the-mother-of_b_530494.html

Jason, L. A., Porter, N., Brown, M., Anderson, V., Brown, A., Hunnell, J., & Lerch, A. (2009). CFS: A review of epidemiology and natural history studies. *Bull IACFS ME*. 17(3): 88–106. Retrieved from: http://www.ncbi.nlm.nih.gov/pmc/articles/PMC3021257/

Johnson, C. (December 10, 2013). Study suggests gut bacteria may be able to trigger autoimmune disorders. Retrieved from: http://www.cortjohnson.org/blog/2013/12/10/study-suggests-specific-gut-bacteria-may-able-provoke-autoimmune-disorder/

Jowit, J. (March 7, 2010). Humans driving extinction faster than species can evolve, say experts. The Guardian, U.S. Edition. Retrieved from: http://www.theguardian.com/environment/2010/mar/07/extinction-species-evolve

Kaiser, J. D. (2014). Chronic fatigue syndrome. Retrieved from: http://jonkaiser.com/

Kaiser, J. D. (2015). Mitochondrial medicine: A clinician's guide [Video File]. Retrieved from: https://vimeo.com/channels/mitochondria?elq=fccf373f1a8b415fa54a1196b7d1ff12&elqCampaignId=75&elqaid=306&elqat=1&elqTrackId=e9ae78473bc24150addc7c9dd4c7770e

Kane, E.A. (May 2015). SOS for pms. Better Nutrition, May 2015, Volume 77, Number 6, 22-26.

Kahn, J. (October 24, 2005). [25th Anniversary Issue]. How our genes interact with foods we eat: Nutritional genomics promises to make diets truly personal. Discover Magaine. Retrieved from: http://discovermagazine.com/2005/oct/nutrition

Kaldveer, Z. (2013, August 7). U.S. and Monsanto dominate global market for GM seeds. Retrieved from: https://www.organicconsumers.org/essays/us-and-monsanto-dominate-global-market-gm-seeds

Kananen, L., Surakka, I., Pirkola, S., Suvisaari, J., Lönnqvist, J., Peltonen, L.; ..., & Hovatta, I. (May 25, 2010). Childhood adversities are associated with shorter telomere length at adult age both in individuals with an anxiety disorder and controls. *PLoS ONE*, 5(5): doi:10.1371/journal.pone.0010826

Kapoor, S. (2013). D-Limonene: an emerging antineoplastic agent. *Hum. Exp Toxicol.* Retrieved from: http://www.ncbi.nlm.nih.gov/pubmed/23716733

Kinnamon, S. C., & Finger, T. E. (December 18, 2013). A taste for ATP: neurotransmission in taste buds. *Front Cell Neurosci* 7:264. doi: 10.3389/fncel.2013.00264. Retrieved from: http://www.ncbi.nlm.nih.gov/pmc/articles/PMC3866518/

Kenner, R., Pearlstein, E. & Roberts, K. (writers). Kenner, R., (director). (2008). *Food, Inc.* [Motion Picture]. Pollan, M. (consultant & appears), Schlosser, E. (co-producer & appears), Kenner, R. (co-producer with others). USA. Magnolia Pictures. Retrieved from: http://www.imdb.com/title/tt1286537/

Kipen, H., & Gochfeld, M. (2002). Mind and matter: OEM and the World Trade Center. *Occupational and Environmental Medicine*, 59(3), 145–146. doi:10.1136/oem.59.3.145

Komak, R. (December 28, 2013). Geologists look into naturally occurring asbestos minerals in the boulder city region. Retrieved from: http://www.mesothelioma.com/news/2013/12/geologists-look-into-naturally-occurring-asbestos-minerals-in-the-boulder-city-region.htm#ixzz3PfPvdUjQ

Komiya, M., Takeuchi, T., & Harada, E. (September 25, 2006). Lemon oil vapor causes an anti-stress effect via modulating the 5-HT and DA activities in mice. *Behav Brain Res.,172*(2), 240-9. Retrieved from: http://www.ncbi.nlm.nih.gov/pubmed/16780969

Koopman, F. A., Stoof, S. P., Straub, R. H., van Maanen, M. A., Vervoordeldonk, M. J., & Tak, P. P. (2011). Restoring the balance of the autonomic nervous system as an innovative approach to the treatment of rheumatoid arthritis. *Mol Med. 2011 Sep-Oct; 17*(9-10), 937–948. doi: 10.2119/molmed.2011.00065

Kristof, N. D. (June 27, 2009). It's time to learn from frogs. *NY Times Opinion*. Retrieved from: http://www.nytimes.com/2009/06/28/opinion/28kristof.html?_r=0

Kongsbak, M., Trine, B., Levring, T. B., Geisler C., & von Essen, M. R. (June 18, 2013). The vitamin D receptor and T cell function. *Front. Immunol.* http://dx.doi.org/10.3389/fimmu.2013.00148. Retrieved from: http://journal.frontiersin.org/article/10.3389/fimmu.2013.00148/full#B108

Lakhan, S., & Kirchgessner, A. (Oct. 12, 2010). Gut inflammation in chronic fatigue syndrome. *Nutr Metab (Lond)*. 2010; 7: 79. doi: 10.1186/1743-7075-7-79 PMCID: PMC2964729 Retrieved from: http://www.ncbi.nlm.nih.gov/pmc/articles/PMC2964729/#B12

Lederberg, J. (Dec. 18, 1986). Forty years of genetic recombination in bacteria. *Nature* 324, 627 – 628. Retrieved from: http://www.nature.com/nature/journal/v324/n6098/abs/324627a0.html doi: 10.1038/324627a0

442

Lehrner, J., Marwinsky, G., Lehr, S., Johren, P., & Deecke, L. (September15, 2005). Ambient odors of orange and lavender reduce anxiety and improve mood in a dental office. *Physiol Behav.* 86(1-2):92-5. Retrieved from: http://www.ncbi.nlm.nih.gov/pubmed/16095639

Levine, P. A. (1997). *Waking the tiger: Healing trauma - The innate capacity to transform overwhelming experiences.* Berkeley, California. North Atlantic Books.

Levine, P. A. (October 1, 2008). [audio]. *Healing trauma: A pioneering program for restoring the wisdom of your body.* Louisville, CO. Sounds True, Inc.

Lewin, R. (September 29, 2005). *Making waves: Irving Dardik and his superwave principle.* Emmaus, PA. Rodale Books.

Lindsley, C. W. (August 15, 2012). The top prescription drugs of 2011 in the United States: antipsychotics and antidepressants once again lead CNS therapeutics. *ACS Chem. Neurosci.* 3(8), 630–631, doi: 10.1021/cn3000923 http://pubs.acs.org/doi/full/10.1021/cn3000923

Lioy, P.J., & Gochfeld, M. (n.d.). Lessons learned on environmental, occupational, and residential exposures from the attack on the WTC. *American Journal of Industrial Medicine.* http://www.isea.rutgers.edu/files/Lessons%20Learned%20Manuscript.pdf

Lioy, P. J., Weisel, C. P., Millette, J., Eisenreich, S., Vallero, D., Offenberg, J.,... Chen, L. C. (2002). Characteristics of the dust/smoke aerosol that settled east of the World Trade Center (WTC) in Lower Manhattan after the collapse of the WTC September 11, 2001. *Environ Health Perspect., 110*(7). 703-714. Retrieved from: http://www.ncbi.nlm.nih.gov/pmc/articles/PMC1240917/

Lipkin, W. I. [head consult], Alter, H. J., Mikovits, J. A., Switzer, W. M., Ruscetti, F. W., Lo, S-C., Hornig, M. (2012, September 18). A multicenter blinded analysis indicates no association between chronic fatigue syndrome/myalgic encephalomyelitis and either xenotropic murine leukemia virus-related virus or polytropic murine leukemia virus. *American Society for Microbiology. mBio,3*(5), e00266-12. doi: 10.1128/mBio.00266-12

Lipkin,W. I. [senior consult], Hornig, M., Montoya, J. G., Klimas, N. G., Levine S., Felsenstein, D., Klimas, N., Komaroff, A. L., Montoya, J.G. Bateman, L., Levine, S., Peterson, D., Levin B., Hanson, M.R., Genfi, A., Bhat, M., Zhen H., Wang, R., Li B., Hung, G.-C., Lee, L. L., Sameroff, S., Heneine, W., ...Coffin J. (2015, February 27). Distinct plasma immune signatures in ME/CFS are present early in the course of illness. *Science Advances, Vol. 1*(1), e1400121 DOI: 10.1126/sciadv.1400121

Lipkin, W. I. & Hornig, M. (February 27, 2015). [News Release from Columbia University Mailman School of Public Health]. Scientists discover robust evidence that chronic fatigue syndrome is a biological illness. Retrieved from: http://www.mailman.columbia.edu/news/scientists-discover-robust-evidence-chronic-fatigue-syndrome-biological-illness

Lipton, B. (2008). *The biology of belief: Unleashing the power of consciousness, matter, & miracles.* Carlsbad, California. Hay House.

Live from Expo West 2016: Watch natural products business school & state of the industry. (March 1, 2016). [Video File]. New Hope Network. Retrieved from: http://m.newhope.com/expo-west-2016-live?utm_rid=CNHNM000000256146&utm_campaign=15621&utm_medium=email&elqTrackId=c4b1472231348c9819c2ab8d55c335d&elq=acf8609d0b54498d93eb329c26718838&elqaid=15621&elqat=1&elqCampaignId=7499

Lopate, L. [Interviewer] & Rossol, M. [Interviewee]. (September 17, 2009). [WNYC radio interview of Monona Rossol on The Leonard Lopate Show]. Retrieved from: http://www.wnyc.org/story/59701-50-million-chemicals/

Lustig, R. H., Schmidt, L. A., & Brindis, C. D. (2012, February 2). Public Health: The toxic truth about sugar. *Nature 482*, (7383) 27–29 doi:10.1038/482027a Retrieved from: http://pdfsr.com/pdf/public-health-the-toxic-truth-about-sugar

Lynch, B. (2015) [Site has current and archived articles and reports; Dr. Lynch conducts research on MTHFR gene mutations]. http://mthfr.net/

Lobo, V., Patil, A., Phatax, A., & Chandra, N. (2010). Free radicals, antioxidants and functional foods: Impact on human health. Retrieved from: http://www.ncbi.nlm.nih.gov/pmc/articles/PMC3249911/

Matute, C., & Ransom, B. R. (2012). Roles of white matter in central nervous system pathophysiologies. *ASN Neuro. vol. 4 no. 2 AN 20110060.* Retrieved from: http://asn.sagepub.com/content/4/2/AN20110060.full

Maes, M., & Leunis, J.C. (December 29, 2008). Normalization of leaky gut in chronic fatigue syndrome (CFS) is accompanied by a clinical improvement: effects of age, duration of illness and the translocation of LPS from gram-negative bacteria. *Neuroendocrinol Lett.* 29 (6): 101–000. Retrieved from:
https://www.researchgate.net/profile/Michael_Maes2/publication/23709068_Normalization_of_lea ky_gut_in_chronic_fatigue_syndrome_CFS_is_accompanied_by_a_clinical_improvement_Effects_of _age_duration_of_illness_and_the_translocation_of_LPS_from_gram-negative_bacteria/links/55c0913f08ae092e9666c31b.pdf

May, J. M., Qu, Z.-C., & Meredith, M. E. (Aug.19, 2012). Mechanisms of ascorbic acid stimulation of norepinephrine synthesis in neuronal cells. *Biochem Biophys Res Commun*; 426(1):148-152. doi: 10.1016/j.bbrc.2012.08.054 Retrieved from:
http://www.ncbi.nlm.nih.gov/pmc/articles/PMC3449284/

Mercola, J. (2013). MSM health benefits may be related to its sulfur content. Retrieved from:
http://articles.mercola.com/sites/articles/archive/2013/03/03/msm-benefits.aspx

McCarthy, J., & Kartzinel, J. (2009). *Healing and preventing autism: A complete guide.* New York, NY. Dutton Adult, Penguin Group (USA),Inc.

McCleery, R. E., & Middendorf, P. J. (2012). [Corporate Authors: National Institute for Occupational Safety and Health; WTC Health Program; WTC Cancer Working Group. Cancer classifications by National Toxicology Program & International Agency for Research on Cancer]. World Trade Center chemicals of potential concern and selected other chemical agents. Retrieved from:
http://stacks.cdc.gov/view/cdc/11780

McEwen, B. S. (1999, March). Stress and hippocampal plasticity. *Annual Review of Neuroscience 22*, 105-122. DOI: 10.1146/annurev.neuro.22.1.105

McEwen, B.S. (2000). Allostasis and allostatic load: Implications for neuropsychopharmacology. Laboratory of Neuroendocrinology, The Rockefeller University, New York, NY USA. Retrieved from: http://www.nature.com/npp/journal/v22/n2/full/1395453a.html

McMillen, M. (2015*).* What you should know if you think you have leaky gut syndrome. Retrieved from:
http://www.webmd.com/digestive-disorders/features/leaky-gut-syndrome

Mackenzie, L. (2006). The healing power of the mind. Retrieved from:
http://www.lindamackenzie.net/HealingMindarticle.htm

Malterre, T. (2013). How foods assit with processing of environmental toxins. *NANP: National Association of Nutrition Professionals.* Retrieved from: http://www.nanp.org/conference/wp-content/uploads/2013/04/Tom-Malterre_How-Foods-Assist-with-the-Processing-of-Environmental-Toxicants-v2.pdf

Matthews, W. (2008, November 23). *Methylation* - A simple explanation. Retrieved from:
http://healthiertalk.com/author/warren-matthews

Maxmen, J. S., Ward, N. G., & Kilgus, M. D. (2009). [third edition]. *Essential psychopathology & it's treatment.* New York, NY: W. W. Norton & Company.

Medical Xpress (February 26, 2014). New research indicates causal link between vitamin D, serotonin synthesis and autism. Retrieved from: http://medicalxpress.com/news/2014-02-causal-link-vitamin-d-serotonin.html

Meyer, N. (2014, June 11). MIT researcher's new warning: At today's rate, half of all U.S. children will be autistic (by 2025). Retrieved from: http://althealthworks.com/2494/mit-researchers-new-warning-at-todays-rate-1-in-2-children-will-be-autistic-by-2025/

Miles, K. (May 2, 2014). Deepak chopra on how to modify your own genes. Retrieved from:
http://www.huffingtonpost.com/2014/05/02/deepak-chopra-genes_n_5249988.html

Miller, G.E, Cohen, S., & Ritchey, A.K. (2002). Chronic psychological stress and the regulation of pro-inflammatory cytokines: A glucocorticoid resistance model. *Health Psychology.* 21:531–541. Retrieved from: http://www.ncbi.nlm.nih.gov/pubmed/1243300

Morris, G., Anderson, G., Galecki, P., Berk, M., & Maes, M. (2013). A narrative review on the similarities and dissimilarities between myalgic encephalomyelitis/chronic fatigue syndrome (ME/CFS) and sickness behavior. *BMC Medicine* 2013, 11:64 doi:10.1186/1741-7015-11-64. Retrieved from:
http://www.biomedcentral.com/1741-7015/11/64

Miller, J. G. (1978 & 1995). *Living systems.* Hardcover, 1978, Texas, Mcgraw-Hill. Paperback, 1995, Boulder, CO, University of Colorado Press.

Module 2: Toxin exposure among children - Introduction: Toxic chemicals. (2014-15). [nonprofit organization; phone: (203) 404-4900; email: ufs@uniteforsight.org]. Unite For Sight. Retrieved from:
http://www.uniteforsight.org/environmental-health/module2

Moore, M. & Tschannen-Moran, B. (2010). *Coaching psychology manual.* Baltimore, MD: Wolters Kluwer/Lippincott Williams & Wilkins.

Moy, D. (2011). Oh my myelin. Retrieved from: http://fascialconnections.com/oh-my-myelin

Ms. S. (2010). Children: Alarming health trends. Retrieved from:
http://www.health.thesfile.com/children/children-alarming-health-trends/

MTHFR: Since an estimated 60% of the population has this condition, and it is the underlying cause for many chronic illnesses, shouldn't we all be getting tested? (2013, April 9). Retrieved from:
http://www.freshideamama.com/mthfr-since-40-60-of-the-population-has-this-condition-and-it-is-the-underlying-cause-for-many-chronic-illnesses-shouldnt-we-all-be-getting-tested.html

Mukherjee, S. (April 19, 2012). Post-Prozac nation: The science and history of treating depression. *The New York Times Magazine*. Retrieved from: http://www.nytimes.com/2012/04/22/magazine/the-science-and-history-of-treating-depression.html?pagewanted=all&_r=0

Mundell, E. J. (2006, September 11). 9/11's grim toll on health continues. HealthDay, News for Healthier Living, a health blog by Scott News. Retrieved from: http://consumer.healthday.com/cancer-information-5/lung-cancer-news-100/9-11-s-grim-toll-on-health-continues-534853.html

Murray, W. H. (1951). The scottish himalayan expedition. London. J.M. Dent & Sons Ltd. Retrieved from:
https://openlibrary.org/books/OL6111279M/The_Scottish_Himalayan_Expedition

Myhill, S. (2014). Fibromyalgia - possible causes and implications for treatment. Retrieved from:
http://drmyhill.co.uk/wiki/Fibromyalgia_-_possible_causes_and_implications_for_treatment

Myers, W., & Malterre, T. (2015). How GMO's affect gut health with Tom Malterre. Retrieved from:
https://liveto110.com/69-gmos-affect-gut-health-tom-malterre/

National Partnership for Women & Families (2009). [Fact sheet compiled by non-profit, non-partisan advocacy group promoting workplace fairness, access to health care, & policies to help meet dual demands of work and family.] Medical Errors Are Not Just a Headline. Retrieved from: http://go.nationalpartnership.org/site/DocServer/Fact_Sheet_Medical_Errors_Not_Just_a_Headline.pdf?docID=5482

Naturally occurring asbestos and what you can do to avoid it. (2014, February 18). Mesothelioma Cancer Aliance Blog. Retrieved from: http://www.mesothelioma.com/blog/authors/staff/naturally-occurring-asbestos-and-what-you-can-do-to-avoid-it.htm

Nishida, C., Uauy, R., Kumanyika, S., & Shetty, P. (2004). The joint WHO/FAO expert consultation on diet, nutrition and the prevention of chronic diseases: process, product and policy implications. *Public Health Nutr. 7*(1A), 245-250. PMID:14972063 Retrieved from:
http://www.ncbi.nlm.nih.gov/pubmed/14972063

Organic Consumers Association (2013, August 7). U.S. and Monsanto dominate global market for GM seeds. Retrieved from: http://www.organicconsumers.org/articles/article_28059.cfm

Organization of American States/Secretariat of Legal Affairs (2012). American convention on human rights. Retrieved from: *http://www.oas.org/dil/treaties_B-32_American_Convention_on_Human_Rights.pdf*

Ornish, D. (2015). *Super genes*. [Review of the book *Super genes* by Deepak Chopra, M.D. & Rudolph E. Tanzi, Ph.D.]. Retrieved from: http://www.chopra.com/book/super-genes

PANNA(Pesticide Action Network of North America). (2011). Pesticides & pollinator decline. Retrieved from: http://www.panna.org/current-campaigns/bees

Park, A. (June 14, 2012). [Online source as follows]: The good bugs: How the germs in your body keep you healthy. Time Magazine, Genetics. Retrieved from:
http://healthland.time.com/2012/06/14/the-good-bugs-how-the-germs-in-your-body-keep-you-healthy/ 100 New Scientific Discoveries (August 9, 2011). [In the magazine *Time*]. p.104; *Time, Inc.*

Park, M. (May 25, 2010). Distress of 9/11 may have led to miscarriages, research says. *CNN*. Retrieved from: http://www.cnn.com/2010/HEALTH/05/25/9.11.miscarriage.bereavement/

Park, S. (2014). [Dr. Simon Park discusses the concept of more bacterial cells than human cells (10:1). The other link is a display of microbiome color visuals in which Park, a "photographer" of sorts, was involved.] Exploring the invisible. Retrieved from: http://exploringtheinvisible.com/about/
[also see]: http://exploringtheinvisible.com/ http://annadumitriu.tumblr.com/Super-organism

FDA to review safety issues surrounding leading birth control pill YAZ. [Video file]. Retrieved from:
http://abcnews.go.com/Health/fda-discuss-safety-issues-surrounding-leading-birth-control/story?id=15099220

Pert, C. B. (1997). *Molecules of Emotion: Why you feel the way you feel*. New York, NY. Scribner.

Pert, C. B. (1999) *Molecules of Emotion: The science behind mind-body medicine*. [paperback]. New York, NY. Simon & Schuster.

Pert, C. B. (May 11, 2000). *Molecules of emotion: Why you feel the way you feel* [Abridged]. [Listen to Dr. Pert who narrates this Audible Audio Edition]. New York, NY. Audiobook, a Division of Simon & Schuster.

Pert, C. B. (September 1, 2004). Your body is your subconscious mind: New insights into the Body-Mind connection [CD and audio download] Sounds True, Inc. Retrieved from:
http://www.soundstrue.com/shop/Your-Body-Is-Your-Subconscious-Mind/336.pd

Phelan, J. (2013). *What is life? DNA, gene expression, and biotechnology, second edition.* Chapter 5, Section 15, Pg. 191. New York, NY. Macmillan.

Phyo, A. (2012). *Ani's raw food essentials: Recipes and techniques for mastering the art of live food.* Boston, MA, Da Capo Lifelong Books.

Pitchot, W., Herrera C., & Ansseau M. (2001). HPA axis dysfunction in major depression: relationship to 5-HT(1A) receptor activity. *Neuropsychobiology*, 44(2): 74-7. Retrieved from: http://www.ncbi.nlm.nih.gov/pubmed/11490174

Pollan, M. (October 25, 1988). Playing god in the garden. NY Times magazine. Retrieved from: http://www.nytimes.com/1998/10/25/magazine/playing-god-in-the-garden.html?pagewanted=1

Polycyclic aromatic hydrocarbons and other semivolatile organic compounds collected in NY city in response to the events of 9/11. (July 23, 2003). *Environ. Sci. Technol.*, 2003, 37 (16), pp 3537–3546 DOI: 10.1021/es030356l.

Poppitt, S. D., Keogh, G., Prentice, A., Williams, D., Sonnemans, H., Valk, E., Schul & Wareham, N. (2002). Long-term effects of ad libitum low-fat, high-carbohydrate diets on body weight and serum lipids in overweight subjects with metabolic syndrome. *Am J Clin Nutr.75*(1), 11-20. Retrieved from: http://ajcn.nutrition.org/content/75/1/11.full#sec-1

Porges, S. W. (January 22, 2001). The polyvagal theory: phylogenetic substrates of a social nervous system. *International Journal of Psychophysiology 42*, 123 -146. Retrieved from: http://wisebrain.org/Polyvagal_Theory.pdf

Prezant, D. J., Weiden, M., Banauch, G. I., McGuinness, G., Rom, W. N., Aldrich, T. K., & Kelly, K. J. (September 12, 2002). Cough and bronchial responsiveness in firefighters at the world trade center site. *N Engl J Med, 347*, 806-815. doi:10.1056/NEJMoa021300

Price, L. H., Kao, H-T., Burgers, D. E., Carpenter, L. L., & Tyrka, A. R. (January 1, 2013). Telomeres and early life stress: An overview. *Biological Psychiatry, A Journal of Psychiatric Neuroscience and Therapeutics, 73*,(1), 15–23. DOI: http://dx.doi.org/10.1016/j.biopsych.2012.06.025

Prochaska, J. O., Norcross, J.C., & DiClemente, C. C. (2007). *Changing for good: A revolutionary six-stage program for overcoming bad habits and moving your life positively forward.* New York, NY. William Morrow Paperbacks.

Radford, T. (March 19, 2004). Warning sounded on decline of species. *The Guardian, US Edition.* Retrieved from: http://www.theguardian.com/science/2004/mar/19/taxonomy.science

Relaxation response can influence expression of stress-related genes. (July 2, 2008). Source: Massachusetts General Hospital. Retrieved from: http://phys.org/news134195926.html#jCp

Richards, B. J. (Dec 3, 2013). Nutrition makes Anti-Aging possible: Secrets of your telomeres. Retrieved from: http://www.wellnessresources.com/health/articles/how_nutrition_makes_anti-aging_possible_secrets_of_your_telomeres/

Robbins, D. (September 22, 2013). [An anthology reflecting the lives of 40 global female leaders as they share their stories of passion, purpose, love, and service]. The return of the divine feminine. USA. Retrieved from: *ReVeolution: The Return of the Divine Feminine.*

Rossol, M. (October 6, 2009). We interact with 100,000+ chemicals, and the dangers are barely understood. Retrieved from: http://www.alternet.org/story/143130/we_interact_with_100,000%2B_chemicals,_and_the_dangers_are_barely_understood

Ruiz, D. M. (1997). *The four agreements: A practical guide to personal freedom (a Toltec wisdom book).* Amber-Allen Publishing: San Rafael, CA.

Rutberg, S. (June 23, 2015). Is vitamin D far more powerful than we thought? Retrieved from: http://newhope360.com/breaking-news/d-far-more-powerful-we-thought

Salazar, M. K., Connon, C. Takaro, T. K., Beaudet, N., & Barnhart, S. (2001). An evaluation of factors affecting hazardous waste workers' use of respiratory protective equipment. *AIHAJ, 62*(2), 236-45. PMID: 11331996. Retrieved from: http://www.ncbi.nlm.nih.gov/pubmed?cmd=retrieve&tool=UWMedicine&dopt=Abstract&list_uid s=11331996

Samsel A., & Seneff S. (2013). Glyphosate's suppression of cytochrome P450 enzymes and amino acid biosynthesis by the gut microbiome: Pathways to modern diseases. *Entropy. 15*(4), 1416-1463; doi: 10.3390/e15041416 Retrieved from: http://www.mdpi.com/1099-4300/15/4/1416

Shuler, C. S. (May 25, 2016). HPA Axis Commentary Part 3. http://thecampractitioner.com/hpa-axis-commentary-part-3/

Schulze, M. B., Manson J. E., Ludwig, D. S., Colditz, G., Stampfer, M., Willett, W., & Hu, F. (August 25, 2004). [updated June 1, 2010]. Sugar-Sweetened beverages, weight gain, and incidence of type 2 diabetes in young and Middle-Aged women. *JAMA, 292*(8), 927-934. doi:10.1001/jama.292.8.927. Retrieved from: http://jama.amaassn.org/cgi/content/full/292/8/927

Science & Environmental Health Network, (2015). [Network Groups: Clean Water Fund, Lowell Center for Sustainable Production, MA Breast Cancer Coalition, & Science & Environmental Health Network]. The Massachusetts precautionary principle project. Retrieved from: http://www.sehn.org/pppra.html

Scolding, N. (2001, November 1). Quote on Bunge et al., 1961 research. Found in Dr. Neil Scolding's

2001 article, Regenerating myelin. DOI: http://dx.doi.org/10.1093/brain/124.11.2129 2129-2130

Scott, S. (2012, August 30). Do you need to give up sugar? *ABC Health and Wellbeing blog.* Retrieved from: http://www.abc.net.au/health/features/stories/2012/08/30/3578541.htm

Selvaraj, N., Bobby, Z. & Sridhar, M. G. (2008). Is euthyroid sick syndrome a defensive mechanism against oxidative stress? *Medical Hypotheses, 71*(3), 404-405 doi:10.1016/j.mehy.2007.11.019

Segerstrom, S. C., & Miller, G. E. (2004). Psychological stress and the human immune system: A meta-analytic study of 30 Years of inquiry. *Psychol Bull.* 130(4): 601-630. Retrieved from: http://www.ncbi.nlm.nih.gov/pmc/articles/PMC1361287/ doi: 10.1037/0033-2909.130.4.601

Seneff, S., Lauritzen, A., Davidson, R., & Lentz-Marino, L. (2013). Is encephalopathy a mechanism to renew sulfate in autism? *Entropy 15*, 372-406. doi:10.3390/e15010372

Seneff, S. (June 5, 2014). Is Roundup the toxic chemical that's making us all sick? Groton School, Campbell Performing Arts Center, Groton MA. Retrieved from https://people.csail.mit.edu/seneff/

Setting Me Free. Beth Hart's music. (2006). Retrieved from: www.bethhart.com

Seyle, H. (1956, Revised 1976). *The stress of life.* New York, NY, McGrawHill.

Seyle, H. (1974). *Stress without distress.* New York, NY. Lippencott & Crowell Publishers.

Shaffer, J. (2012, December). Neuroplasticity and positive psychology in clinical practice: A review for combined benefits. *Psychology. 3*(12A), 1110-1115. Retrieved from: http://www.SciRP.org/journal/psych) DOI:10.4236/psych.2012.312A164

Sheean, G. L., Murray, N. M., Rothwell, J. C., Miller, D. H. & Thompson, A. J. (February 1, 1997). An electrophysiological study of the mechanism of fatigue in multiple sclerosis. DOI: http://dx.doi.org/10.1093/brain/120.2.299

Sheldrake, R. (1987). Part I - Mind, memory, and archetype morphic resonance and the collective unconscious. *Psychological Perspectives, 18*(1) 9-25. Retrieved from: http://www.sheldrake.org/Articles&Papers/papers/morphic/morphic1_paper.html

Sheldrake, R. (1988). *The presence of the past: Morphic resonance and the habits of nature.* New York, NY, Times Books.

Shojai, P. (Producer), & Shojai P. (director). (2014). *Origins* [motion picture]. USA. Retrieved from: http://origins.well.org/movie/

Simpson, S., Ash, C., Pennisi, E., & Travis, J. (March 25, 2005). The gut: inside out, the inner tube of life. *Science: 307*(5717), 1914 *DOI:* 10.1126/science.307.5717.1914a

Sircus, M. (December 8, 2009). Magnesium deficiency, symptoms and diagnosis. Retrieved from: http://drsircus.com/medicine/magnesium/magnesium-deficiency-symptoms-diagnosis

Skolnick, A. (January 4, 2007). [Step 5, by Skolnick, describes Herbert Benson's ideas on stress]. The 5-step self-improvement overhaul. Retrieved from: http://www.outsideonline.com/1928726/5-step-self-improvement-overhaul

Slater, L. (2013). Getting lighter: The transformative power of a little sprucing up. *O, the Oprah Magazine.* Retrieved from: http://www.oprah.com/spirit/Depression-Makeover-Lauren-Slater-Essay#ixzz3be7mAvlv

Neuroscience. (February 28, 2009). How inflammatory disease causes fatigue. ScienceDaily. Retrieved from: www.sciencedaily.com/releases/2009/02/090217173034.htm

Spader, C. (2013). Multiple Sclerosis. Retrieved from: http://www.localhealth.com/article/multiple-sclerosis-1/causes

Stanford University Medical Center (July 29, 2015). Women's immune system genes operate differently from men's. Retrieved from: http://www.eurekalert.org/pub_releases/2015-07/sumc-wis072715.php

Staton, T. (April 30, 2013). Merck wins Bellwether Fosamax femur-fracture trial. Retrieved from: http://www.fiercepharma.com/story/merck-wins-bellwether-fosamax-femur-fracture-trial/2013-04-30

Sternberg, E. M., & Gold, P. W. (2002). The mind-body interaction in disease. *Scientific American.* Retrieved from: http://people.brandeis.edu/~teuber/mind_body.pdf

Study: Gulf war syndrome doesn't exist. (2006, September 12). [Article appeared on Associated Press web page]. Retrieved from: http://www.military.com/NewsContent/0,13319,113282,00.html

Sun, J. (2007). D-limonene: safety and clinical application. *Alternative Medicine Review 12*(3), 259-264. Retrieved from Thorne Research, Inc. at http://altmedrev.com/publications/12/3/259.pdf

Swartz, E., Stockburger, L., & Vallero, D. (2001). Preliminary data of polyaromatic hydrocarbons (PAHs) and other semi-volatile organic compounds collected in New York City in response to the events of September 11, 2001. Research Triangle Park, NC. *Report of U.S. Environmental Protection Agency, National Exposure Research Laboratory.*

Sweet, D. (2015). [paragraphs 4 & 5]. What is trauma? Retrieved from: http://www.drdeborahsweet.com/what-is-trauma.php

Thaler, J. P., Choi S.J., Schwartz M. W., & Wisee, B. E. (January 2010). Hypothalamic inflammation and energy homeostasis: Resolving the paradox. *Frontiers in Neuroendocrinology.*Volume 31, Issue 1. PP. 79-84. Retrieved from: http://www.sciencedirect.com/science/article/pii/S0091302209000685

TEDX Endocrine Disruption Exchange (2015) [Data set. An on-going project]. TEDX list of potential endocrine disruptors. Retrieved from: http://endocrinedisruption.org/endocrine-disruption/tedx-list-of-potential-endocrine-disruptors/overview

Teitelbaum, J. (2009). Effective treatment for chronic fatigue (cfs) and fibromyalgia. Retrived from: http://www.doctoroz.com/blog/jacob-teitelbaum-md/effective-treatment-chronic-fatigue-cfs-and-fibromyalgia

Timms, P. (2012). Tiredness. Royal College of Psychiatrists. Retrieved from: http://www.rcpsych.ac.uk/healthadvice/problemsdisorders/tiredness.aspx

The Blue Water Navy Vietnam Veterans Act of 2013. (2013). [Act of Congress]. Retrieved from: http://www.vva.org/Committees/Resolutions/2013%20Convention%20Resolutions%20Package3%281%29.pdf

The Terrifying Side Effects of Prescription Drugs. (April 12, 2008). Retrieved from: http://articles.mercola.com/sites/articles/archive/2008/04/12/the-terrifying-side-effects-of-prescription-drugs.aspx

Thyroid Disease Manager. (March 28, 2014). Adult hypothyroidism. Wilmar M. Wiersinga, MD. Retrieved from: http://www.thyroidmanager.org/chapter/adult-hypothyroidism/

Tracey, K. J. (2009). Reflex control of immunity. *Nature Reviews Immunology 9(6), 418–28*. doi:10.1038/nri2566. PMID 19461672

Transparency in action. (2015). [e-Guide. Pdf. 1st ed.]. New Hope Network. Retrieved from: http://newhope.com/eguide-transparency-action-0

Tucker, M. E. (February 1, 2015). [Originally aired on NPR News]. Panel says chronic fatigue syndrome is a disease, and renames it. Retrieved from: http://soundmedicine.org/post/panel-says-chronic-fatigue-syndrome-disease-and-renames-it

Understanding the stress response. (March , 2011). Retrieved from: http://www.health.harvard.edu/newsletters/Harvard_Mental_Health_Letter/2011/March/understanding-the-stress-response

UC Davis (2015). White matter matters. UC Davis Health System News. Retrieved from: http://www.ucdmc.ucdavis.edu/welcome/features/20071017_Medicine_whitematter/

US Department of Veterans Affairs (June 3, 2015). Fibromyalgia in gulf war veterans. Retrieved from: http://www.publichealth.va.gov/exposures/gulfwar/fibromyalgia.asp#sthash.7hnGHi5P.dpuf

US Department of Health & Human Services. (2009). [data file]. Heparin deaths. Retrieved from: http://www.fda.gov/Drugs/DrugSafety/PostmarketDrugSafetyInformationforPatientsandProviders/ucm112669.htm

US Department of Veterans Affairs. (October 22, 2013). [How to file claims]. New conditions VA presumes are related to herbicide exposure. Retrieved from: http://www.benefits.va.gov/compensation/claims-postservice-questionnaire-claimherbicide.asp

US Environmental Protection Agency. (n.d.). EPA response to September 11. Retrieved from: http://www.epa.gov/WTC/

University of Maryland Medical Center. (May 7, 2013). Complementary and alternative medicine guide: Supplement: magnesium. Retrieved from: http://umm.edu/health/medical/altmed/supplement/magnesium

Van Konynenburg, R. (August 11, 2003). [NIH CFS workshop Report: Dr. Sternberg on chronic fatigue syndrome and dysregulated stress response.] Retrieved from: http://www.prohealth.com/library/showarticle.cfm?libid=9672

Vio, F., Uauy, R., Pinstrup-Andersen, P., & Cheng, F. (2007). [Food Policy for Developing Countries: Case Studies.] The sugar controversy, case study #9-5. Retrieved from: http://cip.cornell.edu/dns.gfs/1200428197

Walsh, B. (May 13, 2013). Why a hotter world will mean more extinctions. Time, Ecocentric, Endangered Species. Retrieved from: http://science.time.com/2013/05/13/why-a-hotter-world-will-mean-more-extinctions/

Walsh, B. (August 9, 2013). [Shortened version of lead article titled "A World without Bees"]. The trouble with beekeeping in the Anthropocene. Retrieved from: http://science.time.com/2013/08/09/the-trouble-with-beekeeping-in-the-anthropocene/

Walsh, B. (August 19, 2013). Plight of the honeybee. Time, science, agriculture. Retrieved from: http://content.time.com/time/magazine/article/0,9171,2149141,00.html [or] http://time.com/559/the-plight-of-the-honeybee/

Wardrop, M. (April 14, 2009). Forty per cent of children now suffer from food allergies. Retrieved from: http://www.telegraph.co.uk/health/healthnews/5154644/Forty-per-cent-of-children-now-suffer-from-food-allergies.html

Ware, L. (2010). Interview with Herbert Benson: The mind's healing power. A pioneer in meditation reflects on the past and future of research into the mind body connection. Retrieved from: http://archive.protomag.com/assets/herbert-benson-the-minds-healing-power

Watkins, L. R. (2004). When pain goes bad: Might glia be the culprit causing fibromyalgia pain? National Fibromyalgia Research Association. New and Future Directions in FM Pain Management. Symposium: Portland, OR. Retrieved from: https://www.nfra.net/fibromyalgia_watkins.htm

Webster, J. I., Tonelli, L., & Sternberg, E. M. (2002). Neuroendocrine regulation of immunity. *Annual Review of Immunology 20*, 125-163. DOI: 10.1146/annurev.immunol.20.082401.104914

Wernick, A. (July 4, 2015). Scientists have discovered the 'missing link' between the brain and the immune system. Retrieved from: http://www.pri.org/stories/2015-07-04/scientists-have-discovered-missing-link-between-brain-and-immune-system

What if the world's soil runs out? (December 14, 2012). Time, Magazine,World Economic Forum. Retrieved from: http://world.time.com/2012/12/14/what-if-the-worlds-soil-runs-out/

Wiener, N. (1965). [2nd edition]. *Cybernetics: Or control and communication in the animal and the machine*. Cambridge, MA, The MIT Press.

Wilson, G. R., Curry, R. W., Jr. (October 15, 2005). Subclinical thyroid disease. *Am Fam Physician. 72*(8), 1517-24. Retrieved from: http://www.ncbi.nlm.nih.gov/pubmed/16273818

Woese, C. R. (2004). A new biology for a new century. *Microbiol. Mol. Biol. Rev., 68*(2), 173-186. doi: 10.1128/MMBR.68.2.173-186.2004

WHO/FAO. World Health Organization, & Food/Agriculture Organization of the UN. (2003). *Diet, nutrition and the prevention of chronic diseases*. WHO Technical Report Series (TRS 916). Report launched in Rome by WHO & FAO Directors. Retrieved from: http://www.who.int/dietphysicalactivity/publications/trs916/en/

WHO Media Centre. (2014). Dioxins and their effects on human health. Fact sheet N 225. Retrieved from: http://www.who.int/mediacentre/factsheets/fs225/en/

WHO. (2015). Health topics, food, genetically modified. Retrieved from: http://www.who.int/topics/food_genetically_modified/en/

Wolfe, M.M., Lichtenstein D.R., & Gurkirpal S. (Feb. 1, 2006). Gastrointestinal toxicity of nonsteroidal anti-inflammatory drugs. Retrieved from: http://jeffreydachmd.com/wp-content/uploads/2013/03/Gastrointestinal-toxicity-of-nonsteroidal-antiinflammatory-drugs-NSAIDS-Micheal-Wolfe-NEJM-1999.pdf

World trade center indoor environment assessment: Selecting contaminants of potential concern and setting health-based benchmarks. (2003). [Prepared by Contaminants of Potential Concern (COPC) Committee of the WTC Indoor Air Task Force. EPA, NYC Dept. of Mental Health & Hygiene, ATSDR, NY State Dept. of Health, OSHA]. Retrieved from: http://www.epa.gov/wtc/reports/contaminants_of_concern_benchmark_study.pdf

Wu, G., Feder, A., Cohen, H., Kim, J. J., Calderon, S., Charney, D. S., & Mathé, A. A. (2013). Understanding resilience. *Front Behav Neurosci. 7*(10). doi: 10.3389/fnbeh.2013.00010

Wu, S., Patel, K. B., Booth, L. J., Metcalf, J. P., Lin, H-K., & Wu, W. (Nov.15, 2010). Protective essential oil attenuates influenza virus infection: An in vitro study in MDCK cells. *Complement Altern Med.* 2010; 10: 69. doi: 10.1186/1472-6882-10-69 PMCID: PMC2994788

Yang, D. S., Pennisi, S. V., Son, K-C., & Kays, S. J. (2009). Screening indoor plants for volatile organic pollutant removal efficiency. *HortScience, 44*(5), 1377-1381. Retrieved from: http://hortsci.ashspublications.org/content/44/5/1377.abstract

Yasco, A. (2015). The methylation cycle. Retrieved from: http://www.dramyyasko.com/our-unique-approach/methylation-cycle/

Yeanoplos, K. (February 13, 2014). Deepak Chopra discusses "Timeless You": Mind over matter. Retrieved from: http://www.examiner.com/article/deepak-chopra-discusses-timeless-you-mind-over-matter?cid=db_articles

Yun, J. (May, 2014). Limonene inhibits methamphetamine-induced locomotor activity via regulation of 5-HT neuronal function and dopamine release. *Phytomedicine.* 15;21(6):883-7. doi: 10.1016/j.phymed.2013.12.004. Epub 2014 Jan 22. Retrieved from: http://www.ncbi.nlm.nih.gov/pubmed/24462212

Zeineh, M. M., Kang, J., Atlas, S. W., Raman, M. M., Reiss, A. L., Norris, J. L....Montoya, J. G. (2015). Right arcuate fasciculus abnormality in chronic fatigue syndrome. *Radiology. 274*(2):517-26. doi: 10.1148/radiol.14141079. Epub 2014 Oct 29

Zhou, S. F., Liu, J. P., & Chowbay, B. (2009). Polymorphism of human cytochrome P450 enzymes and its clinical impact. *Drug Metab Rev.,41*(2), 89-295. doi: 10.1080/03602530902843483

Zhou, W., Yoshioka, M., & Yokogoshi, H. (2009). Sub-chronic effects of s-limonene on brain neurotransmitter levels and behavior of rats. *Journal of Nutritional Science and Vitaminology.* Retrieved from: https://www.aromaticscience.com/sub-chronic-effects-of-s-limonene-on-brain-neurotransmitter-levels-and-behavior-of-rats-2/

Zuckerman, M. (1999). *Vulnerability to psychopathology: A biopsychosocial model.* Washington, D.C., American Psychological Association.

Additional Resources

http://weheal.org/ - Tools, Patient Advocacy, Support

This article is in the references too, but I am highlighting it again, as it discusses tight junctions, mucosal barrier function, stress and hyperactive immune response,CFS/SEID, IBS, etc. Great research. Please note: The XMRV virus has been ruled out.

Gut inflammation in chronic fatigue syndrome:
http://www.ncbi.nlm.nih.gov/pmc/articles/PMC2964729/#B12

Increased d-lactic Acid intestinal bacteria in patients with chronic fatigue syndrome:
http://www.ncbi.nlm.nih.gov/pubmed/19567398

Detection of Herpesviruses and Parvovirus B19 in Gastric and Intestinal Mucosa of Chronic Fatigue Syndrome Patients:
http://iv.iiarjournals.org/content/23/2/209.long

Activation of human herpesviruses 6 and 7 in patients with chronic fatigue syndrome:
http://www.journalofclinicalvirology.com/article/S1386-6532%2806%2970011-7/abstract

Low stomach acid: The risks, the symptoms, and the solutions:*
http://bodyecology.com/articles/low_stomach_acid_symptoms.php
*This article has supplements recommended with it. I am not endorsing the supplements, just the research and information included in this article, as I feel it may be relevant for some people.

Becoming a Conscious Consumer

I became a *conscious consumer* in my quest of seeking answers to my health challenges. *Quality and efficacy of product* mattered to me, as it made a difference in my well-being. It also mattered to me the *values* of the companies to whom I gave my business. These days, conscious consumers are *seeking transparency* in the companies they choose to buy from as well as s*afety and traceability* of ingredients.

Issues to consider are GMO's, animal welfare, pesticides, sustainability, the well-being of *farmers/workers*, quality of ingredients, allergen cross-contamination, responsible ingredient sourcing, and third-party testing from laboratories like USP and NSF International ("Transparency in Action," 2015). While not regulated, there are many outstanding companies in the supplements industry that seek to and do offer safe, high-quality products. Do your own research and make your own conclusions. This is what being a conscious consumer is really all about: making conscious, informed choices that benefit not only you but the planet as a whole. *Mainstream companies like Kraft, Panera, Nestle, Campbell's, and General Mills are stepping up too, and taking out artificial colors and flavors, sourcing organics, etc.* ("General Mills Accelarates Plan to Double Organic Acerage," 2016 & "Live from Expo West,"2016).

Vitamin D – (Autism, Immunity, Social Behavior, Mood)

Research points to how crucial Vitamin D may be for mood (it is needed to produce serotonin), immunity, and even Autism. The research around Autism again points to serotonin production and social behavior (Medical Xpress, 2014). See page 189 for more information. *When I lived in San Jose, my well-being improved dramatically, quite possibly from being in a sunnier climate and lower latitude than Portland.*

Microbiome & Mycobacterium Vaccae

The NIH Human Microbiome Project is emerging research that studies microbes living in and on humans in order to study what may contribute to health or disease. Here is a landmark study that defines what is considered the normal bacterial makeup in our bodies:
http://www.genome.gov/27549144
Also, check out this article on top-soil: https://goo.gl/t2oeZd

Microbes outnumber human cells by 10:1 and make up part of our genome as well. We are also connected to and influenced by bacteria that live outside of us, like mycobacterium vaccae, that may influence mood via the immune system (in other words, dirt smells good, and there's a reason): http://www.ncbi.nlm.nih.gov/pmc/articles/PMC1868963/

Another thing to consider might be what are known as tight junctions. Tight junctions are cells whose membranes are so close together there is no liquid in-between them. They act as barriers and gates in your body. They can be found in your gut, blood vessels, your kidneys, and the blood-brain barrier. Pro-inflammatory cytokines may weaken tight junctions, leading to not only increased gut inflammation, but the translocation of gram negative bacteria and activation of microglia. This scenario could be triggered by acute or severe stress - often found in CFS - including surgery, trauma, and infections (Maes & Leunis, 2008). Is a similar mechanism occurring in other disease states where a loss of bio-diversity from over-use of antibiotics, NSAID's, pesticides, etc. may lead to interference in communication between gut bacteria inhabit us and the tight junction signaling pathway? Does this activate microglia and auto-immunity?

Recap of My Protocol & Stress, EBV, HSP's

My game-changers: deep nutrition, mindful living, conscious choices. I emphasize real, whole, fresh food and to avoid irritants to my body: caffeine, alcohol, sugar, gluten, synthetics. For strategic stimulation I use acai (small amounts), Korean Ginseng, etc. I use high-quality natural products & supplements like raw & food-based vitamins for nutritional support (see Ch. 4). I pay attention to my body's signals, and address inflammation first to eliminate fatigue. A big one for me, as an HSP (pg.204), was realizing I was overstimulated by stress/irritants and low in electrolytes and/or vital minerals. My cortisol levels were low during the day and high when I was sleeping, resulting in fatigue and chronic inflammation. I solved this (see pg. 291). Watch your stress levels, as it may lead to lower HCl levels, which may possibly leave one vulnerable to latent viruses such as EBV (pp.431/450) and/or an overgrowth of candida. My mother had mono as a child and was often sick, out of school for months at a time. Having me made her well. Did I inherit any genetic vulnerabilities from her? We know there are immune markers that point to SEID being biological and research points to white matter atrophy/inflammation and the presence of EBV anti-bodies ("Chronic Fatigue Syndrome," 2012). I focus on what is going right, manage and reinterpret stress as positive, and practice mind-body fitness like yoga. All is connected and behaves as such. Wishing you much peace, love, & success on your journey to well-being.

Who looks outside, dreams; who looks inside, awakes. ~Carl Gustav Jung

The more you lose yourself in something bigger than yourself, the more energy you will have. ~Norman Vincent Peale

*See page 431 for New York Times Article. EBV anti-bodies have been found in the blood of people with SEID.

About the Author

Edie Summers is an author, executive, top-rated radio host, wellness coach/consultant, and yoga/mind-body fitness instructor.

The Memory of Health is her third non-fiction book. Her other books include *Frozen Light* and *Self-Coach Your Way to More Energy*. She is pursuing her Ph.D. in Health Psychology and certifications in Clinical Nutrition and Functional Medicine.

1-800-536-1322
ediesummers@hotmail.com
support@portlandwellnesscoach.com

Wellness Retreats, Self & Group Coaching, Yoga Videos:
www.ConnektWell.com

http://portlandwellnesscoach.com/

http://www.blogtalkradio.com/TheWellnessCoach

Chronic Fatigue Support on Facebook:
https://www.facebook.com/ChronicFatigueSupport?ref=hl

http://ediesummers.wix.com/author

http://ediesummers.wix.com/yoga

EmpowerPreneur ™ - Empowering people to make a living no matter what their circumstances – see www.ConnektWell.com for details

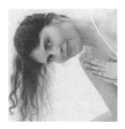

For bulk orders of <u>The Memory of Health</u>, *or other inquiries, please contact:*
ediesummers@hotmail.com